Cochlear Hearing Loss

Cochlear Hearing Loss

Brian C.J. Moore

Department of Experimental Psychology,
University of Cambridge,
Cambridge, UK

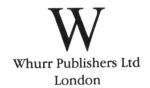

Whurr Publishers Ltd
London

British Library Cataloguing in Publication Data
A catalogue record for this book is available from the
British Library.

ISBN 1 86156 091 5

Printed and bound in the UK by Athenæum Press Ltd,
Gateshead, Tyne & Wear

Contents

Preface

In 1995 I published a book called *Perceptual Consequences of Cochlear Damage* (Oxford University Press). The book reviewed the perceptual changes associated with cochlear hearing loss and related these to the underlying physiological mechanisms. A compact disc (CD) containing simulations of several of these perceptual changes was produced at the same time, but sold separately from the book (Moore, 1997a). The book was aimed primarily at researchers in the field, and much of the material contained in it was rather technical. The book was well reviewed, and I received favourable comments from colleagues, but it became clear that it was not ideal as a textbook for students.

This new book covers similar topics to *Perceptual Consequences of Cochlear Damage*, but some of the more technical material has been omitted, and much more effort has been made to explain basic concepts. I have attempted to write at a level that is accessible and comprehensible to students in audiology and in speech and hearing science. I hope, therefore, that the book will be considered suitable as a textbook for such students.

The book is intended to impart an understanding of the changes in perception that take place when a person has a cochlear hearing loss. I have tried to interrelate physiological data and perceptual data. The book aims to present both data and concepts in an integrated way. The main goal is to convey an understanding of the perceptual changes associated with cochlear hearing loss, of the difficulties faced by the hearing-impaired person and of the limitations of current hearing aids. The reader should come away with an impression not only of what happens, but also of why it happens.

The book assumes some prior knowledge about sound. For example, it assumes familiarity with the decibel and the concept of the spectrum of a sound. However, an extensive glossary is provided to give brief explanations of technical terms used in the book. The concept of linear and non-linear systems is also explained in some detail as this concept is crucial for understanding this book, but it is often poorly explained in textbooks on hearing.

Listening to simulations of the perceptual effects of cochlear hearing loss can help appreciation of these effects. A compact disc containing simulations of different aspects of cochlear damage can be obtained by writing to the author at:

Department of Experimental Psychology, University of Cambridge, Downing Street, Cambridge CB2 3EB, England.

The price of the disc is £12 sterling or 20 US dollars. Payment (a cheque payable to B.C.J. Moore) should be enclosed with the order. The disc also illustrates the effectiveness of various types of amplification and compression in compensating for the effects of cochlear hearing loss.

I would like to thank the colleagues and research students who commented on preliminary drafts of chapters of this book. They include Joseph Alcántara, Thomas Baer, Lianne Cartee, Brian Glasberg, Robert Peters, Marina Rose, Aleksander Sek, Michael Stone, Deborah Vickers and Joyce Vliegen. Michael Stone in particular went through the whole text with a fine-tooth comb, and contributed greatly to improving the clarity of the book. I would also like to thank Ian Cannell, Brian Glasberg and Aleksander Sek for considerable assistance in producing new figures.

Brian C. J. Moore
March, 1998

Chapter 1
Physiological Aspects of Cochlear Hearing Loss

Introduction

Hearing loss caused by damage to the cochlea is probably the most common form of hearing loss in the developed countries. Its most obvious symptom, and the one that is almost always assessed in the clinic, is an elevation of the threshold for detecting sounds. However, it is also accompanied by a variety of other changes in the way that sound is perceived. Even if sounds are amplified (for example by a hearing aid) so that they are well above the threshold for detection, the perception of those sounds is usually abnormal; the person with cochlear hearing loss often reports that the sounds are unclear and distorted and that it is hard to hear comfortably over a wide range of sound levels. A common complaint is difficulty in understanding speech, especially when background sounds or reverberations are present. One of the main aims of this book is to explain why these problems occur and why current hearing aids are of limited benefit in compensating for the problems.

The book assumes that the reader has a basic knowledge of physics and acoustics, for example an understanding of what is meant by terms such as sinusoid, spectrum, frequency component, and the decibel. The reader who is not familiar with these terms should consult a textbook such as *An Introduction to the Psychology of Hearing* (Moore, 1997b) or *Signals and Systems for Speech and Hearing* (Rosen and Howell, 1991). For the reader who knows these things but needs a 'reminder', many of the key terms are defined briefly in the glossary. Most of the terms that appear in italics in the text are defined in the glossary. One concept that may not be familiar is that of a *linear system*. This topic is of importance, since the normal peripheral auditory system shows significant *non-linearities,* whereas the system becomes more linear when cochlear damage occurs. Hence, this chapter starts with a description of the properties of linear and non-linear systems. It then goes on to consider the physiology and the function of the normal and damaged cochlea.

Linear and non-linear systems

The auditory system is often thought of as a series of stages, the output of a given stage forming the input to the next. Each stage can be considered as a device or system, with an input and an output. For a system to be linear, certain relationships between the input and output must hold true. The following two conditions must be satisfied:

(1) If the input to the system is changed in magnitude by a factor k, then the output should also change in magnitude by a factor k, but be otherwise unaltered. This condition is called homogeneity. For example, if the input is doubled, then the output is doubled, but without any change in the form of the output. Thus, a plot of the output as a function of the input would be a straight line passing through the origin (zero input gives zero output) - hence the term 'linear system'. Such a plot is called an *input-output function*. An example of such a function is given in panel (a) of Figure 1.1.

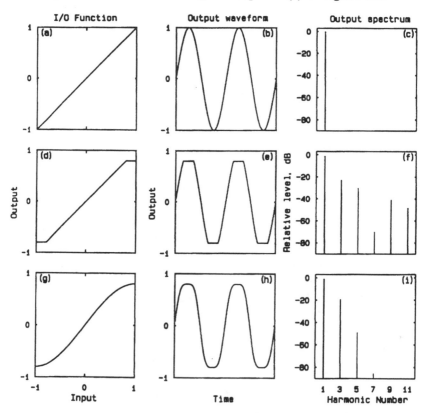

Figure 1.1: The left column shows input-output functions for a linear system (a), a non-linear system with 'hard' peak clipping (d), and a non-linear system with more progressive 'saturation' (g). The middle column shows outputs from these systems in response to a sinusoidal input. The third column shows spectra of the outputs.

(2) The output of the system in response to a number of independent inputs presented simultaneously should be equal to the sum of the outputs that would have been obtained if each input were presented alone. For example, if the response to input A is X, and the response to input B is Y, then the response to A and B together is simply X + Y. This condition is known as 'superposition'.

When describing a system as linear, it is usually assumed that the system is *time invariant*. This means that the input-output function does not change over time. For example, if the input is I, and the output is O, the relationship between the input and the output would be:

$$O = cI$$

$$(1.1)$$

where c is a constant that does not vary with time.

When a sinusoid is used as an input to a linear system, the output is a sinusoid of the same frequency. This is illustrated in panel (b) of Figure 1.1. The amplitude and phase of the output may, however, be different from that of the input. Assume that the input is a single sinusoid, whose waveform as a function of time, $I(t)$, can be described by:

$$I(t) = A\sin(2\pi ft)$$

$$(1.2)$$

where A is the peak amplitude of the input and f is the frequency in Hz (cycles per second). The output as a function of time, $O(t)$, could then be represented by:

$$O(t) = G \times A\sin(2\pi ft + \phi)$$

$$(1.3)$$

where G is a constant representing the amplitude ratio between the input and output, and ϕ is a constant representing the phase shift between the input and output. G is sometimes referred to as the *gain* of the system.

The output of a linear system in response to a sinusoidal input is itself sinusoidal so the spectrum of the output, by definition, consists of a single frequency component. This is illustrated in panel (c) of Figure 1.1. More generally, the output of a linear system never contains frequency components that were not present in the input signal. The response of a linear system may, however, vary with the frequency of the input sinusoid. This is equivalent to saying that the constants G and ϕ in Eq. 1.3 can vary with the input frequency.

In practice, many devices or systems are linear as long as the input is not too large. Excessive inputs may cause the system to become non-linear; more details are given later on. Such a system is usually called linear, even though it can become non-linear under extreme conditions. As an example, consider a loudspeaker. The input is a voltage and the output is a movement of the cone of the loudspeaker, which can produce audible sound waves. For the types of inputs that are typically used for a loudspeaker, the response is approximately linear; the conditions of homogeneity and superposition are obeyed. If the input voltage varies in a sinusoidal manner, the movement of the cone is almost sinusoidal. However, if the frequency of the input is changed, holding the magnitude of the input constant, the magnitude of the movement of the cone may vary. In this case, we would say that the loudspeaker does not have a 'flat' frequency response; G may vary with frequency. Similarly, ϕ may vary with frequency. Other examples of systems that usually operate in a nearly linear way are microphones, amplifiers and the output transducers used in hearing aids (often called 'receivers').

When waveforms other than sinusoids are applied as the input to a linear system, the output waveform will often differ from that of the input. For example, if the input to a linear system is a square wave, the output is not necessarily a square wave. This is one reason for the popularity of sinusoids in auditory research; sinusoids are the only waveforms that are always 'preserved' by a linear system. However, if a system is linear, then it is relatively easy to predict its output for any arbitrary complex input. As a first step, the output is measured as a function of frequency for a sinusoidal input. Essentially, the values of G and ϕ are determined as a function of the input frequency. To predict the output for a complex input, a *Fourier analysis* of the input is performed. This gives a description of the input in terms of the amplitudes and phases of its sinusoidal components. The output for each of the sinusoidal components comprising the input can then be calculated. Finally, using the principle of superposition, the output in response to the whole complex can be calculated as the sum of the outputs in response to its individual sinusoidal components. This is a powerful method and it gives another reason for using sinusoids as stimuli.

As mentioned earlier, many linear systems become non-linear if the input is made large enough. An example is shown in panel (d) of Figure 1.1. The input-output function is linear over a large part of its range, but it flattens out for large positive or negative values of the input. This is sometimes called 'saturation' or 'peak clipping' and it can occur in systems such as transistor amplifiers and condenser microphones. In the example shown, the clipping is symmetrical, in that it occurs at the same absolute value for positive and negative values of the input. When a sinusoid is used as input to such a system, and the peak amplitude of the sinusoid, A, is sufficiently large, the output is no longer sinusoidal. This is illustrated in panel (e) of Figure 1.1. The output is periodic, with the same period as the input sinusoid, but the waveform is distorted. In this case, the output contains frequency components that are not present in the input. This is illustrated in panel (f) of Figure 1.1 In general, the output of a non-linear system in response to a single sinusoid at the input contains one or more components (sinusoids) with frequencies that are integer multiples of the frequency of the input. These components are referred to as *harmonics,* and the non-linear system is said to introduce *harmonic distortion.* For example, if the input was a sinusoid with a frequency of 500 Hz, the output might still contain a component with this frequency, but components with other frequencies might be present too - for example 1000, 1500, 2000 . . . Hz.

Another example of a non-linear input-output function is shown in panel (g) of Figure 1.1. In this case, the function does not show 'hard' clipping, but the slope becomes shallower when the absolute value of the input or output exceeds a certain value. This type of input-output function can occur in valve (tube) amplifiers, moving coil microphones, and loudspeakers, and it can also occur in the auditory system. The output waveform, shown in panel (h) of Figure 1.1, is less distorted than when hard clipping occurs, and the output spectrum, shown in panel (i), reveals less harmonic distortion.

If the input to a non-linear system consists of two sinusoids, then the output may contain components with frequencies corresponding to the sum and difference of the two input frequencies, and their harmonics, as well as the original sinusoidal components that were present in the input. These extra components are said to result from *inter-modulation distortion.* For example, if the input contains two sinusoids with frequencies f_1 and f_2, the output may contain components with frequencies $f_1 - f_2, f_1 + f_2, 2f_1 - f_2, 2f_2 - f_1$, etc. These components are referred to as inter-modulation distortion products, and, in the case of the auditory system, they are also called *combination tones.*

When a system is non-linear, the response to complex inputs cannot generally be predicted from the responses to the sinusoidal components comprising the inputs. Thus the characteristics of the system must be investigated using both sinusoidal and complex inputs.

Often, the input and output magnitudes of a system are plotted on logarithmic axes (the decibel scale is an example). In that case, the input and output magnitudes are not specified as instantaneous values (for example as the instantaneous voltage in the case of an electrical signal). Generally, instantaneous magnitudes can have both positive and negative values, but it is not possible to take the logarithm of a negative number. Instead, the input and output are averaged over a certain time, and the magnitude is expressed as a quantity that cannot have a negative value. Typically, both the input and output are specified in terms of their *power* (related to the *mean-square* value) or their *root-mean-square value*. Sometimes, the peak amplitude may be used. For a linear system, the condition of homogeneity still applies to such measures. For example, if the input power is doubled, the output power is also doubled. When plotted on 'log-log' axes, the input-output function of a linear system is a straight line with a slope of unity. To see why this is the case, we take the logarithm of both sides of Eq. 1.1 ($O = cI$). This gives:

$$\log(O) = \log(cI) = \log(c) + \log(I)$$

$$(1.4)$$

The value of $\log(c)$ is itself a constant. Therefore, since $\log(O)$ is simply equal to $\log(I)$ plus a constant, the slope of the line relating $\log(O)$ to $\log(I)$ must be unity. In a non-linear system, the slope of the input-output function on logarithmic axes differs from unity. Say, for example, that the output is proportional to the square of the input:

$$O = cI^2$$

$$(1.5)$$

Taking logarithms of both sides gives:

$$\log(O) = \log(cI^2) = \log(c) + 2\log(I)$$

$$(1.6)$$

In this case, the slope of the input-output function on logarithmic axes is two. When the slope of the input-output function is greater than one, the non-linearity is referred to as *expansive*. If the output were proportional to the square root of the input ($O = cI^{0.5}$), the slope of the function would be 0.5. When the slope of the input-output function is less than one, the non-linearity is referred to as *compressive*. Examples of input-output functions plotted on log-log axes will be presented later in this chapter, in connection with the response of the basilar membrane within the cochlea.

Structure and function of the outer and middle ears

Figure 1.2 shows the structure of the peripheral part of the human auditory system. It is traditionally considered as composed of three parts, the outer, middle and inner ear. The outer ear is composed of the pinna and the auditory canal or meatus. The pinna and meatus together create a broad resonance which enhances sound levels at the eardrum, relative to those obtained at the same point in free space (i.e. when the head is not present), over the frequency range from about 1.5 to 5 kHz. This is illustrated in Figure 1.3. The maximum boost is typically about 12-15 dB in the region around 2.5 kHz. When a hearing aid is fitted so as to block the meatus, this broad resonance is lost for a behind-the-ear aid,

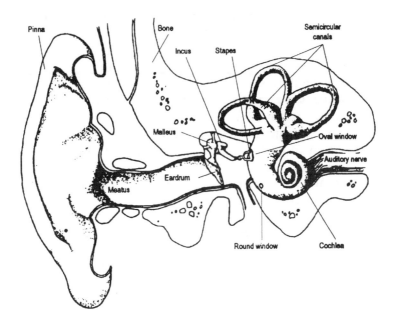

Figure 1.2: Illustration of the structure of the peripheral auditory system showing the outer, middle and inner ear. Redrawn from Lindsey and Norman (1972).

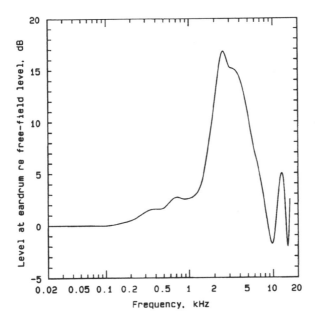

Figure 1.3: The difference between the sound level measured at the eardrum (for a sound coming from the frontal direction) and the sound level in the free field at the point corresponding to the centre of the listener's head. Data from Shaw (1974).

reduced in magnitude for a concha aid, and shifted to higher frequencies for a completely-in-the-canal aid. This has to be taken into account when fitting hearing aids. The pinna, head and upper torso significantly modify the incoming sound at medium and high frequencies. Specifically, when the sound contains a broad range of frequencies, the pinna introduces a complex pattern of peaks and notches into the spectrum. This pattern varies systematically with the direction of the sound source relative to the head, and the spectral patterns thus provide important information about the location of sound sources (see Chapter 7 for more details).

Sound travels down the meatus and causes the eardrum, or tympanic membrane, to vibrate. The eardrum forms the boundary between the outer and middle ear. These vibrations are transmitted through the middle ear by three small bones, the ossicles, to a membrane-covered opening in the bony wall of the spiral-shaped structure of the inner ear - the cochlea. This opening is called the oval window and it forms the boundary between the middle and inner ear. The three bones are called the *malleus, incus* and *stapes* (popularly known as the hammer, anvil and stirrup), the stapes being the lightest and smallest of these and the one which actually makes contact with the oval window.

The major function of the middle ear is to ensure the efficient transfer of sound energy from the air to the fluids in the cochlea. If the sound were to impinge directly on to the oval window, most of it would simply be reflected back, rather than entering the cochlea. This happens because the resistance of the oval window to movement is very different from that of air. This is described as a difference in acoustical impedance. The middle ear acts as an impedance-matching device or transformer that improves sound transmission and reduces the amount of reflected sound. This is accomplished mainly by the 27:1 ratio of effective areas of the eardrum and the oval window, and to a small extent by the lever action of the ossicles. Transmission of sound energy through the middle ear is most efficient at middle frequencies (500-4000 Hz), which are the ones most important for speech perception - see Chapter 8. This is illustrated in Figure 1.4, taken from Moore, Glasberg and Baer (1997) which shows an estimate of the relative effectiveness of transmission through the middle ear as a function of frequency.

The ossicles have minute muscles attached to them that contract when we are exposed to intense sounds. This contraction, known as the *middle ear reflex* or *acoustic reflex*, is probably mediated by neural centres in the brain stem. The reflex can be triggered by sound of any frequency, but it reduces the transmission of sound through the middle ear only at low frequencies. It may help to prevent damage to the delicate structures inside the cochlea. However, the activation of the reflex is too slow to provide any protection against impulsive sounds, such as gunshots or hammer blows.

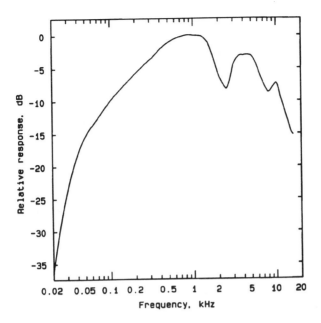

Figure 1.4: The transfer function of the middle ear, plotted as relative response versus frequency. The response was arbitrarily labelled as 0 dB at 1 kHz. The estimate comes from Moore, Glasberg and Baer (1997).

For moderate sound levels (below about 90 dB SPL), the outer ear and middle ear behave essentially as linear systems; they do not introduce significant harmonic or inter-modulation distortion. However, at high sound levels both the tympanic membrane and the ossicles may vibrate in a non-linear manner, and the acoustic reflex also introduces non-linearity. These non-linearities may result in audible harmonic and inter-modulation distortion.

Structure and function of the normal cochlea

The cochlea, the basilar membrane and the organ of Corti

The inner ear is also known as the cochlea. It is shaped like the spiral shell of a snail. However, the spiral shape does not appear to have any functional significance, and the cochlea is often described as if the spiral had been 'unwound'. The cochlea is filled with almost incompressible fluids, and it has bony rigid walls. It is divided along its length by two membranes, Reissner's membrane and the *basilar membrane* (BM) (see Figure 1.5). The start of the spiral, where the oval window is situated, is known as the *base*; the other end, the inner tip, is known as the *apex*. It is also common to talk about the 'basal end' and the 'apical end'. At the apex there is a small opening (the helicotrema) between the BM and the walls of the cochlea, which connects the two outer chambers of the cochlea, the *scala vestibuli* and the *scala tympani*. Inward movement of the oval window results in a corresponding outward movement in a membrane covering a second opening in the cochlea - the round window. Such movements result in pressure differences between one side of the BM and the other (i.e. the pressure is applied in a direction perpendicular to the BM) and this results in movement of the BM (see below for details). The helicotrema eliminates any pressure differences between the scala vestibuli and the scala tympani at very low frequencies. This prevents the BM from moving significantly in response to movements of the oval window caused by jaw movements or by slow changes in air pressure (such as occur when changing altitude). The helicotrema also reduces movement of the BM in response to low-frequency sounds.

A third membrane, called the *tectorial membrane*, lies above the BM, and also runs along the length of the cochlea. Between the BM and the tectorial membrane are hair cells, which form part of a structure called the *organ of Corti* (see Figures 1.5 and 1.6). They are called hair cells because they appear to have tufts of hairs, called *stereocilia*, at their apexes. The hair cells are divided into two groups by an arch known as the tunnel of Corti. Those on the side of the arch closest to the outside of the spiral shape are known as *outer hair cells* (OHCs), and they are arranged in three rows in the cat and up to five rows in humans. The hair cells on the other side of the arch form a single row, and are known as *inner hair cells* (IHCs). The stereocilia on each OHC form a V or W-shaped pattern, and they are arranged in rows (usually about three) that are graded in height, the tallest stereocilia lying on the outside of the W or V. The stereocilia on each IHC are also arranged in rows graded in height, but the arrangement is more like a straight line or a broad arc. In humans, there are about 25 000 OHCs (per ear), each with about 140 stereocilia protruding from it, whereas there are about 3500 IHCs, each with about 40 stereocilia.

The tectorial membrane, which has a gelatinous structure, lies above the hairs. It appears that the stereocilia of the OHCs actually make contact with the tectorial membrane, but this may not be true for the IHCs. The tectorial membrane appears to be effectively hinged at one side (the left in Fig. 1.6). When the BM moves up and down, a shearing motion is created; the tectorial membrane moves sideways (in the left-right direction in Figure 1.6) relative to the tops of the hair cells. As a result the stereocilia at the tops of the hair cells are moved sideways. The movement occurs via direct contact in the case of the OHCs, but in the case of the IHCs it may be produced by the viscous drag of fluid streaming between the upper part of the organ of Corti and the tectorial membrane. The movement of the stereocilia of the IHCs leads to a flow of electrical current through the IHCs, which in turn leads to the genera-

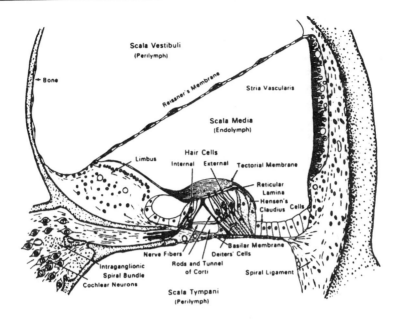

Figure 1.5: Cross-section of the cochlea, showing the basilar membrane, Reissner's membrane, and the organ of Corti. Redrawn from Davis (1962).

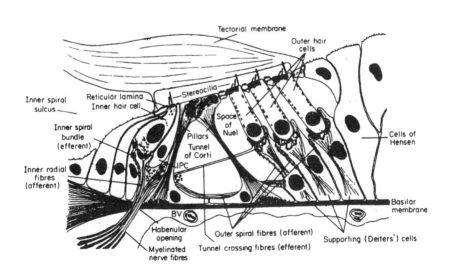

Figure 1.6: Cross section of the organ of Corti as it appears in the basal turn of the cochlea. Adapted from Ryan and Dallos (1984).

tion of action potentials (nerve spikes) in the neurones of the auditory nerve. Thus, the IHCs act to transduce mechanical movements into neural activity.

The IHCs and OHCs have very different functions. The great majority of afferent neurones, which carry information from the cochlea to higher levels of the auditory system, connect to IHCs; each IHC is contacted by about 20 neurones (Spoendlin, 1970). Thus, most information about sounds is conveyed via the IHCs. The main role of the OHCs is probably actively to influence the mechanics of the cochlea. The OHCs have a motor function, changing their length, shape and stiffness in response to electrical stimulation (Ashmore, 1987; Yates, 1995), and they can there-fore influence the response of the BM to sound. The OHCs are often described as being a key element in an *active mechanism* within the cochlea. The function of this active mechanism is described in more detail below.

The action of the OHCs is partly under the control of higher centres of the auditory system. There are about 1800 efferent nerve fibres that carry information from the auditory system to the cochlea, most of them originating in the superior olivary complex of the brain stem. Many of these efferent fibres make contact with the OHCs, and thus can affect their activity. Thus, even the earliest stages in the analysis of auditory signals are partly under the control of higher centres.

Tuning on the basilar membrane

When the oval window is set in motion by a sound, a pressure difference occurs between the upper and lower surface of the BM. The pressure wave travels almost instantaneously through the incompressible fluids of the cochlea. Consequently, the pressure difference is applied essen-tially simultaneously along the whole length of the BM. This causes a pattern of motion to develop on the BM. The pattern does not depend on which end of the cochlea is stimulated. Sounds that reach the cochlea via the bones of the head rather than through the air do not produce atypical responses.

The response of the BM to stimulation with a sinusoid takes the form of a travelling wave, which moves along the BM from the base towards the apex. The amplitude of the wave increases at first and then decreases rather abruptly. The basic form of the wave is illustrated in Figure 1.7, which shows schematically the instantaneous displacement of the BM for four successive instants in time in response to a low-frequency sinusoid. The four successive peaks in the wave are labelled 1, 2, 3 and 4. This figure also shows the line joining the amplitude peaks, which is called the envelope. The envelope shows a peak at a particular position on the BM.

The response of the BM to sounds of different frequencies is strongly affected by its mechanical properties, which vary progressively from base to apex. At the base the BM is relatively narrow and stiff. This causes the base to respond best to high frequencies. At the apex the BM is wider

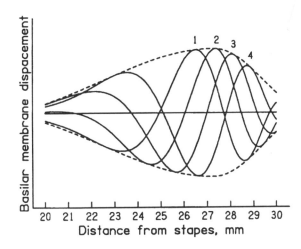

Figure 1.7: The solid lines show the instantaneous displacement of the BM at four successive instants in time (labelled 1 to 4), derived from a cochlear model. The pattern moves from left to right, building up gradually with distance, and decaying rapidly beyond the point of maximal displacement. The dashed line represents the envelope traced out by the amplitude peaks in the waveform.

and much less stiff, which causes the apex to respond best to low frequencies. Each point on the BM is *tuned*; it responds best (with greatest displacement) to a certain frequency, called the characteristic frequency (CF) or best frequency, and responds progressively less as the frequency is moved away from the CF. It is now believed that the tuning of the BM arises from two mechanisms. One is referred to as the *passive* system or passive mechanism. This depends on the mechanical properties of the BM and surrounding structures and it operates in a roughly linear way. The other mechanism is the *active* mechanism. This depends on the operation of the OHCs, and it operates in a non-linear way. The active mechanism depends on the cochlea being in good physiological condition, and it is easily damaged.

Figure 1.8 shows the envelopes of the patterns of vibration for several different low-frequency sinusoids (data from Von Békésy, 1960). Sounds of different frequencies produce maximum displacement at different places along the BM, i.e. there is a frequency-to-place transformation. If two or more sinusoids with different frequencies are presented simultaneously, each produces maximum displacement at its appropriate place on the BM. In effect, the cochlea behaves like a frequency analyser, although with less than perfect resolution. The resolution is often described in terms of the sharpness of tuning. This refers to the 'narrowness' of the response patterns on the BM. In the case of responses to a single tone, as shown in Figure 1.7, it refers to the spread of the

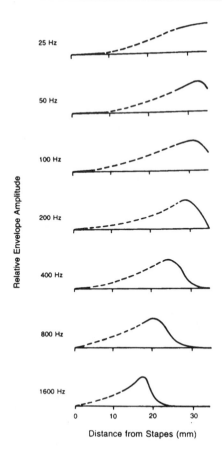

Figure 1.8: Envelopes of patterns of vibration on the BM for a number of low-frequency sounds. Solid lines indicate the results of actual measurements, while the dashed lines are von Békésy's extrapolations. Redrawn from von Békésy (1960).

response along the BM; sharp tuning would be associated with a narrow spread.

Most of the pioneering work on patterns of vibration along the BM was done by Von Békésy (1960). The vibration patterns found by Von Békésy were rather broad; for example, the pattern for a 400 Hz sinusoid extended along almost the whole length of the BM (see Figure 1.8). However, these patterns probably reflect only the passive mechanism. The active mechanism would not have been functioning in Von Békésy's experiments, for two reasons. Firstly, he had to use very high sound levels - about 140 dB SPL; such high levels are known to damage the active mechanism. Secondly, he used cadaver ears and the active mechanism ceases to function after death.

Recent work measuring BM responses to sound differs from that of Von Békésy in several ways. Firstly, living animals have been used. Great care has been taken to keep the animals in good physiological condition during the measurements and to minimise trauma caused by the necessary surgery. Secondly, the techniques themselves are designed to be minimally invasive. Finally, rather than measuring the response of several different points on the BM to a single frequency, measurements have been made of the responses of a single point to sinusoids of differing frequency. In this case, the sharpness of tuning is often measured by adjusting the level at each frequency to produce a fixed response on the BM. If a point on the BM is sharply tuned, then the sound level has to be increased rapidly as the frequency is moved away from the CF. If the tuning is broad, then the sound level has to be increased only gradually as the frequency is moved away from the CF.

The results show that the sharpness of tuning of the BM depends critically on the physiological condition of the animal; the better the condition, the sharper is the tuning (Khanna and Leonard, 1982; Sellick, Patuzzi and Johnstone, 1982; Leonard and Khanna, 1984; Robles, Ruggero and Rich, 1986; Ruggero, 1992). The health of the cochlea is often monitored by placing an electrode in or near the auditory nerve and measuring the combined responses of the neurones to tone bursts or clicks; this response is known as the *compound action potential* (AP or CAP). The lowest sound level at which an AP can be detected is called the AP threshold. Usually, the BM is sharply tuned when the AP threshold is low, indicating that the cochlea is in good physiological condition and the active mechanism is functioning.

An example is given in Figure 1.9, which shows the input sound level (in dB SPL) required to produce a constant velocity of motion at a particular point on the BM, as a function of stimulus frequency (Sellick, Patuzzi and Johnstone, 1982). This is sometimes called a *constant velocity tuning curve*. It is not yet clear whether the effective stimulus to the IHCs is BM vibration amplitude (equivalent to displacement) or BM velocity. However, for a given frequency, velocity is directly proportional to displacement; the greater the amplitude the faster the movement. At the start of the experiment, when AP thresholds were low, a very sharp tuning curve was obtained (open circles). This curve reflects the contribution of both the passive and the active mechanism. As the condition of the animal deteriorated, the active mechanism ceased to function. The tuning became broader, and the sound level required to produce the criterion response increased markedly around the tip. The broad tuning curve recorded after death (filled squares) reflects the tuning produced by the passive mechanism alone.

The frequency at the tip of the tuning curve (the CF - where the sound level was lowest) shifted downwards when the condition of the animal deteriorated. This occurred because the active mechanism gives maximum gain for a frequency that is somewhat above the best frequency determined by the passive mechanics. In a healthy ear, the CF

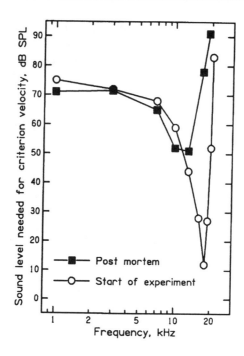

Figure 1.9: Tuning curves measured at a single point on the BM. Each curve shows the input sound level required to produce a constant velocity on the BM, plotted as a function of stimulus frequency. The curve marked by open circles was obtained at the start of the experiment when the animal was in good physiological condition. The curve marked by filled squares was obtained after the death of the animal. Data from Sellick, Patuzzi and Johnstone (1982).

is determined mainly by the active mechanism. When the active mechanism ceases to function, the sharply tuned tip of the tuning curve is lost, and the CF shifts to a lower frequency determined by the passive mechanics.

Even in a healthy ear, the balance between the active and passive mechanics can change with sound level. If the input level of a sinusoid is held constant, and its frequency is varied, then the response of the BM (velocity or amplitude) at a specific point shows a peak for a specific frequency. However, the frequency that gives the maximum response often varies with the input sound level (Ruggero, Rich, Recio et al., 1997). Typically, this frequency decreases with increasing sound level as the relative contribution of the active mechanism decreases. This implies that, for a fixed input frequency, the place on the BM showing the maximum response shifts towards the base with increasing sound level. Usually, the CF is specified for a low input sound level.

In summary, in a normal healthy ear each point along the BM is sharply tuned, responding with high sensitivity to a limited range of frequencies, and requiring higher and higher sound intensities to produce a response as the frequency is moved outside that range. The sharp tuning and high sensitivity reflect the active process mediated by the OHCs.

The non-linearity of input-output functions on the BM

In a normal healthy ear, the response of the BM is non-linear; when the input magnitude is increased, the magnitude of the response does not grow directly in proportion to the magnitude of the input (Rhode, 1971; Rhode and Robles, 1974; Sellick, Patuzzi and Johnstone, 1982; Robles, Ruggero and Rich, 1986; Ruggero, 1992; Ruggero, Rich, Recio et al., 1997). This is illustrated in Figure 1.10, which shows input-output functions of the BM for a place with a CF of 8 kHz (from Robles, Ruggero and Rich, 1986). A series of curves is shown; each curve represents a particular stimulating frequency indicated by a number (in kHz) close to the curve. The output (velocity of vibration) is plotted on a logarithmic scale as a function of the input sound level (in dB SPL - also a logarithmic scale). If the responses were linear, the functions would be parallel to the dashed line. Two functions are shown for a CF tone (8 kHz), one (at higher levels) obtained about one hour after the other. The slight shift between the two was probably caused by deterioration in the condition of the animal. An 'idealised' function for a CF tone, with the ordinate scaled in dB units (i.e. as $20\log_{10}$(velocity)) is shown in Figure 1.11.

The function for the CF tone is almost linear for very low input sound levels (below 20-30 dB) and approaches linearity at high input sound

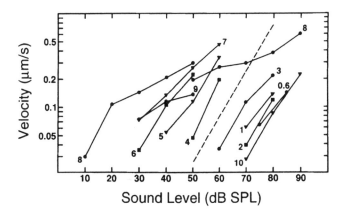

Figure 1.10: Input-output functions for a place on the BM with CF = 8 kHz. The stimulating frequency, in kHz, is indicated by a number close to each curve. The dashed line indicates the slope that would be obtained if the responses were linear (velocity directly proportional to sound pressure). Redrawn from Robles, Ruggero and Rich (1986)

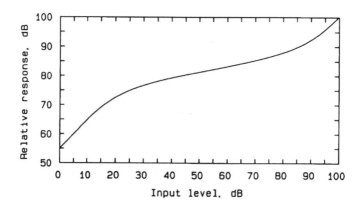

Figure 1.11: Schematic input-output function of the BM for a sinusoid at CF. A decibel scale is used for both axes. The ordinate is scaled (arbitrarily) so that an input of 100 dB gives an output of 100 dB

levels (above 90 dB); the function has a very shallow slope at mid-range levels. This indicates a compressive non-linearity; a large range of input sound levels is compressed into a smaller range of responses on the BM. The form of this function can be explained in the following way. At low and medium sound levels the active mechanism amplifies the response on the BM. The amplification may be 50 dB or more (Ruggero, Rich, Recio et al., 1997). At very low sound levels, below about 30 dB, the amplification is roughly constant and is at its maximal value. As the sound level increases the amplification progressively reduces. Thus the response grows more slowly than it would in a linear system. When the sound level is sufficiently high, around 90 dB SPL, the active mechanism is unable to contribute any amplification, and the response becomes linear. Hence, at high levels, the 'passive' response becomes dominant.

The non-linearity mainly occurs when the stimulating frequency is close to the CF of the point on the BM whose response is being measured. For stimuli with frequencies well away from the CF, the responses are more linear. Hence the curves for frequencies of 7 and 9 kHz (close to CF) show shallow slopes, whereas the curves for frequencies below 7 kHz and above 9 kHz show steeper (linear) slopes. Effectively, the compression occurs only around the peak of the response pattern on the BM. As a result, the peak in the distribution of vibration along the BM flattens out at high sound levels, which partly accounts for the broad tuning observed by Von Békésy.

Given that the BM response at moderate sound levels is highly non-linear, one might expect that, in response to a single sinusoid, harmonics would be generated and the waveform on the BM would be significantly distorted. In fact this does not seem to happen (Cooper and Rhode, 1992; Ruggero, Rich, Recio et al., 1997). The reason why is not

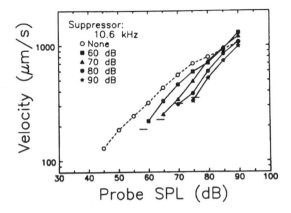

Figure 1.12: An example of two-tone suppression for a place on the BM with CF = 8.6 kHz. The dashed curve with open circles shows an input-output function for an 8.6 kHz tone alone, referred to as the 'probe'. The solid curves show input-output functions when a suppressor tone was added to the probe. The suppressor was presented at each of several overall levels, from 60 to 90 dB SPL, as indicated by the key in the Figure. The solid curves are truncated at the level where the suppressor led to an increase in response rather than a decrease. Redrawn from Ruggero, Robles and Rich (1992)

fully understood. Perhaps the active mechanism involves feedback on to the BM in such a way that potential harmonic distortion is filtered out by the passive mechanism. However, in response to inputs containing more than one sinusoidal component, significant distortion can occur. This is described later on in this chapter.

Two-tone suppression

Experiments using two tones have revealed another aspect of non-linearity on the BM, namely *two-tone suppression*. The effect is analogous to an effect that was first discovered from measurements of the responses of single neurones in the auditory nerve (see below for details). The response to a tone (called the 'probe' tone) with frequency close to the CF of the place on the BM being studied can be reduced by a second tone with a higher or lower frequency, especially when the second tone is higher in level than the probe tone (Rhode, 1977; Patuzzi, Sellick and Johnstone, 1984; Ruggero, Robles and Rich, 1992). The effect is illustrated in Figure 1.12 for a probe tone of 8.6 kHz (close to the CF) and a suppressor tone at 10.6 kHz. Ruggero, Robles and Rich (1992) provided a detailed comparison of the properties of mechanical two-tone suppression on the BM and two-tone suppression measured in the auditory nerve. They concluded that all of the properties match qualitatively (and mostly quantitatively) and that two-tone suppression in the auditory nerve probably originates from two-tone suppression on the BM.

Combination tone generation

Another aspect of BM non-linearity is the generation of distortion products in response to two or more sinusoidal inputs. These products are often called *combination tones*. When two sinusoids are presented simultaneously, and their frequency separation is not too great, their response patterns overlap on the BM. It appears that, at the point of overlap, distortion products are generated that behave like additional sinusoidal tones. For example, if the two primary tones presented to the ear have frequencies f_1 and f_2 ($f_2 > f_1$), the distortion products have frequencies such as $2f_1 - f_2$ and $f_2 - f_1$. The distortion products appear to propagate along the BM to the locations tuned to their own frequencies (Robles, Ruggero and Rich, 1991). For example, the combination tone with frequency $2f_1 - f_2$ produces a local maximum on the BM at the place tuned to $2f_1 - f_2$.

Human listeners can sometimes hear these additional tones. The one with frequency $2f_1 - f_2$ is especially easy to hear. It is audible even at relatively low levels of the primary tones when f_2 is about 1.2 times f_1 (Smoorenburg, 1972a; 1972b). For example, if the two primary tones have frequencies of 1000 and 1200 Hz, then a tone is heard with a frequency of 800 Hz. The combination tone with frequency $2f_1 + f_2$ is much harder to hear. This may be the case because this tone has a higher frequency than the two primary tones. Although $2f_1 + f_2$ is probably generated at the point where the response patterns of f_1 and f_2 overlap, it does not propagate to the location on the BM tuned to $2f_1 + f_2$; this would involve propagation in the 'wrong' direction, from the apex towards the base.

Responses of the BM to complex sounds

Consider the response of the BM to two sinusoids, of different frequencies, presented simultaneously. Assume that the sinusoids are equal in level, so that two-tone suppression is small. The kind of pattern of vibration that occurs depends on the frequency separation of the two sinusoids. If this is very large, then the two sinusoids produce two, effectively separate, patterns of vibration on the BM. Each produces a maximum at the place on the BM that would have been excited most had that component been presented alone. Thus the response of the BM to a low-frequency sinusoid of moderate intensity is essentially unaffected by a high-frequency sinusoid, and vice versa. In this case, the BM behaves like a frequency analyser, breaking down the complex sound into its sinusoidal components. Correspondingly, when we listen to two sinusoids with widely spaced frequencies, we hear two separate tones, with two different pitches. When the two sinusoids are relatively close in frequency, however, the patterns of vibration on the BM interact, so that some points on the BM respond to both of the sinusoids. At those points the displacement of the BM as a function of time is not sinusoidal, but is a complex waveform resulting from the interference of the two sinusoids. When the two sinusoids are sufficiently close in frequency, each of the component sinusoids no longer gives a separate maximum in the pattern of vibration; instead there is a single, broader, maximum. Thus, the BM has failed to separate (resolve) the individual frequency components. Correspondingly, when two sinusoids are very closely spaced in frequency, we cannot hear two separate tones, each with its own pitch; rather, we hear a single sound corresponding to the mixture. This is described more fully in Chapter 3.

Consider, now, the more complex case of the pattern of responses on the BM to a periodic complex tone, such as a voiced vowel or an instrument playing a note. Such a tone typically contains many harmonics of a common fundamental frequency. For example, a note of 'A5' would have a fundamental component with a frequency of 440 Hz, and higher harmonics with frequencies of 880, 1320, 1760 . . . Hz. The harmonics are equally spaced on a linear frequency scale. However, the mapping of CF to distance along the BM roughly follows a *logarithmic* scale. For example, sinusoids with frequencies of 400, 800, 1600 and 3200 Hz would produce peaks that were roughly equally spaced along the BM (see Figure 1.8). When a harmonic complex tone is presented to the ear, the lower harmonics each give rise to a separate peak on the BM whereas the higher harmonics give responses that overlap, so that there are not distinct peaks corresponding to the individual harmonics. A perceptual consequence of this is that individual low harmonics can often be 'heard out' as separate tones whereas higher harmonics cannot be individually heard; this is described more fully in Chapter 3. These factors play a crucial role in the perception of complex tones, as is explained in Chapter 6.

Evoked otoacoustic emissions

Evidence supporting the idea that there are active biological processes influencing cochlear mechanics has come from a remarkable phenomenon first reported by Kemp (1978). If a low-level click is applied to the ear, then it is possible to detect sound being reflected from the ear, using a microphone sealed into the ear canal. The early part of this reflected sound appears to come from the middle ear, but some sound can be detected for delays from 5 to 60 ms following the instant of click presentation. These delays are far too long to be attributed to the middle ear, and they almost certainly result from activity in the cochlea itself. The reflected sounds are known as evoked *otoacoustic emissions*. They have also been called *Kemp echoes* and *cochlear echoes*.

Although the input click in Kemp's experiment contained energy over a wide range of frequencies, only certain frequencies were present in the reflected sound. Kemp suggested that the reflections are generated at points on the BM, or in the IHC/OHC transduction mechanism, where there is a gradient or discontinuity in the mechanical or electrical properties. The response is non-linear, in that the reflected sound does not have an intensity in direct proportion to the input intensity. In fact, the relative level of the reflection is greatest at low sound levels; the emission grows about 3 dB for each 10 dB increase in input level. This non-linear behaviour can be used to distinguish the response arising from the cochlea from the linear middle-ear response.

Sometimes the amount of energy reflected from the cochlea at a given frequency may exceed that which was present in the input sound (Burns, Keefe and Ling, 1998). Kemp and others have suggested that the emissions are a by-product of the active mechanism. Indeed, many ears emit sounds in the absence of any input and these can be detected in the ear canal (Zurek, 1981). Such sounds are called *spontaneous otoacoustic emissions,* and their existence indicates that there is a source of energy within the cochlea that is capable of generating sounds.

Cochlear emissions can be very stable in a given individual, both in waveform and frequency content, but each ear gives its own characteristic response. Responses tend to be strongest between 500 and 2500 Hz, probably because transmission from the cochlea back through the middle ear is most efficient in this range, as described earlier. Cochlear emissions can be measured for brief tone bursts as well as clicks, and it is even possible to detect a reflected component in response to continuous stimulation with pure tones.

When the ear is stimulated with two tones, an emission may be detected at the frequency of one or more combination tones, particularly $2f_1 - f_2$. Such emissions are called *distortion-product otoacoustic emissions.* This confirms that the combination tone is present as a mechanical disturbance in the cochlea, as a travelling wave on the BM.

Sometimes the transient stimulation used to evoke a cochlear echo induces a sustained oscillation at a particular frequency, and the subject may report hearing this oscillation as a tonal sensation. The phenomenon of hearing sound in the absence of external stimulation is known as *tinnitus.* It appears that tinnitus may arise from abnormal activity at several different points in the auditory system, but in a few cases it corresponds to mechanical activity in the cochlea.

In summary, several types of otoacoustic emissions can be identified, including evoked emissions, spontaneous emissions and distortion-product emissions. While the exact mechanism by which otoacoustic emissions are generated is not understood, there is agreement that it is connected with the active mechanism inside the cochlea.

Neural responses in the normal auditory nerve

Most studies of activity in the auditory nerve have used electrodes with very fine tips, known as microelectrodes. These record the nerve impulses, or spikes, in single auditory nerve fibres (often called single units). The main findings, summarised below, seem to hold for most mammals.

Spontaneous firing rates and thresholds

Most neurones show a certain baseline firing rate, called the spontaneous rate, in the absence of any external stimulus. Liberman (1978) presented evidence that auditory nerve fibres could be classified into three groups on the basis of their spontaneous rates. About 61% of fibres have high spontaneous rates (18 to 250 spikes per second); 23% have medium rates (0.5 to 18 spikes per second); and 16% have low spontaneous rates (less than 0.5 spike per second). The spontaneous rates are correlated with the position and size of the synapses of the neurones on the IHCs. High spontaneous rates are associated with large synapses, primarily located on the side of the IHCs facing the OHCs. Low spontaneous rates are associated with smaller synapses on the opposite side of the hair cells. The spontaneous rates are also correlated with the thresholds of the neurones. The threshold is the lowest sound level at which a change in response of the neurone can be measured. High spontaneous rates tend to be associated with low thresholds and vice versa. The most sensitive neurones may have thresholds close to 0 dB SPL, whereas the least sensitive neurones may have thresholds of 80 dB SPL or more.

Tuning curves and iso-rate contours

The tuning of a single nerve fibre is often illustrated by plotting the fibre's threshold as a function of frequency. This curve is known as the *tuning curve* or *frequency-threshold curve* (FTC). The stimuli are usually tone bursts, rather than continuous tones. This avoids effects of long-term adaptation (a decrease in response over time that can occur with continuous stimulation) and also makes it easier to distinguish spontaneous from evoked neural activity. The frequency at which the threshold of the fibre is lowest is called the *characteristic frequency* (CF) (the same term is used to described the frequency to which a given place on the BM is most sensitive). Some typical tuning curves are presented in Figure 1.13. On the logarithmic frequency scale used, the tuning curves are usually steeper on the high-frequency side than on the low-frequency side. It is generally assumed that the tuning seen in single auditory nerve fibres occurs because those fibres are responding to

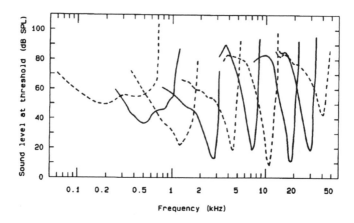

Figure 1.13: A sample of tuning curves (also called frequency-threshold curves) obtained from single neurones in the auditory nerve of anaesthetised cats. Each curve shows results for one neurone. The sound level required for threshold is plotted as a function of the stimulus frequency (logarithmic scale). Redrawn from Palmer (1987).

activity at a particular point on the BM. Iso-velocity tuning curves on the BM are similar in shape to neural FTCs (Khanna and Leonard, 1982; Sellick, Patuzzi and Johnstone, 1982; Robles, Ruggero and Rich, 1986; Ruggero, Rich, Recio et al., 1997).

The CFs of single neurones are distributed in an orderly manner in the auditory nerve. Fibres with high CFs are found in the periphery of the nerve bundle, and there is an orderly decrease in CF towards the centre of the nerve bundle (Kiang, Watanabe, Thomas et al., 1965). This kind of arrangement is known as *tonotopic organisation* and it indicates that the place representation of frequency along the BM is preserved as a place representation in the auditory nerve.

In order to provide a description of the characteristics of single fibres at levels above threshold, iso-rate contours can be plotted. To determine an iso-rate contour the intensity of sinusoidal stimulation required to produce a predetermined firing rate in the neurone is plotted as a function of frequency. The resulting curves are generally similar in shape to tuning curves, although they sometimes broaden at high sound levels. The frequency at the tip (the lowest point on the curve) may also decrease slightly with increases in the predetermined firing rate. This reflects the change in BM tuning with level, described earlier.

Rate-versus-level functions

Figure 1.14 shows schematically how the rate of discharge for three auditory nerve fibres changes as a function of stimulus level. The curves

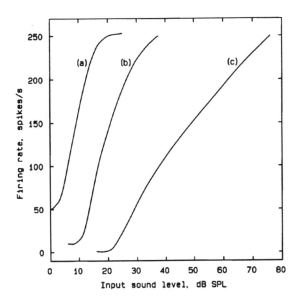

Figure 1.14: Schematic examples of how the discharge rates of single auditory neurones vary as a function of stimulus level. The curves are called *rate-versus-level functions*. In each case, the stimulus was a sinusoid at the CF of the neurone. Curves (a), (b) and (c) are typical of what is observed for neurones with high, medium and low spontaneous firing rates, respectively.

are called *rate-versus-level functions*. In each case, the stimulus was a sinusoid at the CF of the neurone. Consider first the curve labelled (a). This curve is typical of what is observed for neurones with high spontaneous firing rates. Above a certain sound level the neurone no longer responds to increases in sound level with an increase in firing rate; the neurone is said to be *saturated*. The range of sound levels between threshold and the level at which saturation occurs is called the *dynamic range*. For neurones with high spontaneous rates, this range is often quite small, about 15-30 dB. Curve (b) is typical of what is observed for neurones with medium spontaneous rates. The threshold is slightly higher than for (a) and the dynamic range is slightly wider. Curve (c) is typical of what is observed for neurones with low spontaneous rates. The threshold is higher than for (b). The firing rate at first increases fairly rapidly with increasing sound level, but then the rate of increase slows down. The firing rate continues to increase gradually with increasing sound level over a wide range of levels. This has been called 'sloping saturation' (Sachs and Abbas, 1974).

The shapes of rate versus level functions can be understood in terms of two functions (Yates, 1990; Patuzzi, 1992). This is illustrated in Figure 1.15. The first function is the input-output function of the BM, illustrated schematically in the top-right panel. The second is the function

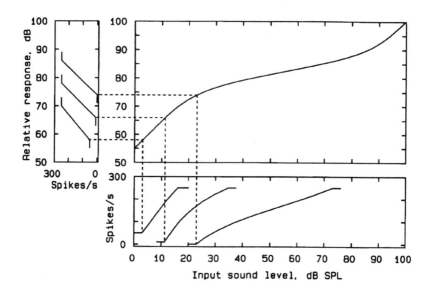

Figure 1.15: Schematic illustration of how the shapes of rate-versus-level functions can be accounted for in terms of the BM input-output function (top-right panel), and the functions relating neural firing rate (spikes/sec) to amount of vibration on the BM (top-left panel). Three such functions are shown, corresponding to synapses with different sensitivities. The resulting three rate-versus-level functions are shown in the bottom panel. Adapted from Patuzzi (1992).

relating the spike rate in a specific neurone to the magnitude of the BM response. This second function is similar in form for different neurones, showing saturation when the BM amplitude is a certain factor above the value required for threshold, but it varies in the magnitude required for threshold. Three such functions are illustrated schematically in the top-left panel of Figure 1.15. The rate-versus-level functions corresponding to these three functions are shown in the bottom-right panel.

The variation across neurones depends mainly on the type of synapse, as discussed earlier. Neurones with low thresholds have large sensitive synapses. They start to respond at very low sound levels, where the input-output function on the BM is nearly linear. As the sound level increases, the BM displacement increases in a nearly linear manner, and the neurone saturates relatively early, giving a small dynamic range, as shown by the left-most curve in the lower panel. Neurones with higher thresholds have less sensitive synapses. They respond over the range of sound levels where the BM input-output function shows a strong compressive non-linearity. Hence a large increase in sound level is needed to increase the BM displacement to the point where the neurone saturates, and the neurone has a wide dynamic range, as shown by the right-most curve in the lower panel.

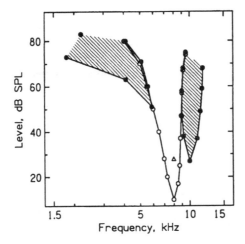

Figure 1.16: Neurophysiological data from Arthur, Pfeiffer and Suga (1971). The open circles show the tuning curve (threshold versus frequency) of a single neurone with a CF at 8 kHz. The neurone was stimulated with a tone at CF, and just above threshold (indicated by the open triangle). A second tone was then added and its frequency and intensity varied. Any tone within the shaded areas bounded by the solid circles reduced the response to the tone at CF by 20% or more. These are the suppression areas.

Two-tone suppression

Auditory neurones show an effect that is exactly analogous to the two-tone suppression on the BM that was described earlier. Indeed, the neural effect was discovered long before the BM effect. The tone-driven activity of a single fibre in response to one tone can be suppressed by the presence of a second tone. This was originally called 'two-tone inhibition' (Sachs and Kiang, 1968), although the term *two-tone suppression* is now generally preferred as the effect does not appear to involve neural inhibition. The phenomenon is typically investigated by presenting a tone at, or close to, the CF of a neurone. A second tone is then presented, its frequency and intensity are varied, and the effects of this on the response of the neurone are noted. When the frequency and intensity of the second tone fall within the excitatory area bounded by the tuning curve, this usually produces an increase in firing rate. However, when it falls just outside that area, the response to the first tone is reduced or suppressed. The suppression is greatest when the suppressor falls in one of two frequency regions on either side of the excitatory response area, as illustrated in Figure 1.16. The suppression begins very quickly when the suppressor is turned on, and ceases very quickly when it is turned off (Arthur, Pfeiffer and Suga, 1971). This is consistent with the probable origin of the suppression as a mechanical effect on the BM.

Phase locking

In response to a sinusoid with a frequency below about 5 kHz, the nerve firings tend to be *phase locked* or synchronised to the stimulating waveform. A given nerve fibre does not necessarily fire on every cycle of the stimulus but, when firings do occur, they occur at roughly the same phase of the waveform each time. Thus, the time intervals between firings are (approximately) integer multiples of the period of the stimulating waveform. For example, a 500-Hz tone has a period of 2 ms; the waveform repeats regularly every 2 ms. The intervals between nerve firings in response to a 500-Hz tone are approximately 2 ms, or 4 ms, or 6 ms, or 8 ms, etc. Neurones do not fire in a completely regular manner, so that there are not exactly 500, or 250 or 125 spikes/s. However, information about the period of the stimulating waveform is carried unambiguously in the temporal pattern of firing of a single neurone.

One way to demonstrate phase locking in a single auditory nerve fibre is to plot a histogram of the time intervals between successive nerve firings. Several such *interspike interval histograms* are shown in Figure 1.17, for a neurone with a CF of 1.6 kHz. For each of the different stimulating frequencies (from 0.408 to 2.3 kHz in this case) the intervals between nerve spikes lie predominantly at integer multiples of the period of the stimulating tone. These intervals are indicated by dots below each abscissa. Thus, although the neurone does not fire on every cycle of the stimulus, the distribution of time intervals between nerve firings depends very much on the frequency of the stimulating waveform.

Phase locking does not occur over the whole range of audible frequencies. In most mammals it becomes progressively less precise for stimulus frequencies above 1 kHz, and it disappears completely at about 4-5 kHz (Rose, Brugge, Anderson et al., 1968), although the exact upper limit varies somewhat across species (Palmer and Russell, 1986). Phase locking improves in precision with increasing sound level at low levels, and then stays roughly constant in precision over a very wide range of sound levels.

Information from phase locking contributes to the ability to localise sounds in space and it probably also plays a role in the perception of pitch. These aspects of auditory perception are discussed more fully in Chapters 6 and 7.

Types of hearing loss

A *conductive* hearing loss is caused by reduced efficiency of sound transmission through the outer and/or middle ear. This may be caused by wax (cerumen) in the ear canal, damage to the eardrum produced by infection or trauma, damage to the ossicles in the middle ear, or fluid in the middle ear caused by infection. It results in an attenuation of sound reaching the cochlea, so that sounds appear quieter than normal. The amount of loss may vary with frequency, so sounds may appear to have a

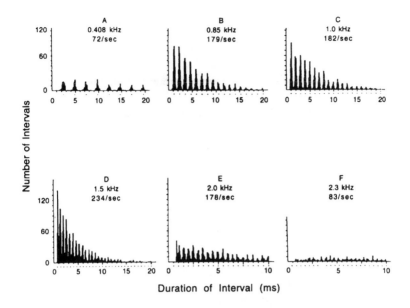

Figure 1.17: Interspike interval histograms for a single auditory neurone (in the squirrel monkey) with a CF of 1.6 kHz. The frequency of the sinusoidal input and the mean response rate in spikes per second are indicated above each histogram. All tones had a level 80 dB SPL. Notice that the time scales in E and F differ from those in A to D. Redrawn from Rose, Brugge, Anderson and Hind (1968).

somewhat different tonal quality from normal. However, these are the main perceptual consequences of a conductive loss. Unlike cochlear hearing loss, it does not generally result in marked distortions or abnormalities in other aspects of sound perception. Conductive hearing loss can often be treated by drugs (to cure infections) or surgery.

Cochlear hearing loss involves damage to the structures inside the cochlea. It can arise in many ways - for example by exposure to intense sounds or to ototoxic chemicals (such as certain antibiotics, drugs used to treat high blood pressure or solvents), by infection, by metabolic disturbances, by some allergies and as a result of genetic factors. These agents can produce a variety of types of damage to the cochlea and, to complicate matters further, the damage may extend beyond the cochlea. For example, an infection may produce damage at several sites, such as the auditory nerve and higher centres in the auditory pathway. When both cochlear and neural structures are involved, the more general term *sensorineural hearing loss* is used.

Finally, hearing loss can occur through damage to structures or neural systems occurring at a level in the auditory system beyond the cochlea, for example in the auditory nerve or the auditory cortex. Such types of hearing loss are given the general name *retrocochlear* loss. A

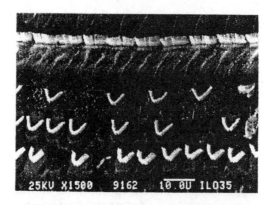

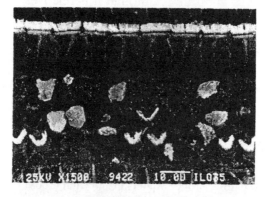

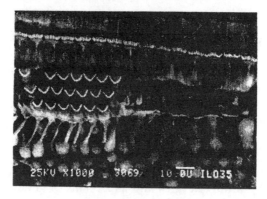

Figure 1.18: Examples of patterns of damage to the OHCs. For the top two panels, the damage was caused by administration of aminoglycosides. For the bottom panel, the damage was of unknown origin. In the upper panel the stereocilia of some OHCs are missing. In the middle panel the stereocilia of the OHCs are mostly either missing or grossly deformed. In the bottom panel, the stereocilia of the OHCs are completely missing over a certain region. The bottom panel also shows expansion of the supporting cells to replace lost hair cells. The electronmicrographs were supplied by Dr. Andrew Forge of the Institute of Laryngology and Otology, University College London Medical School.

common cause of retrocochlear loss is the growth of a tumour that presses on the auditory nerve.

Although sensorineural hearing loss can involve structures other than the cochlea, it is common for the most serious damage to occur within the cochlea. This is probably true for the majority of cases of *presbyacusis*, the hearing loss that is associated with ageing. Furthermore, it is common for the damage to be largely confined to certain specific structures within the cochlea. This book is concerned with cases where the hearing loss arises primarily from damage to the cochlea. Henceforth, when the phrase 'hearing impairment' is used, it should be taken to imply hearing impairment caused by cochlear damage. However, it should be borne in mind that, although it is relatively easy to produce 'pure' cochlear damage in animal models, such 'pure' damage may be relatively rare in hearing-impaired humans.

In the last 20 years there has been a considerable increase in understanding of the physiology and function of the normal cochlea. Along with this has come improved understanding of the changes in function that are associated with cochlear hearing loss. The rest of this chapter reviews the structure and function of the impaired cochlea.

Physiology of the damaged cochlea

There is strong evidence that the functioning of the normal cochlea depends upon the operation of an active mechanism that is linked to the integrity of the OHCs. This mechanism may involve feedback of energy on to the BM, via the OHCs, and it plays an important role in producing the high sensitivity of the BM to weak sounds and the sharp tuning on the BM. The normal BM has a strongly non-linear response that results in compressive input-output functions, two-tone suppression and combination-tone generation.

Cochlear hearing loss often involves damage to the OHCs and IHCs; the stereocilia may be distorted or destroyed, or entire hair cells may die. The OHCs are generally more vulnerable to damage than the IHCs. Some examples of OHC damage are shown in Figure 1.18. When OHCs are damaged, the active mechanism tends to be reduced in effectiveness or lost altogether. As a result, several changes occur. Sensitivity to weak sounds is reduced, so sounds need to be more intense to produce a given magnitude of response on the BM. The tuning curves on the BM become much more broadly tuned. All of the frequency-selective non-linear effects weaken or disappear altogether.

BM responses

There have been many studies showing that the responses on the BM are highly physiologically vulnerable. One example has already been given; see Figure 1.9. Generally, the tuning on the BM becomes less sharp and

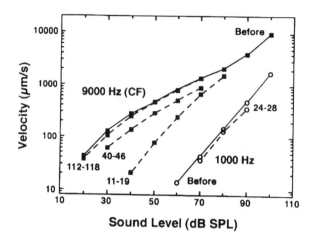

Figure 1.19: Input-output functions on the BM immediately preceding (solid lines) and following (broken lines) an intravenous furosemide injection. See text for details. Redrawn from Ruggero and Rich (1991).

the sensitivity around the tip is reduced when the cochlea is damaged. In the great majority of studies the changes in BM responses have been associated with some form of damage to the OHCs, either directly or via some form of metabolic disturbance.

The effects of cochlear damage on the input-output functions of the BM of a chinchilla are illustrated in Figure 1.19 (Ruggero and Rich, 1991). The solid curve with black squares, labelled 'Before', shows the input-output function obtained when the cochlea was in good condition; the stimulus was a sinusoid with frequency corresponding to the CF of 9000 Hz. The curve shows a compressive non-linearity for input sound levels between about 30 and 90 dB SPL. In contrast, the response to a sinusoid with a frequency of 1000 Hz, well below the CF, is steeper and is almost linear (solid curve with open circles).

To manipulate the functioning of the cochlea, the animal was injected with furosemide (also known as frusemide), a diuretic that is known to disrupt hair cell potentials. The dashed curves in Figure 1.19 were obtained at various times after injection of the drug - the time is indicated by a range in minutes next to each curve. Shortly after the injection (11-19 minutes) the input-output function for the CF tone was markedly altered. The biggest alteration was at low sound levels. To produce a given response on the BM (say, 40 μm/s), the input level had to be increased by about 25 dB relative to the level measured before the injection. However, the response to a CF tone at a high level (80 dB SPL) was almost normal. This is consistent with the idea that the contribution of the active mechanism reduces progressively as the sound level is increased above about 40 dB. After a sufficiently long time (112-118 minutes), the input-output function returned to normal. In this case, the cochlear damage was reversible. Larger doses of the drug, or treatment with other drugs, can result in permanent cochlear damage.

Note that injection of the drug did not change the input-output function for the 1000-Hz tone (see the curve with open symbols labelled 24-28). This is consistent with the idea that the active mechanism mainly influences responses around the peak of the response pattern evoked by a sinusoidal tone. Responses to tones with frequencies well away from the CF are linear, and remain so when the active mechanism is damaged.

Neural responses

Some of the first evidence for a physiologically vulnerable active mechanism came from studies of the responses of single neurones in the auditory nerve. Robertson and Manley (1974) showed that the normal, sharp tuning seen in auditory neurones could be altered by reducing the oxygen supply to the animal. The tuning curves became less sharp and at the same time the sensitivity around the tip decreased. These changes were similar to those found subsequently in BM responses with similar manipulations (see Figure 1.9). The changes in BM tuning and sensitivity found by Robertson and Manley were reversible. Similar effects were reported by Evans (1975), who also found that a reversible degradation in tuning could be produced by the ototoxic agents cyanide and furosemide. Evans and Harrison (1976) used the drug Kanamycin to produce selective damage to the OHCs. They found that the threshold and tuning properties of auditory nerve fibres were dependent on the integrity of the OHCs.

Structure-function correlation

Liberman and his colleagues used noise exposure and ototoxic drugs, separately or in combination, to produce a variety of types of damage to the hair cells in the cochlea. They then measured neural responses and compared them with structural changes in the cochlea (for a review, see Liberman, Dodds and Learson, 1986). After studying the properties of a given single neurone, the neurone was injected with horseradish peroxidase. This labelled the neurone so that it could be traced to the IHC with which it synapsed in the organ of Corti. In this way, the neural response properties could be directly compared with the structural changes in the hair cells and the immediately surrounding structures in the organ of Corti.

Figure 1.20 shows the situation when there is partial destruction of the OHCs, with intact IHCs. This pattern of damage is typical of that associated with moderate doses of ototoxic drugs, but is less typical of noise exposure. The left part of the figure schematically illustrates the

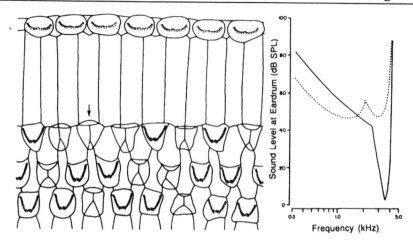

Figure 1.20: The left part shows a schematic diagram of an organ of Corti with sub-total loss of OHCs and intact IHCs. The right part shows a normal neural tuning curve (solid) and an abnormal tuning curve (dotted) associated with this kind of damage. Adapted from Liberman, Dodds and Learson (1986).

pattern of structural damage. The view is looking down on to the tops of the hair cells, so each stereocilium appears as a small dot. The three rows of OHCs appear at the bottom. In the figure, some OHCs are missing or lack stereocilia (see arrow).

The right-hand part of Figure 1.20 shows a typical normal tuning curve (solid curve) and a tuning curve associated with this type of damage (dotted curve). The normal tuning curve shows a sharply tuned 'tip' and a broadly tuned 'tail'. The abnormal tuning curve also appears to have two sections, but the tip is elevated, and the tail is hypersensitive (i.e. thresholds in the region of the tail are lower than normal). The elevated tip may reflect the operation of the active mechanism at reduced effectiveness. The pattern of results suggests that the active mechanism is tuned to a frequency slightly above the resonance frequency of the passive mechanical BM at that place. This is consistent with the observation that, in a normal ear, the peak response on the BM shifts towards the base of the cochlea with increasing sound level (see above).

Figure 1.21 shows the situation when there is total loss of OHCs with intact IHCs. This pattern of damage is most easily produced with large doses of ototoxic drugs. The bowl-shaped abnormal tuning curve completely lacks the sharp tip, because the active mechanism is completely destroyed. The broad tuning of the curve probably depends largely on the passive mechanical properties of the BM.

Figure 1.22 shows the situation where there is severe damage to the stereocilia of the IHCs and the stereocilia of the first row of OHCs (the row closest to the IHCs). The OHC damage is sufficient to eliminate completely the sharply tuned tip of the tuning curve, suggesting that the

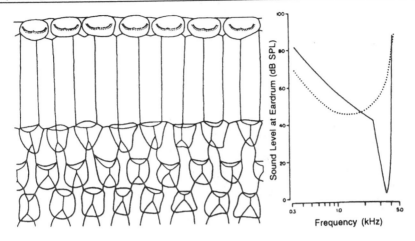

Figure 1.21: As Figure 1.20, but for the situation with total loss of OHCs with intact IHCs.

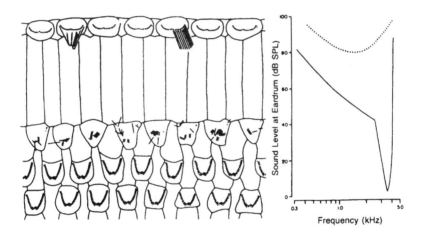

Figure 1.22: As Figure 1.20, but for the situation with severe damage to both OHC and IHC stereocilia. Most of the damage to the OHC stereocilia is confined to the first row of hair cells.

active mechanism is particularly dependent on the first row of OHCs. In addition the whole curve is shifted upwards, i.e. sensitivity is much less than normal. This overall loss of sensitivity (compare the tuning curves in Figures 1.20 and 1.21) can probably be attributed to the IHC damage. According to Liberman et al., significant damage to the IHC stereocilia is always associated with reduced sensitivity on the tail of the tuning curve.

Liberman et al. did not find any cases of pure IHC damage, without OHC damage. It appears that the OHCs are generally more vulnerable to damage than the IHCs, and so damage to the IHCs is nearly always

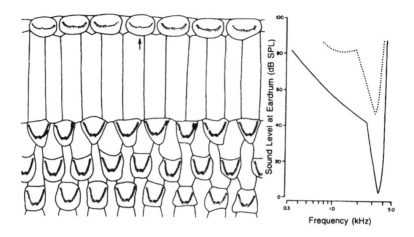

Figure 1.23: As Figure 1.20, but for a situation with moderate damage to IHC stereocilia and minimal damage to OHC stereocilia.

associated with damage to the OHCs. However, cases approximating pure IHC damage were sometimes found. Figure 1.23 shows an example of a neurone contacting an IHC missing the entire tall row of stereocilia (see arrow) in a region with only modest disarray of OHC stereocilia. The tuning curve shows a tip that is almost normal in shape, but the tip and tail are both shifted upwards by about 40 dB. It appears that the active mechanism was operating, but the transduction mechanism had greatly reduced sensitivity.

These findings can be summarised as follows. The OHCs are responsible for the sharp tips of the tuning curves. When the OHCs are damaged the sharp tip becomes elevated, or may disappear altogether. This can cause a threshold elevation around the tip of the tuning curve of 40-50 dB. The condition of the OHCs determines the ratio of tip to tail thresholds. Damage to the IHCs causes an overall loss of sensitivity. This is apparent in the tail of the tuning curve, whether or not the OHCs are damaged. Pure OHC damage either leaves the tail unaffected or causes hypersensitivity (lower thresholds) in the tail. When both OHCs and IHCs are damaged, thresholds are usually greatly elevated by 80 dB or more and the tuning curve is broad, without any sign of a sharp tip.

Liberman et al. found that they could 'account for' most of the threshold shift in the neurones by evaluating the presence or absence of OHCs and IHCs and the condition of their stereocilia. Furthermore, behavioural thresholds after noise exposure have been found to be correlated with patterns of damage in hair cell stereocilia (Slepecky, Hamernik, Henderson et al., 1982). It seems likely that, for many types of cochlear hearing loss, the primary cause of the loss is damage to the OHCs and/or IHCs. For moderate losses, where thresholds are elevated by less than 50 dB, it may often be the case that the main cause of the loss is damage to the OHCs, with consequent impairment of the active mechanism. In this case, the loss of absolute sensitivity (elevation of threshold) occurs mainly because of reduced responses on the BM to low-level sounds. For more severe losses, it is likely that both OHCs and IHCs are damaged. When the IHCs are damaged, a greater response on the BM is needed to produce a 'threshold' amount of neural activity.

Evoked otoacoustic emissions

Evoked otoacoustic emissions are reduced in magnitude by cochlear hearing loss. Human ears with hearing losses exceeding 40 to 60 dB (see Chapter 2 for the definition of 'hearing loss') usually show no detectable emissions (Gorga, Neely, Ohlrich et al., 1997). The emissions appear to be particularly associated with OHC function. The emissions are abolished in ears that have been exposed to intense sounds or to drugs that adversely affect the operation of the cochlea. In the former case, the emissions may return after a period of recovery. This suggests that the emissions are linked to the active mechanism. The measurement of cochlear emissions provides a sensitive way of monitoring the physiological state of the cochlea and it is now being commonly applied in clinical situations, especially for assessing cochlear function in the very young.

Phase locking

The effect of cochlear damage on phase locking is not entirely clear. Harrison and Evans (1979) used the ototoxic drug kanamycin to produce hair cell damage (mainly to OHCs) in the guinea pig and found that phase locking was not affected. However, Woolf, Ryan and Bone (1981) carried out a similar experiment using the chinchilla and found that phase locking was adversely affected by damage to the OHCs. For neurones with CFs corresponding to frequencies where the behavioural thresholds were elevated by 40 dB or more compared to normal, phase locking was significantly reduced. There was a reduction in the highest frequency at which phase locking could be observed, and the precision of phase locking over the range 0.4-3 kHz was reduced.

The reason for the discrepancy between studies is unclear. It could be related to a species difference. Another possibility is that the data of Harrison and Evans are atypical. Woolf et al. pointed out that the upper limit of phase locking reported by Harrison and Evans (5-7 kHz) was higher than usually observed in the guinea pig. The reason why phase locking should deteriorate as a consequence of cochlear damage is also unclear. Woolf et al. suggested that it could be connected with poorer mechanical coupling between the tallest stereocilia of the OHCs and the tectorial membrane. Whatever the reason, it seems clear that phase locking can be affected by cochlear damage, and this may have important perceptual consequences.

Cochlear damage can certainly affect phase locking to complex sounds such as speech. Vowel sounds contain peaks in their spectral envelope at certain frequencies called formants; these correspond to resonances in the vocal tract (see Chapter 8 and Figure 8.2). Each formant is actually defined by several harmonics, whose amplitudes exceed those of adjacent harmonics. The formants are numbered, the lowest in frequency being called F1, the next F2, and so on. The frequencies of the formants, and especially the first two formants, are believed to be important for determining the identities of vowel sounds. At low levels in a normal auditory system, each neurone shows phase locking to a single harmonic or a small group of harmonics whose frequencies lie close to the CF of the neurone. Hence, the temporal response patterns vary markedly across neurones with different CFs. However, at higher levels, the temporal response patterns show a 'capture' phenomenon in which the first two formant frequencies dominate the responses; neurones with CFs that are somewhat removed from a formant frequency may nevertheless show strong phase locking to that formant. Most of the neurones with mid-range CFs show phase locking either to F1 or to F2. This may partly depend upon a suppression effect, related to two-tone suppression, whereby the relatively strong harmonics close to the formant frequencies suppress the responses to weaker harmonics at adjacent frequencies. Whatever the mechanism, the temporal information coded in the phase locking may be used by the auditory system to determine the formant frequencies.

Miller, Schilling, Franck and Young (1997) studied the effect on this phenomenon of cochlear damage caused by exposure to intense sound. After the acoustic trauma, capture by the second formant (which fell in the region of threshold elevation) was not observed; neurones with CFs adjacent to F2 did not show clear phase locking to F2 but showed more complex response patterns. The phase locking to formant frequencies observed in the normal auditory nerve may play an important role in the coding of the formant frequencies in the auditory system. If so, the reduced phase locking associated with cochlear damage might contribute to problems in understanding speech.

Conclusions

The functioning of the normal cochlea is strongly dependent on an active mechanism that is physiologically vulnerable. This mechanism depends upon the integrity of the OHCs, and particularly their stereocilia. The active mechanism is responsible for the high sensitivity and sharp tuning of the BM. It is also responsible for a variety of non-linear effects that can be observed in BM responses and neural responses. These effects include: the non-linear input-output functions on the BM;

the reduction in sharpness of tuning with increasing sound level; and combination-tone generation. Finally the active mechanism is probably responsible for the generation of evoked and spontaneous otoacoustic emissions. The active mechanism strongly influences responses on the BM at low and medium sound levels, but its contribution progressively reduces as the sound level increases.

The OHCs are easily damaged by noise exposure, ototoxic chemicals, infection, and metabolic disturbances. When they are damaged, the active mechanism is reduced in effectiveness or destroyed completely. This has several important consequences: (1) sensitivity is reduced, so that the tips of tuning curves are elevated by up to 40-50 dB; (2) the sharpness of tuning on the BM is greatly reduced. The tip of the tuning curve may be elevated or may disappear altogether, leaving only the broad tuning of the passive BM; (3) non-linear effects such as compressive input-output functions on the BM, two-tone suppression and combination tone generation are reduced or disappear altogether; (4) evoked and spontaneous otoacoustic emissions are reduced or disappear, at least in the frequency range corresponding to the damaged place.

The IHCs are the transducers of the cochlea converting the mechanical vibrations on the BM into neural activity. They are less susceptible to damage than the OHCs. When they are damaged, sensitivity is reduced. Damage primarily to the IHCs, with intact OHCs, is rare. When it does occur, sharp tuning may be preserved, but the whole tuning curve is elevated (less sensitive). More commonly, damage occurs both to the OHCs and IHCs. In this case the whole tuning curve is elevated, with a greater elevation around the tip than around the tail.

Damage to the hair cells can also result in a reduction in phase locking; the precision with which neural impulses are synchronised to the cochlear-filtered stimulating waveform is reduced. The reason why this occurs is unclear, but it may have important perceptual consequences.

Chapter 2
Absolute Thresholds

Introduction

The absolute threshold of a sound is the minimum detectable level of that sound in the absence of any other external sounds. The most obvious result of cochlear damage is reduced sensitivity to weak sounds; absolute thresholds are higher than normal. When measuring absolute thresholds, it is important to define the way in which the physical intensity of the threshold stimulus is measured. This chapter first describes the three common methods for specifying the threshold intensity. It then considers the origins of the loss of sensitivity associated with cochlear damage.

Measures of absolute threshold

Minimum audible pressure (MAP)

The first method requires the measurement of the sound pressure at some point close to the entrance of the ear canal or inside the ear canal, using a small 'probe' microphone. Such probe microphones are now often incorporated in 'real-ear' measurement systems that are used in fitting hearing aids. Ideally, the measurement of sound level is made very close to the eardrum. In all cases it is necessary to specify the exact position of the probe, since small changes in position can markedly affect the results at high frequencies. The threshold so determined is called the *minimum audible pressure* (MAP). The sounds are usually, but not always, delivered by headphone.

Minimum audible field (MAF)

A second method uses sounds delivered by loudspeaker, preferably in a room whose walls are highly sound absorbing. When reflections of sound from the walls, floor and ceiling are negligible, the listening conditions are described as *free field*. The measurement of sound level is made after the listener is removed from the sound field, at the point that had been occupied by the centre of the listener's head. The threshold determined in this way is called the *minimum audible field* (MAF). Usually, the sound is assumed to be coming from directly in front of the listener. Considerable errors can occur using this method if the reflections from the walls, floor and ceiling are not negligible, especially when sinusoids are used as stimuli. The errors can be reduced by the use of signals covering a wider frequency range, such as bands of noise or frequency modulated tones, which are also called 'warble tones'.

Comparison of MAP and MAF

Figure 2.1 shows estimates of the MAP, with sound level measured close to the eardrum, published by Killion (1978), and estimates of the MAF published in an ISO standard (ISO 389-7, 1996). Note that the MAP estimates are for monaural listening and the MAF estimates are for binaural listening. On average, thresholds are about 2 dB lower when two ears are used as opposed to one. Both curves represent the average data from many young listeners with normal hearing. It should be noted, however, that individual subjects may have thresholds as much as 20 dB above or below the mean at a specific frequency and still be considered as 'normal'.

The 'audibility curves' for the MAP and MAF are somewhat differently shaped, since the physical presence of the head, the pinna and the meatus influences the sound field. The MAP curve shows only minor peaks and dips (± 5 dB) for frequencies between about 0.2 kHz and 13 kHz, whereas the MAF curve shows a distinct dip around 3-4 kHz and a peak around 8-9 kHz. The difference derives mainly from a broad *resonance* produced by the meatus and pinna (see Figure 1.3).

Another factor which contributes to the shapes of the audibility curves is the transmission characteristic of the middle ear. Transmission is most efficient for mid-range frequencies and drops off markedly for very low and very high frequencies (see Figure 1.4). This can account for the rapid rise in threshold at low and high frequencies.

To a first approximation, the cochlea in humans is equally sensitive to all frequencies from about 500 Hz up to 15,000 Hz; variations in absolute threshold with frequency over this range probably reflect primarily the transmission characteristics of the outer and middle ear (Moore, Glasberg and Baer, 1997; Puria, Rosowski and Peake, 1997). Below 500 Hz, the sensitivity of the cochlea appears to decrease. This may reflect reduced gain from the active mechanism at low frequencies (Yates, 1995), internal noise produced by blood flow (Zwicker and Fastl, 1990) and/or an effect of the helicotrema (Dallos, 1973) (recall that this is a small opening which connects the two outer chambers of the cochlea, the *scala vestibuli* and the *scala tympani* at the apical end of the cochlea). The helicotrema reduces the pressure difference applied across the BM for very low-frequency sounds.

The highest audible frequency varies considerably with age. Young children can often hear sinusoids with frequencies as high as 20 kHz, but for most adults threshold rises rapidly above about 15 kHz. The loss of sensitivity with increasing age (presbyacusis) is much greater at high frequencies than at low, and the variability between people is also greater at high frequencies.

The audiogram

A third method of specifying absolute thresholds is commonly used in audiology; thresholds are specified relative to the average threshold at each frequency for young, healthy listeners with 'normal' hearing. In this case, the sound level is usually specified relative to standardised values produced by a specific earphone in a specific coupler. A coupler is a device that contains a cavity or series of cavities, and a microphone for measuring the sound produced by the earphone. The preferred earphone varies from one country to another. For example, the Telephonics TDH49 is often used in the USA, whereas the Beyer DT48 is used in Germany. Thresholds specified in this way have the units dB HL (hearing level) in Europe or dB HTL (hearing threshold level) in the

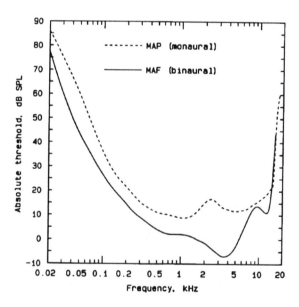

Figure 2.1: The absolute threshold expressed as the minimum audible pressure (MAP) and the minimum audible field (MAF) plotted as a function of frequency for young normally hearing subjects.

USA. For example, a threshold of 40 dB HL at 1 kHz would mean that the person had a threshold that was 40 dB higher than 'normal' at that frequency. In psychoacoustic work, thresholds are normally plotted with threshold increasing upwards, as in Figure 2.1. However, in audiology, threshold elevations are shown as hearing losses, plotted downwards. The average 'normal' threshold is represented as a horizontal line at the top of the plot, and the degree of hearing loss is indicated by how much the threshold falls below this line. This type of plot is called an *audiogram*. Figure 2.2 compares an audiogram for a hypothetical hearing-impaired person with a 'flat' hearing loss with a plot of the same thresholds expressed as MAP values. Notice that although the audiogram is flat, the corresponding MAP curve is not flat. Note also that thresholds in dB HL can be negative. For example, a threshold of −10 dB simply means that the individual is 10 dB more sensitive than the average.

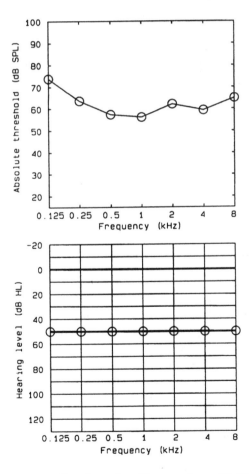

Figure 2.2: Comparison of a clinical audiogram for a 50 dB hearing loss at all frequencies (bottom), and the absolute threshold curve for the same hearing loss plotted in terms of the MAP (top).

Sensation level (abbreviated SL) describes the level of a sound relative to the absolute threshold of the subject for that sound. For example, if the absolute threshold is 23 dB SPL, and the sound is presented at 33 dB SPL, then its level is 10 dB SL.

Descriptions of the severity of hearing loss

The measurement of absolute thresholds provides the easiest way of detecting and measuring damage to the auditory system. Often, the hearing loss varies with frequency. However, it is useful to have a way of describing the overall severity of a hearing loss. A common way of quantifying hearing loss is in terms of the absolute threshold for sinusoids, expressed in dB HL, and averaged over the frequencies 500, 1000 and 2000 Hz; this is often known as the pure-tone average (PTA) hearing loss. Goodman (1965) proposed the following classification:

PTA -10 to 26 dB	normal limits
PTA 27 to 40 dB	mild hearing loss
PTA 41 to 55 dB	moderate hearing loss
PTA 56 to 70 dB	moderately severe hearing loss
PTA 71 to 90 dB	severe hearing loss
PTA over 90 dB	profound hearing loss

A similar classification is still used, although nowadays the boundary between normal hearing and mild hearing loss is usually put at a PTA of 16 dB. Generally, the categories are indicative of the severity of the problems that are likely to be experienced in everyday life; greater losses are associated with greater problems. However, individuals with similar absolute thresholds may vary considerably in this respect.

Causes of hearing loss due to cochlear damage

Elevation of absolute threshold due to cochlear damage can occur in two main ways. Firstly, damage to the OHCs impairs the active mechanism, resulting in reduced BM vibration for a given low sound level. Hence, the sound level must be larger than normal to give a just-detectable amount of vibration. Secondly, IHC damage can result in reduced efficiency of transduction, so the amount of BM vibration needed to reach threshold is larger than normal. In principle, it is possible to partition the overall hearing loss at a given frequency into a component due to OHC damage and a component due to IHC (and neural) damage (Moore and Glasberg, 1997):

$$HL_{OHC} + HL_{IHC} = HL_{TOTAL}$$

$$(2.1)$$

where all quantities are in decibels. For example, if the total hearing loss at a given frequency is 60 dB, 40 dB of that loss might be due to OHC damage and 20 dB to IHC damage. It is not possible to determine the balance between the two components from measures of absolute threshold alone. However, the balance can be estimated in other ways, as will be described later in this book. Probably, the hearing loss due to OHC damage alone cannot be greater than about 50 dB at low frequencies and 65 dB at high frequencies. Note that the proportion of a hearing loss that is attributed to OHC or IHC damage is not the same as the relative proportion of OHC and IHC physiological damage. In the above example, 40 dB of the hearing loss was attributed to OHC damage and 20 dB to IHC damage, but this does *not* imply that damage to the OHCs was twice as great as damage to IHCs.

In extreme cases, the IHCs at certain places along the BM may be completely non-functioning. In such cases, vibration at those places is not detected by the neurones directly innervating that place. Say, for example, the IHCs at the basal end of the cochlea are non-functioning. Neurones innervating the basal end, which would normally have high CFs, will not respond. However, if a high-frequency sinusoid is presented, it may be detected if it produces sufficient BM vibration at a more apical region; this corresponds to downward spread of excitation. In other words, a high-frequency sound may be detected via neurones that are tuned to lower frequencies. Similarly, if there are no functioning IHCs at an apical region of the cochlea, a low-frequency sound may be detected via neurones that are tuned to higher frequencies. Because of this possibility, the 'true' hearing loss at a given frequency may be greater than suggested by the audiometric threshold at that frequency.

A region of the BM over which there are no functioning IHCs will be referred to as a *dead region* (Moore and Glasberg, 1997). Often it is described in terms of the range of characteristic frequencies (CFs) that would normally be associated with the dead region. Say, for example, that the IHCs are non-functioning over a region of the BM having CFs in the range 4000 to 10 000 Hz. One might then describe this as a dead region extending from 4000 to 10 000 Hz. Dead regions are not necessarily easily identified from the pure-tone audiogram. For example, when there is a low-frequency dead region, low-frequencies will be detected using the responses of neurones with CFs above the dead region (Thornton and Abbas, 1980; Florentine and Houtsma, 1983) - see Chapter 3. However, audiometric thresholds at low frequencies may not be markedly higher than audiometric thresholds at higher frequencies, because the neurones with high CFs may have tuning curves with shallow low-frequency 'tails' (see Figure 1.22). There is, at present, no simple clinical procedure for determining the extent of dead regions.

Perceptual consequences of elevated absolute thresholds

Loss of sensitivity to weak sounds is one of the main causes of the problems experienced by people with cochlear hearing loss. Weak sounds, and especially the weaker sounds in speech, like p, t and k, are simply not heard. The effect of this on speech perception is discussed in Chapter 8.

As mentioned earlier, individuals with similar absolute thresholds may vary considerably in terms of the difficulty that they experience in everyday life. These individual differences are partly explicable in terms of differing patterns of OHC and IHC loss. The most severe situation is when there are one or more extensive dead regions. Tones with frequencies corresponding to a dead region are often described as sounding noise-like or distorted (Villchur, 1973; Moore, Laurence and Wright, 1985; Murray and Byrne, 1986). It is likely that when complex sounds such as speech are presented very little information can be extracted from the frequencies in the speech corresponding to the dead region.

Chapter 3
Masking, Frequency Selectivity and BM Non-linearity

Introduction

Although loss of sensitivity caused by cochlear damage is of major importance in creating hearing difficulty in everyday life, it is not the only factor involved. Cochlear damage produces a variety of changes in the perception of sounds that are well above the threshold for detection. This chapter considers the reduced frequency selectivity associated with cochlear hearing loss. Frequency selectivity refers to the ability of the auditory system to separate or resolve (to a limited extent) the components in a complex sound. For example, if two tuning forks, each tuned to a different frequency, are struck simultaneously, two different tones can usually be heard, one corresponding to each frequency. This ability is also known as frequency analysis and frequency resolution; these terms will be used interchangeably in this book.

Frequency selectivity probably depends largely on the filtering that takes place in the cochlea (see Chapter 1). The sinusoidal components of a complex sound each lead to a peak in the vibration pattern at a specific place on the BM, and the components are coded independently in the auditory nerve, provided that their frequency separation is sufficiently large. Damage to the cochlea, and particularly to the OHCs, leads to reduced sharpness of tuning on the BM and in single neurones of the auditory nerve. Hence, it is to be expected that frequency selectivity is poorer than normal in people with cochlear hearing loss.

This chapter starts by describing how frequency selectivity can be measured in normally hearing subjects, using *masking* experiments. Typically, the subject is required to detect a signal such as a sinusoid in the presence of a background (masking) sound. The results are used to provide a description of frequency selectivity in the normal auditory system. The description is based on two complementary concepts. One is called the auditory filter shape. This characterises the tuning or selectivity available at a particular centre frequency. It can be thought of as analogous to measures of tuning at a single point on the BM (for example, the constant velocity tuning curve described in Chapter 1; see Figure 1.9) or in single neurones of the auditory nerve (for example, the frequency-threshold curve described in Chapter 1; see Figure 1.13). The second concept is that of the excitation pattern. This represents the distribution of activity produced by a given sound at different places (corresponding to different characteristic frequencies) in the auditory system. It can be considered as analogous to measures of the magnitude of response at different points along the BM; see, for example, Figure 1.8.

The chapter also describes *non-simultaneous masking*, when a brief signal is presented either before or after a masker. Non-simultaneous masking can be used as a tool for measuring the effects of non-linearities on the BM, such as compressive input-output functions and two-tone suppression (see Chapter 1).

The remainder of the chapter is concerned with the measurement of frequency selectivity in people with cochlear hearing loss. It describes how frequency selectivity is reduced by cochlear hearing loss. It also describes how non-linearities are reduced by cochlear hearing loss. Finally, the perceptual consequences of reduced frequency selectivity and reduced non-linearity are described.

The measurement of frequency selectivity using masking

Introduction

We are all familiar with the fact that sounds we want to hear are sometimes made inaudible by other sounds. This is called masking. For example, it may be impossible to hear the doorbell ringing when music is being played at high volume on a stereo system. Masking may be defined as the process by which the threshold for detecting one sound (the signal) is raised in the presence of another sound (the masker). Masking reflects the limits of frequency selectivity; if a signal with a given frequency is masked by a masker with a different frequency, then the auditory system has failed to resolve the signal and the masker. Hence, by measuring the conditions necessary for one sound just to mask another, it is possible to characterise the frequency selectivity of the auditory system.

It should be noted that the tuning on the BM has often been measured using sinusoids whose frequency and intensity have been systematically varied. At any one time, only a single sinusoid is present. In contrast, measurements of masking usually involve the presentation of more than one sinusoid at the same time. This may be important in interpreting the results, as will be described later.

The power spectrum model

To explain the properties of auditory masking, Fletcher (1940) suggested that the peripheral auditory system behaves as if it contained an array of bandpass filters, with overlapping passbands (the passband of a given filter refers to the range of frequencies passed by the filter). These filters are now called the 'auditory filters'. Each filter can be thought of as corresponding to a particular place on the BM. Fletcher and subsequent researchers (Patterson and Moore, 1986) proposed a model of masking known as the *power-spectrum model*, which is based on the following assumptions:

- The peripheral auditory system contains an array of linear overlapping bandpass filters.
- When trying to detect a signal in a noise background, the listener makes use of just one filter with a centre frequency close to that of the signal. Usually, it is assumed that the filter used is the one that has the highest signal-to-masker ratio at its output; this filter has the 'best' representation of the signal.
- Only the components in the noise which pass through the filter have any effect in masking the signal.
- The threshold for detecting the signal is determined by the amount of noise passing through the auditory filter; specifically, threshold is assumed to correspond to a certain signal-to-noise ratio at the output of the filter. The stimuli are represented by their long-term power spectra, i.e. by the average power plotted as a function of frequency. The relative phases of the components and the short-term fluctuations in the masker are ignored.

We now know that none of these assumptions is strictly correct: the filters are not linear but are level-dependent (Moore and Glasberg, 1987), as would be expected from the properties of the filtering that takes place on the BM; listeners can combine information from more than one filter to enhance signal detection, especially when the signal contains components with frequencies spread over a wide range (Spiegel, 1981; Buus, Schorer, Florentine et al., 1986); noise falling outside the passband of the auditory filter centred at the signal frequency can affect the detection of that signal (Hall, Haggard and Fernandes, 1984); and short-term fluctuations in the masker can play a strong role (Patterson and Henning, 1977; Kohlrausch, 1988; Moore, 1988).

These failures of the model do not mean that the basic concept of the auditory filter is wrong. Indeed, the concept is widely accepted and will be used extensively in the rest of this book. Nevertheless, it should be remembered that simplifying assumptions are often made in attempts to characterise and model the auditory filter.

Estimating the shape of a filter

The relative response of a filter as a function of the input frequency, is often called the filter *shape*. For a physical device, such as an electronic filter, the filter shape can be measured in two ways:

(1) A sinusoid is applied to the input of the filter, keeping its magnitude constant, and the output magnitude is measured as a function of the input frequency. A plot of the output magnitude as a function of frequency then gives the desired filter shape.

(2) A sinusoid is applied to the input of the filter, its frequency is systematically varied, and its input magnitude is adjusted so as to hold the output magnitude constant. A method similar to this is used to determine tuning curves on the BM or in the auditory nerve (see Chapter 1).

If a filter is linear, the shapes resulting from these two methods are simply related; if the two curves are plotted on a decibel scale, then one is simply an inverted version of the other. For example, if the filter is a bandpass filter, then method (1) will give a curve with a peak at a certain frequency (the centre frequency of the filter), whereas method (2) will give a minimum at that same frequency. For a linear filter, it does not matter which method is used; the same end result can be obtained by either method.

The determination of the auditory filter shape at a particular centre frequency is complicated by several factors. Firstly, the auditory filter is *not* linear. Hence, different results may be obtained depending on overall level and depending on whether the input to the filter is held constant or the output from the filter is held constant. In practice, it may be difficult to hold either the input or the output constant in a masking experiment, although one can attempt to approximate these conditions. Secondly, in humans, the input to and output from the filter cannot be measured directly. Hence, the filter shape has to be derived from experimental data on masking, using certain assumptions.

Most methods for estimating the shape of the auditory filter at a given centre frequency are based on the assumptions of the power-spectrum model of masking. The signal frequency is held constant and the spectrum of the masker is manipulated in some way. By analogy with methods (1) and (2) above, two basic methods can be used:

(1) The masker level is held constant and the signal level is varied to determine the threshold for detection of the signal. This is analogous to holding the input level to a filter constant and measuring its output; the signal threshold is assumed to be proportional to the masker level at the output of the filter.

(2) The signal level is held constant and the masker level is varied to determine the value required just to mask the signal. This is analogous to holding the output of the filter constant and varying its input to achieve a fixed output.

Both of these approaches will be described.

Estimating frequency selectivity from masking experiments

Psychophysical tuning curves

The measurement of *psychophysical tuning curves* (PTCs) involves a procedure that is analogous in many ways to physiological methods for determination of a tuning curve on the BM or a neural tuning curve (Chistovich, 1957; Small, 1959); see chapter 1. The signal is fixed in level, usually at a very low level, say, 10 dB sensation level (SL). The masker can be either a sinusoid or a narrow band of noise. For each of several masker centre frequencies, the level of the masker needed just to mask the signal is determined. Because the signal is at a low level it is assumed that it will produce activity primarily at the output of one auditory filter. It is assumed further that, at threshold, the masker produces a constant output from that filter, in order to mask the fixed signal. If these assumptions are valid, then the PTC indicates the masker level required to produce a fixed output from the auditory filter as a function of frequency; this is why the procedure is analogous to the determination of a tuning curve on the BM or a neural tuning curve. Both physiological procedures involve adjusting the input level for each frequency to produce a constant response. In the case of the BM, the response is a constant amplitude or velocity of vibration on the BM. In the case of a neural tuning curve, the response is a fixed number of neural spikes per second.

Two PTCs are shown in Figure 3.1; the data are taken from Moore and Glasberg (1986b). The circles show results from the normal ear of a subject with a unilateral cochlear hearing loss. The squares show results from the impaired ear of the same subject. It is obvious that the PTC is broader for the impaired ear.

One complication in interpreting these results is that the auditory filter giving the highest signal-to-masker ratio is not necessarily centred at the signal frequency. The process of detecting the signal through a filter which is not centred at the signal frequency is called *off-frequency listening*. In this context, it is the centre frequency of the filter that is 'off frequency'. There is good evidence that off-frequency listening can

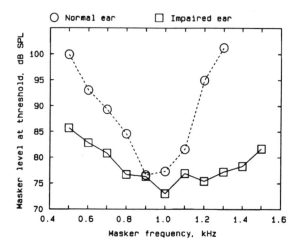

Figure 3.1: Psychophysical tuning curves (PTCs) determined in simultaneous masking for the normal ear (circles and dashed line) and the impaired ear (squares and continuous line) of a subject with a unilateral cochlear hearing loss. The signal frequency was 1 kHz. The variable masker was a narrowband noise. A fixed notched noise was gated with the variable masker, to restrict off-frequency listening. The signal was presented at a level 10 dB above its masked threshold in the notched noise alone.

influence PTCs. When the masker frequency is above the signal frequency, the highest signal-to-masker ratio occurs for a filter centred below the signal frequency. This happens because the filter has a rounded tip, but steeply sloping 'skirts'. For a filter centred just below the signal frequency, the response to the signal is only slightly smaller than would be the case for a filter centred at the signal frequency. However, the response to the masker is markedly reduced by using the 'off-frequency' filter. Similarly, when the masker frequency is below the signal frequency, the highest signal-to-masker ratio occurs for a filter centred above the signal frequency. Assuming that human listeners always select the 'best' filter, then, in both these cases, the masker level required for threshold is higher than would be the case if off-frequency listening did not occur. When the masker frequency equals the signal frequency, the signal-to-masker ratio is similar for all auditory filters that are excited, and off-frequency listening is not advantageous. The overall effect is that the PTC has a sharper tip than would be obtained if only one auditory filter were involved (Johnson-Davies and Patterson, 1979; O'Loughlin and Moore, 1981a; 1981b).

One way to limit off-frequency listening is to add to the main masker (the sinusoid or narrow-band noise) a fixed broad-band noise with a reasonably narrow spectral notch centred at the signal frequency

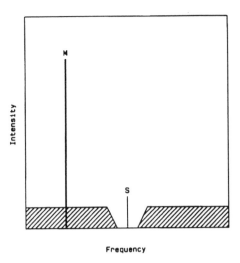

Figure 3.2: Schematic spectra of stimuli used to determine a PTC under conditions where off-frequency listening is restricted. The low-level notched noise is shown as the shaded regions. The signal is indicated by S and the masker by M.

(O'Loughlin and Moore, 1981a; Moore, Glasberg and Roberts, 1984; Patterson and Moore, 1986). The signal is usually presented at a level of about 10 dB above its threshold when the notched noise alone is presented. For example, if the masked threshold of the signal in the notched noise is 15 dB SPL, then the signal would be presented at a level of 25 dB SPL. Schematic spectra of stimuli like this are shown in Figure 3.2. The notched noise makes it disadvantageous to use an auditory filter whose centre frequency is shifted much from the signal frequency; for such a shifted filter, more of the noise would pass through the filter. The notched noise level is kept constant throughout the experiment, and the PTC is determined as before by finding the level of the main masker necessary to mask the signal, as a function of masker frequency. The effect of using such a noise, in addition to the variable masker, is illustrated in Figure 3.3. The main effect is to broaden the tip of the PTC; the slopes of the skirts are relatively unaffected.

The PTCs shown in Figure 3.1 were gathered in the presence of a notched noise of this type. For both the normal and impaired ears, the signal was at a level about 10 dB above masked threshold in the notched noise alone, and the notched-noise level was the same in the two ears. As well as reducing off-frequency listening, the noise had the advantage that it led to equal levels of the tips of the PTCs in the normal and impaired ears. Thus, the comparison of frequency selectivity between the two ears was not confounded by differences in overall level.

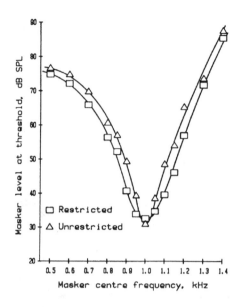

Figure 3.3: Comparison of PTCs where off-frequency listening is not restricted (tri-angles) and where it is restricted using a low-level notched noise centred at the signal frequency (squares). Data from Moore, Glasberg and Roberts (1984)

The notched-noise method

To satisfy the assumptions of the power-spectrum model, it is necessary to use a masker that limits the extent to which off-frequency listening is useful, and that limits the range of filter centre frequencies over which the signal-to-masker ratio is sufficiently high to be useful; this promotes the use of just one auditory filter. This can be achieved using a noise masker with a spectral notch around the signal frequency. For such a masker, the highest signal-to-masker ratio occurs for a filter that is centred reasonably close to the signal frequency, and performance is not improved (or is improved very little) by combining information over filters covering a range of centre frequencies (Patterson, 1976; Patterson and Moore, 1986; Moore, Glasberg and Simpson, 1992). The filter shape can then be estimated by measuring signal threshold as a function of the width of the notch. The noise level is usually kept constant and the signal level is varied to determine threshold, although some measure-ments have been performed with the signal level fixed and the masker level varied (Glasberg, Moore and Nimmo-Smith, 1984; Rosen, Baker and Kramer, 1992; Rosen, Baker and Darling, 1998).

For moderate noise levels, the auditory filter is almost symmetrical on a linear frequency scale (Patterson, 1974; 1976; Patterson and Nimmo-Smith, 1980; Moore and Glasberg, 1987). Hence the auditory filter shape can be estimated using a fixed-level notched-noise masker with the

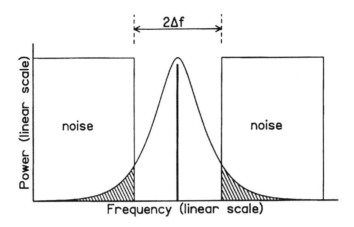

Figure 3.4: Schematic illustration of the notched-noise technique used by Patterson (1976) to determine the shape of the auditory filter. The threshold of the sinusoidal signal is measured as a function of the width of a spectral notch in the noise masker (overall width = 2Δf). The amount of noise passing through the auditory filter centred at the signal frequency is proportional to the shaded areas.

notch placed symmetrically about the signal frequency. The method is illustrated in Figure 3.4. The signal (indicated by the bold vertical line) is fixed in frequency, and the masker is a noise with a bandstop or notch centred at the signal frequency. The deviation of each edge of the noise from the centre frequency is denoted by Δf. The width of the notch is varied, and the threshold of the signal is determined as a function of notch width. As the notch is symmetrically placed around the signal frequency, the method cannot reveal asymmetries in the auditory filter, and the analysis assumes that the filter is symmetric on a linear frequency scale. This assumption appears not unreasonable, at least for the top part of the filter and at moderate sound levels, since PTCs are quite symmetric around the tips. For a signal symmetrically placed in a notched noise, the highest signal-to-masker ratio at the output of the auditory filter is achieved with a filter centred at the signal frequency, as illustrated in Figure 3.4. Using a filter that is not centred at the signal frequency reduces the amount of noise passing through the filter from one of the noise bands, but this is more than offset by the increase in noise from the other band.

As the width of the spectral notch is increased, less and less noise passes through the auditory filter. Thus the threshold of the signal drops. Figure 3.4 is plotted with linear power (not decibels) on the ordinate. With such an ordinate, the total noise power passing through the auditory filter is proportional to the area under the filter in the frequency range covered by the noise. This is shown as the shaded areas in Figure 3.4. Assuming that threshold corresponds to a constant signal-

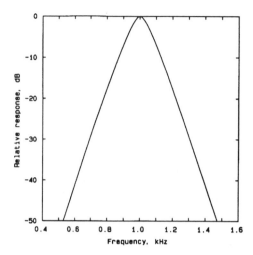

Figure 3.5: An example of an auditory filter shape obtained using the notched-noise method. The filter was centred at 1 kHz. The response is plotted relative to the response at the tip, which was arbitrarily called 0 dB.

to-masker ratio at the output of the filter, the change in signal threshold with notch width indicates how the area under the filter varies with Δf. The area under a function between certain limits is obtained by integrating the value of the function over those limits. Hence by differentiating the function relating threshold (in linear power units) to Δf, the relative response of the filter at that value of Δf is obtained. In other words, the relative response of the filter (in linear power units) for a given deviation, Δf, from the centre frequency is equal to the slope of the function relating signal threshold to notch width, at that value of Δf. If the threshold decreases rapidly with increasing notch width, that indicates a sharply tuned filter. If the threshold decreases slowly with increasing notch width, that indicates a broadly tuned filter. An example of an auditory filter shape obtained with this method is shown in Figure 3.5. Note that, although the derivation is based on the use of linear power units, the relative response of the filter is usually plotted on a decibel scale, and this has been done in Figure 3.5. The response of the filter at its tip was arbitrarily called 0 dB; in other words, it was assumed that for a signal at the centre frequency of the filter, the output magnitude was equal to the input magnitude.

When the auditory filter is asymmetric, as it is when high masker levels are used (see later), then the filter shape can still be measured using a notched-noise masker if some reasonable assumptions are made and if the range of measurements is extended to include conditions where the notch is placed asymmetrically about the signal frequency.

The reader is referred elsewhere for details (Patterson and Nimmo-Smith, 1980; Glasberg and Moore, 1990).

One limitation of the notched-noise method occurs when the auditory filter is markedly asymmetric, as it is in some hearing-impaired people. In such cases, the method does not define the sharper side of the filter very well.

Characteristics of the auditory filter in normal hearing

Variation with centre frequency

A bandpass filter is often characterised by its bandwidth, which is a measure of the 'effective' range of frequencies passed by the filter. The bandwidth of a filter is often defined as the difference between the two frequencies at which the response has fallen by a factor of two in power (i.e. by 3 dB) relative to the peak response; this is known as the *half-power bandwidth* or *–3 dB bandwidth*. For example, if a filter has its peak response at 1000 Hz, and the response is 3 dB below the peak response at 900 Hz and at 1120 Hz, then the –3 dB bandwidth is 220 Hz. An alternative measure is the *equivalent rectangular bandwidth (ERB)*. The ERB of a given filter is equal to the bandwidth of a perfect rectangular filter (a filter whose shape has a flat top and vertical edges) which has a transmission in its passband equal to the maximum transmission of the specified filter and transmits the same power of white noise as the specified filter. In other words, if we take a rectangular filter and scale it to have the same maximum height and area as our filter, then the bandwidth of the rectangular filter is the ERB of our filter. The equalisation of height and area is done with the filter characteristic plotted in linear power co-ordinates. For auditory filters, the ERB is usually about 11% larger than the –3 dB bandwidth. The ERB is related to what is sometimes referred to as the 'critical bandwidth' (Fletcher, 1940; Zwicker, 1961; Scharf, 1970).

Figure 3.6 shows the ERBs of the auditory filters estimated in various studies (Moore and Glasberg, 1983c; Glasberg and Moore, 1990; Moore, 1997b). The solid line in Figure 3.6 provides a good fit to the ERB values over the whole frequency range tested. It is described by the following equation:

$$ERB = 24.7(4.37F + 1)$$

$$(3.1)$$

where the ERB is in Hertz and F is centre frequency in kHz. This equation is a modification of one originally suggested by Greenwood

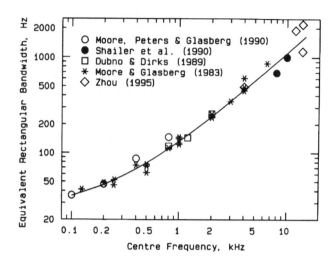

Figure 3.6: Estimates of the auditory filter bandwidth from a variety of experiments, plotted as a function of centre frequency. The solid line represents the equation suggested by Glasberg and Moore (1990). Two points are shown for a centre frequency of 14 kHz, as filter bandwidths were estimated for two different noise spectrum levels, 40 and 50 dB; the ERB was greater at the higher level.

(1961). He based it on the assumption that each ERB corresponds to a constant distance along the basilar membrane. Although the constants in equation 3.1 differ from those given by Greenwood, the form of the equation is the same as his. Each ERB corresponds to a distance of about 0.89 mm on the BM.

Auditory filter shapes for young normally hearing subjects vary relatively little across subjects; the standard deviation of the ERB is typically about 10% of its mean value (Moore, 1987b; Moore, Peters and Glasberg, 1990). However, the variability tends to increase at very low frequencies (Moore, Peters and Glasberg, 1990) and at very high frequencies (Patterson, Nimmo-Smith, Weber et al., 1982; Shailer, Moore, Glasberg et al., 1990).

Sometimes it is useful to plot psychoacoustical data on a frequency scale related to the ERB. Essentially, the ERB is used as the unit of frequency. For example, the value of the ERB for a centre frequency of 1 kHz is about 130 Hz, so an increase in frequency from 935 to 1065 Hz represents a step of one ERB. A formula relating ERB number to frequency can be derived from equation 3.1 (Glasberg and Moore, 1990):

$$\text{ERB number} = 21.4\log_{10}(4.37F + 1)$$

$$(3.2)$$

where F is frequency in kHz. This *ERB scale* is comparable to a scale of distance along the BM, starting at the apical end. A frequency of 100 Hz produces peak activity near the apex; the corresponding ERB number is 3.36. A frequency of 15 000 Hz produces peak activity near the base; the corresponding ERB number is 38.9. A frequency of 1635 Hz produces peak activity about half-way along the BM; the corresponding ERB number is 19.5.

Variation with level

If the auditory filter were linear, then its shape would not vary with the level of the stimuli used to measure it. Unfortunately, this is not the case, as would be expected from measurements of the filtering on the BM. Moore and Glasberg (1987) presented a summary of measurements of the auditory filter shape using notched-noise maskers with notches placed both symmetrically and asymmetrically about the signal frequency. They concluded that the lower skirt of the filter becomes less sharp with increasing level, whereas the higher skirt becomes slightly steeper. Glasberg and Moore (1990) re-analysed the data from the studies summarised in that paper, and they also examined the data presented in Moore, Peters and Glasberg (1990) and Shailer, Moore, Glasberg et al. (1990). The re-analysis led to the following conclusions:

- The auditory filter for a centre frequency of 1 kHz is roughly symmetric on a linear frequency scale when the level of the noise (in a notched-noise experiment) is approximately 51 dB/ERB. This corresponds to a noise spectrum level of about 30 dB (spectrum level is the level of a sound in decibels measured in a 1-Hz wide band). The auditory filters at other centre frequencies are approximately symmetric when the effective input levels to the filters are equivalent to the level of 51 dB/ERB at 1 kHz (after making allowance for changes in relative level produced by passage of the sound through the outer and middle ear).
- The low-frequency side of the auditory filter becomes less sharp with increasing level.
- Changes in slope of the high-frequency side of the filter with level are less consistent. At medium centre frequencies (1-4 kHz) there is a trend for the slope to increase with increasing level, but at low centre frequencies there is no clear trend with level, and the filters at high centre frequencies show a slight decrease in slope with increasing level.

The statements above are based on the assumption that, although the auditory filter is not linear, it may be considered as approximately linear at any given noise level. Furthermore, the sharpness of the filter is assumed to depend on the input level to the filter, not the output level

(Moore and Glasberg, 1987). This may not be strictly accurate (Rosen, Baker and Kramer, 1992; Rosen, Baker and Darling, 1998). Nevertheless, it appears that the lower side of the auditory filter broadens with increasing level whatever assumptions are made in analysing the data (Rosen, Baker and Darling, 1998).

Figure 3.7 illustrates how the shape of the auditory filter varies with input level for a centre frequency of 1 kHz. In this figure, the output of the filter is plotted in decibels as a function of frequency, with the level of the input as parameter. At the centre frequency, the output level in dB was assumed to be equal to the input level in dB. In other words, the gain (the output level minus the input level) at the centre frequency was assumed to be 0 dB. The gain for frequencies well below the centre frequency is negative (the output level is lower than the input level), but the gain at these frequencies *increases* with increasing level. However, it would be more in accord with the functioning of the cochlea to assume that the gain is fixed for frequencies well below the centre frequency, and that the gain at the centre frequency decreases with increasing level (Ruggero, Rich, Recio et al., 1997; Rosen, Baker and Darling, 1998). Recall that the input-output function of the BM is linear for frequencies well below CF, but is compressive for frequencies close to CF (see Figure 1.10).

Figure 3.8 shows auditory filters with the same shapes as in Figure 3.7. However, in Figure 3.8 the shapes are plotted in terms of the relative filter *gain,* and the gain is assumed to be invariant with level for low frequencies; this is consistent with linear BM input-output functions for frequencies well below CF. When plotted in this way, the gain at the centre frequency is seen to decrease with increasing input level, consistent with a progressively reducing gain from the active mechanism with increasing level (see chapter 1). The dashed regions of the curves are based on extrapolations. For example, when the input level is 20 dB, the filter response cannot be determined experimentally for regions more than 20 dB down from the tip.

A discrepancy with BM responses is observed for frequencies well above the centre frequency: BM input-output functions become nearly linear for input frequencies well above CF, whereas the filter gains shown in Figure 3.8 decrease with increasing level, indicating a compressive non-linearity. It is possible that the discrepancy reflects errors of measurement. As mentioned earlier, the notched-noise method does not give a precise estimate of the slope of the steeper side of the auditory filter when the filter is markedly asymmetric. This is a particular problem at high sound levels, where the lower branch becomes very shallow. Thus, at high levels, there may well be significant errors in the estimates of the sharpness of the high-frequency side of the filter. Also, BM responses to tones well above CF are very small in amplitude making it hard to measure the responses accurately. BM responses at these frequencies often show a 'plateau', a range of frequencies where the

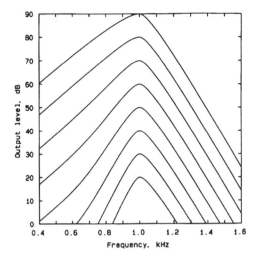

Figure 3.7: The shape of the auditory filter centred at 1 kHz, plotted for input sound levels ranging from 20 to 90 dB SPL/ERB in 10-dB steps. The output of the filter is plotted as a function of frequency, assuming that the gain at the centre frequency is 0 dB. On the low-frequency side, the filter becomes progressively less sharply tuned with increasing sound level. At moderate sound levels the filter is approximately symmetric on the linear frequency scale used.

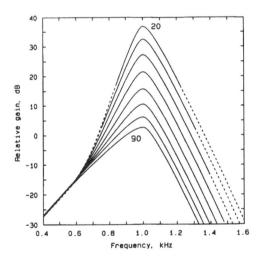

Figure 3.8: Auditory filters for the same input levels as in Figure 3.7: Here, the shapes are plotted in terms of the filter gain, and the gain is assumed to be invariant with level for low frequencies; this is consistent with linear BM input-output functions for frequencies well below CF. When plotted in this way, the gain at the centre frequency is seen to decrease with increasing input level, consistent with a progress-ively reducing gain from the active mechanism with increasing level. Regions of the curves that are dashed are based on extrapolation; the experimental data do not allow these regions of the filter responses to be determined.

response hardly varies with frequency (Ruggero, Rich, Recio et al., 1997). Such a plateau is not evident in neural tuning curves, so the effect in BM measurements may reflect an artefact of some kind.

Summary

In summary, the properties of auditory filters measured in masking experiments using notched noise are broadly consistent with the filtering measured on the BM, in terms of variation with centre frequency and level. The variation of auditory filter shape with level can be interpreted as indicating a fixed gain on the low-frequency tail of the auditory filter and a gain that decreases with increasing level around the centre frequency. As a result, the filter broadens with increasing level.

Masking patterns and excitation patterns

Masking patterns

In the masking experiments described so far, the frequency of the signal was held constant while the masker frequency was varied. These experiments are most appropriate for estimating the shape of the auditory filter at a given centre frequency. However, in many experiments on masking, the signal frequency has been varied while the masker frequency was held constant. Typically, the masker level has been held constant and the signal level required for threshold has been measured as a function of the signal frequency (Wegel and Lane, 1924). The function relating masked threshold to the signal frequency is known as a *masking pattern*, or sometimes as a *masked audiogram*.

A typical set of results is shown in Figure 3.9. The data are taken from Egan and Hake (1950). In this figure, the signal threshold is expressed as the amount of masking. This is the amount by which the masked threshold exceeds the absolute threshold, both thresholds being expressed in decibels. Notice that on the high-frequency sides of the patterns the slopes become shallower at high levels. Thus, if the level of a low-frequency masker is increased by, say, 10 dB, the masked threshold of a high-frequency signal is elevated by more than 10 dB; the amount of masking grows non-linearly (in an *expansive* way) on the high-frequency side. This has been called the 'upward spread of masking'.

Masking patterns do not reflect the use of a single auditory filter. Rather, for each signal frequency, the listener uses a filter centred close to the signal frequency. Thus the auditory filter is shifted as the signal frequency is altered. One way of interpreting the masking pattern is as a crude indicator of the *excitation pattern* of the masker. The excitation pattern of a sound is a representation of the activity or excitation evoked by that sound as a function of CF or 'place' in the auditory system

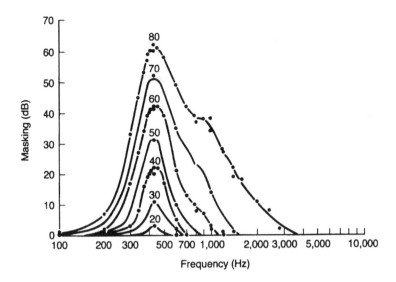

Figure 3.9: Masking patterns (masked audiograms) for a narrow band of noise centred at 410 Hz. Each curve shows the elevation in threshold of a sinusoidal signal as a function of signal frequency. The overall noise level for each curve is indicated in the Figure. Data from Egan and Hake (1950).

(Zwicker, 1970). It can be thought of as a kind of internal representation of the spectrum of the sound. In the case of a masking pattern, one might assume that the signal is detected when the excitation it produces is some constant proportion of the excitation produced by the masker in the frequency region of the signal; 'frequency region' here refers to places on the BM, or neurones, that have CFs close to the signal frequency. Thus, the threshold of the signal as a function of frequency is proportional to the masker's excitation level. The masking pattern should be parallel to the excitation pattern of the masker, but shifted vertically by a small amount. In practice, the situation is not so straightforward, since the shape of the masking pattern is influenced by factors such as off-frequency listening and the detection of combination tones produced by the interaction of the signal and the masker (Greenwood, 1971).

Relationship of the auditory filter to the excitation pattern

Moore and Glasberg (1983c) have described a way of deriving the shapes of excitation patterns using the concept of the auditory filter. They suggested that the excitation pattern of a given sound can be thought of as the output of the auditory filters as a function of their centre frequency. This idea is illustrated in Figure 3.10. The upper portion of the figure shows schematic auditory filter shapes for five centre frequencies. For each filter, the gain is plotted relative to the gain at the centre frequency, which was assumed to be 0 dB (as in Figure 3.5). A moderate

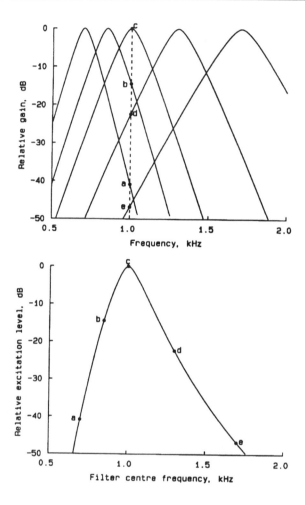

Figure 3.10: An illustration of how the excitation pattern of a 1 kHz sinusoid (dashed line) can be derived by calculating the outputs of the auditory filters as a function of their centre frequency. The top panel shows five auditory filters, centred at different frequencies, and the bottom half shows the calculated excitation pattern.

input level was assumed, so each filter is symmetrical on the linear frequency scale used, but the bandwidths of the filters increase with increasing centre frequency. The dashed line represents a 1 kHz sinusoidal signal whose excitation pattern is to be derived. The lower panel shows the relative response of each filter in response to the 1 kHz signal, plotted as a function of the centre frequency of each filter; this is the desired excitation pattern.

To see how this pattern is derived, consider the output from the filter with the lowest centre frequency. This has a relative response to the 1 kHz tone of about −40 dB, as indicated by point 'a' in the upper panel.

In the lower panel, this gives rise to the point 'a' on the excitation pattern; the point has an ordinate value of -40 dB and is positioned on the abscissa at a frequency corresponding to the centre frequency of the lowest filter illustrated. The relative responses of the other filters are indicated, in order of increasing centre frequency, by points 'b' to 'e', and each leads to a corresponding point on the excitation pattern. The complete excitation pattern was actually derived by calculating the filter outputs for filters spaced at 10 Hz intervals.

In deriving the excitation pattern, excitation levels were expressed relative to the level at the tip of the pattern, which was arbitrarily labelled as 0 dB. To calculate the excitation pattern for a 1 kHz tone with a level of, say, 60 dB, the level at the tip would be labelled as 60 dB, and all other excitation levels would correspondingly be increased by 60 dB. However, for the calculation to be valid, the filter shapes would have to be appropriate for an input level of 60 dB.

Note that, although the auditory filters were assumed to be symmetric on a linear frequency scale, the derived excitation pattern is asymmetric. This happens because the bandwidth of the auditory filter increases with increasing centre frequency.

Changes in excitation patterns with level

In the normal auditory system, the low-frequency side of the auditory filter becomes less steep with increasing sound level (Figures 3.7 and 3.8). Correspondingly, the excitation patterns evoked by narrowband sounds (such as sinusoids) become less steep on the high-frequency side. This is illustrated in Figure 3.11, which shows excitation patterns for a 1 kHz sinusoid at levels from 20 to 90 dB, calculated in a manner similar to that described above, but this time plotted on a logarithmic frequency scale. The excitation patterns have the same general form as the masking patterns shown in Figure 3.9, and show the same non-linear expansive growth on the high-frequency side.

In calculating the excitation patterns in this figure, it was assumed that the auditory filters had a gain of 0 dB at their tips for all input levels, as in Figure 3.7. However, as argued earlier, the gain at the tip probably decreases with increasing input level, as in Figure 3.8. In a sense, the excitation patterns in Figure 3.11 are misleading; probably they do not directly reflect the magnitude of BM responses. On the BM, the magnitude of response at the tip of the excitation pattern grows in a compressive manner with increasing sound level whereas the magnitude of response on the high-frequency side grows linearly. This effect is not directly revealed in simultaneous masking experiments because the masked threshold depends mainly on the signal-to-masker *ratio* at the output of the auditory filter.

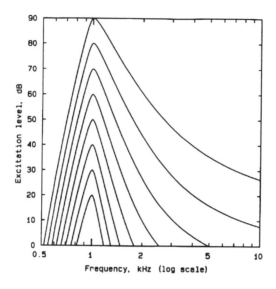

Figure 3.11: Excitation patterns calculated according to the procedure described in the text for 1 kHz sinusoids ranging in level from 20 to 90 dB SPL in 10-dB steps. The frequency scale is logarithmic.

Possible effects of suppression

As pointed out earlier, physiological measures of the tuning of the BM have usually been obtained using sinusoids whose frequency and intensity have been systematically varied. At any one time, only a single sinusoid is present. In contrast, the psychophysical measures of masking described above involved the presentation of more than one sinusoid at the same time. If the filtering on the BM were linear, and if the assumptions of the power spectrum model of masking were correct, this should not matter; estimates of the auditory filter shape derived using complex stimuli should correspond well to the frequency-response shape measured with single sinusoids. However, the filtering on the BM is *not* linear, as described in Chapter 1.

In the power spectrum model of masking, the masking of a signal by a masker with a different centre frequency is assumed to be caused by spread of the excitation produced by the masker to the 'place' corresponding to the signal frequency (Wegel and Lane, 1924; Fletcher, 1940; Zwicker, 1970; Zwicker and Fastl, 1990). The masking of the signal is assumed to occur because the masker excites auditory filters tuned close to the signal frequency. However, an alternative possibility is that the masker suppresses the signal (Wightman, McGee and Kramer, 1977; Weber, 1983; Pickles, 1984; Delgutte, 1988; 1990; Moore and Vickers, 1997). A masker may suppress the response to a signal that is remote in frequency without itself producing excitatory activity at the signal place

(Hind, Rose, Brugge et al., 1967; Sachs and Kiang, 1968), a phenomenon described in Chapter 1 as two-tone suppression.

At present, the relative importance of spread of excitation and suppression remains somewhat controversial. Overall, the results suggest that simultaneous masking might result from a *combination* of suppression and spread of excitation (Delgutte, 1990; Beveridge and Carlyon, 1996; Moore and Vickers, 1997). Spread of excitation probably dominates when the masker contains frequency components reasonably close to the signal frequency, whereas suppression plays a greater role when the masker frequency is remote from the signal frequency, and especially when it is well below the signal frequency.

As pointed out by Delgutte (1990, 1996), the evidence indicating that strong suppression can occur for masker frequencies well below the signal frequency has important implications for the interpretation of masking patterns, such as those shown in Figure 3.7. The signal threshold may seriously overestimate the excitation produced by the masker at the place corresponding to the signal frequency when the masker is much lower in frequency than the signal. Put another way, the high-frequency sides of excitation patterns may be more restricted, and have steeper slopes, than indicated by masking patterns.

Non-simultaneous masking

Basic properties of non-simultaneous masking

The phrase 'simultaneous masking' is used to describe situations where the masker is present for the whole time that the signal occurs. Masking can also occur when a brief signal is presented just before or after the masker; this is called non-simultaneous masking. This type of masking is introduced here since it can be used as a tool to measure the effects of suppression on the internal representation of sounds.

Two basic types of non-simultaneous masking can be distinguished:

* *backward masking,* in which the signal precedes the masker (also known as pre-stimulatory masking); and
* *forward masking,* in which the signal follows the masker (also known as post-stimulatory masking).

The emphasis here will be on forward masking, since it is generally the greater of the two types of masking, at least in well-trained subjects, and since it is better understood than backward masking. Forward masking might occur via two different mechanisms. One is a reduction in sensitivity of recently stimulated neurones; the neurones stimulated by the masker may be 'fatigued' and this reduces the response to a signal that comes just after the masker. A second possible mechanism is based on persistence in the pattern of neural activity evoked by the masker at some level above the auditory nerve. The response to the masker may take some time to decay when the masker is turned off. If the signal is presented during this decay time, the persisting response to the masker may mask the response to the signal.

A third mechanism may sometimes come into operation. The response of the BM to the masker takes a certain time to decay, and for small intervals between the signal and the masker this may result in forward masking (Duifhuis, 1973). This mechanism is probably only important for low frequencies (for which the decay time on the BM is longer) and when the masker-signal interval is less than a few milliseconds.

Figure 3.12 shows the results of an experiment on forward masking using broadband white noise as the masker (Moore and Glasberg, 1983a). The noise level is plotted in terms of the level within the ERB of the auditory filter centred at the signal frequency. The signal was a brief burst of a 4 kHz sinusoid, and the delay, D, of the signal after the end of the masker could have one of three values. In the figure, D is specified as the time from the end of the masker to the end of the signal. The signal threshold was measured for several different levels of the masker. The main properties of forward masking are as follows:

- Forward masking is greater the nearer in time to the masker that the signal occurs. This is illustrated in the left panel of Figure 3.12. When the delay D of the signal is plotted on a logarithmic scale, the data fall roughly on a straight line. In other words, the amount of forward masking, in dB, is a linear function of $\log(D)$.
- The rate of recovery from forward masking is greater for higher masker levels. Thus, regardless of the initial amount of forward masking, the masking decays to zero after 100-200 ms.
- Increments in masker level do not produce equal increments in amount of forward masking. For example, if the masker level is increased by 10 dB, the masked threshold may only increase by 3 dB. This contrasts with simultaneous masking, where, for broadband noise maskers, threshold usually corresponds to a constant signal-to-masker ratio (Hawkins and Stevens, 1950). This effect can be quantified by plotting the signal threshold as a function of masker level. The resulting function is called a *growth-of-masking* function. Several such functions are shown in the right panel of Figure 3.12. In simultaneous masking such functions would have slopes close to one (for a broadband noise masker); this slope is indicated by the dashed line. In forward masking the slopes are less than one, and the slopes decrease as the value of D increases.
- The amount of forward masking increases with increasing masker duration for durations up to at least 20 ms. The results for greater masker durations vary somewhat across studies. Some studies show

an effect of masker duration for durations up to 200 ms (Kidd and Feth, 1982), while others show little effect for durations beyond 50 ms (Fastl, 1976).

Evidence for suppression from non-simultaneous masking

Chapter 1 described how the response to a tone of a given frequency can sometimes be suppressed by a tone with a different frequency, a phenomenon known as two-tone suppression. For other complex signals, similar phenomena occur and are given the general name lateral suppression or suppression. This can be characterised in the following way. Strong activity at a given characteristic frequency (CF) can suppress weaker activity at adjacent CFs.

The question now arises as to what are the perceptual consequences of suppression, and how its effects can be measured. It was suggested above that suppression may have some influence on simultaneous masking, when the masker frequency is well below the signal frequency. However, Houtgast (1972) has argued that simultaneous masking is not an appropriate tool for detecting the effects of suppression. In simultaneous masking, the masking stimulus and the signal are processed

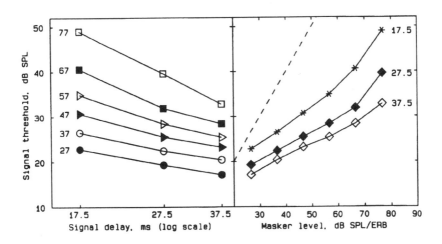

Figure 3.12: The left panel shows the threshold of a brief 4 kHz signal, plotted as a function of the time delay of the signal after the end of the noise masker. Each curve shows results for a different noise level; the noise level is specified in terms of the level within the ERB of the auditory filter centred at the signal frequency. The right panel shows the same thresholds plotted as a function of masker level. Each curve shows results for a different signal delay time (17.5, 27.5 or 37.5 ms). The dashed line has a slope of 1, indicating linear growth of masking. Note that the slopes of the growth-of-masking functions decrease with increasing signal delay. The data are taken from Moore and Glasberg (1983a).

simultaneously in the same auditory filter. He argued that any suppression applied to that filter will affect the neural activity caused by both the signal and the masker. In other words, the signal-to-masker ratio in a given frequency region (corresponding to a given place on the BM) will be unaffected by suppression, and thus the threshold of the signal will remain unaltered.

This argument may not be correct in all cases. Suppression might change the signal-to-masker ratio at the output of a given auditory filter if the signal and masker are widely separated in frequency. However, Houtgast's argument certainly seems reasonable when applied to cases where the signal and masker have coincident or near coincident frequency components. Say, for example, that the masker consists of two frequency components, at 500 and 2000 Hz, while the signal is a sinusoid at 2000 Hz. If the signal and masker are presented simultaneously, then the 500 Hz component in the masker may produce suppression at the place on the BM tuned to 2000 Hz, but that suppression will be applied equally to the 2000 Hz component of the masker and to the 2000 Hz signal, without changing their ratio. If the masking of the signal is determined mainly by the 2000 Hz component of the masker, then the suppression produced by the 500 Hz component will have no measurable effects.

Houtgast suggested that the effects of suppression could be measured by presenting the masker and the signal successively, for example, by using forward masking. It is assumed that the masked threshold of the signal is monotonically related to the excitation evoked by the masker in neurones tuned close to the signal frequency. Thus, increases in masker-evoked excitation will lead to increases in the signal threshold, while decreases in masker-evoked excitation (produced, for example, by suppression) will lead to decreases in signal threshold. It is assumed also that any suppression effects occurring within the masker (e.g. suppression of one frequency component in the masker by another frequency component within the masker) cease as soon as the masker is turned off.

Following the pioneering work of Houtgast (1972; 1973; 1974) many workers have reported that there are systematic differences between the results obtained using simultaneous and non-simultaneous masking techniques. An extensive review is provided by Moore and O'Loughlin (1986). One major difference is that non-simultaneous masking reveals effects that can be directly attributed to suppression. A good demonstration of this involves a psychoacoustical analogue of two-tone suppression. Houtgast (1973; 1974) measured the threshold for a 1 kHz signal and a 1 kHz non-simultaneous masker. He then added a second tone to the masker and measured the threshold again. He found that sometimes the addition of this second tone produced a reduction in the threshold, an effect that has been called *two-tone unmasking*. He attributed this to suppression of the 1 kHz component in the masker by the second component. If the 1 kHz component is suppressed, then there will be less excitation in the frequency region around 1 kHz, producing a drop in the threshold for detecting the signal. Houtgast mapped out the combinations of frequency and intensity over which the 'suppressor' produced a reduction in signal threshold exceeding 3 dB. He found two regions, one above 1 kHz and one below, as illustrated in the right panel of Figure 3.13. The regions found were similar to the suppression areas that can be observed in single neurones of the auditory nerve, as illustrated in the left panel of Figure 3.13 (these data were also shown in Chapter 1). Similar results have been obtained by Shannon (1976).

Under some circumstances, the reduction in threshold (unmasking) produced by adding one or more extra components to a masker can be partly explained in terms of additional cues provided by the added components, rather than in terms of suppression. Specifically, in forward masking the added components may reduce 'confusion' of the signal with the masker by indicating exactly when the masker ends and the signal begins (Moore, 1980, 1981; Moore and Glasberg, 1982, 1985;

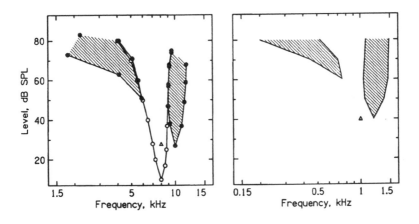

Figure 3.13: The left panel shows neurophysiological data from Arthur, Pfeiffer and Suga (1971). The open circles show the tuning curve (threshold versus frequency) of a single neurone with a CF at 8 kHz. The neurone was stimulated with a tone at CF, and just above threshold (indicated by the open triangle). A second tone was then added and its frequency and intensity varied. Any tone within the shaded areas bounded by the solid circles reduced the response to the tone at CF by 20% or more. These are the suppression areas. The right panel shows the psychoacoustical data of Houtgast (1974) using non-simultaneous masking. The signal was a 1 kHz sinusoid. The masker contained two components. One was a 1 kHz sinusoid which was fixed in level at 40 dB (indicated by the open triangle). The second component (the 'suppressor') was a sinusoid that was varied both in frequency and in level. The shaded areas indicate combinations of frequency and level where the second tone reduced the threshold by 3 dB or more.

Neff, 1985; Moore and O'Loughlin, 1986). This may have led some researchers to overestimate the magnitude of suppression as indicated in non-simultaneous masking experiments. However, not all unmasking can be explained in this way.

The enhancement of frequency selectivity revealed in non-simultaneous masking

A second major difference between simultaneous and non-simultaneous masking is that the frequency selectivity revealed in non-simultaneous masking is greater than that revealed in simultaneous masking. A well-studied example of this is the psychophysical tuning curve (PTC). PTCs determined in forward masking, are typically sharper than those obtained in simultaneous masking (Moore, 1978). An example is given in Figure 3.14. A low-level notched-noise masker was gated with the main narrowband noise masker to restrict off-frequency listening and to provide a consistent detection cue in forward masking. The difference between the two curves is particularly marked on the high-frequency side.

Two different explanations have been proposed for the sharper tuning found in forward masking. According to Houtgast (1974) the sharper tuning arises because the internal representation of the masker (its excitation pattern) is sharpened by a suppression process, with the greatest sharpening occurring on the low-frequency side. In simultaneous masking, the effects of suppression are not seen, since any reduction of the masker activity in the frequency region of the signal is accompanied by a similar reduction in signal-evoked activity. In other words, the signal-to-masker ratio in the frequency region of the signal is unaffected by the suppression. In forward masking, on the other hand, the suppression does not affect the signal. For maskers with frequencies above that of the signal, the effect of suppression is to sharpen the excitation pattern of the masker, resulting in an increase of the masker level required to mask the signal. Thus the suppression is revealed as an increase in the slopes of the PTC.

An alternative explanation is that described earlier; in simultaneous masking, the signal may be suppressed by the masker, and this increases the effectiveness of the masker for masker frequencies well above and below the signal frequency. In non-simultaneous masking the masker does not suppress the signal and so the masker is less effective (Delgutte, 1988, 1990). Hence, when determining a PTC, the masker level has to be increased on the skirts of the PTC.

Whichever of these two explanations is correct, the same inference can be drawn; the tuning curve measured in non-simultaneous masking gives a more accurate indication of the tuning that occurs for single sinusoids. Thus, the PTC measured in non-simultaneous masking is

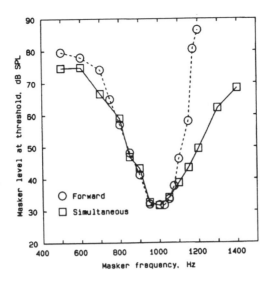

Figure 3.14: Comparison of psychophysical tuning curves (PTCs) determined in simultaneous masking (squares) and forward masking (circles). A low-level notched noise was gated with the masker to provide a consistent detection cue in forward masking and to restrict off-frequency listening. Data from Moore, Glasberg and Roberts (1984).

likely to be closely related to BM tuning curves and neural tuning curves, while the PTC measured in simultaneous masking is likely to be broader than those curves.

Relation between the growth of forward masking and the BM input-output function

As described earlier, growth-of-masking functions in forward masking usually have slopes less than one; when the masker level is increased by X dB, the signal level at threshold increases by less than X dB. Oxenham and Moore (1995) have suggested that the shallow slopes of the growth-of-masking functions can be explained, at least qualitatively, in terms of the compressive input-output function of the BM. Such an input-output function is shown schematically in Figure 3.15. It has a shallow slope for medium input levels, but a steeper slope for very low input levels. Assume that, for a given time delay of the signal relative to the masker, the response evoked by the signal at threshold is directly proportional to the response evoked by the masker. Assume, as an example, that a masker with a level of 40 dB produces a signal threshold of 10 dB. Consider now what happens when the masker level is increased by 30 dB. The increase in masker level, denoted by ΔM in Figure 3.15, produces a relatively small increase in response, ΔO. The small increase

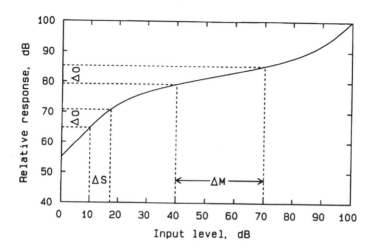

Figure 3.15: The curve shows a schematic input-output function on the BM. When the masker is increased in level by ΔM, this produces an increase in response of ΔO. To restore signal threshold, the response to the signal also has to be increased by ΔO. This requires an increase in signal level, ΔS, which is markedly smaller than ΔM.

occurs because the masker level falls in a range where the input-output function of the BM is highly compressive (it has a shallow slope). To restore the signal to threshold, the signal has to be increased in level so that the response to it increases by ΔO. However, this requires a relatively small increase in signal level, ΔS, as the signal level falls in the range where the input-output function is relatively steep. Thus, the growth-of-masking function has a shallow slope.

According to this explanation, the shallow slope arises from the fact that the signal level is lower than the masker level, so the masker is subject to more compression than the signal. The difference in compression applied to the masker and signal increases with increasing difference in level between the masker and signal. Hence the slope of the growth-of-masking function should also decrease with increasing difference in level between the masker and signal. This can account for the progressive decrease in the slopes of the growth-of-masking functions with increasing time delay between the signal and masker (see Figure 3.12); longer time delays are associated with greater differences in level between the signal and masker.

A prediction of this explanation is that the growth-of-masking function for a given signal time delay should increase in slope if the signal level is high enough to fall in the highly compressive region of the input-output function. Such an effect can be seen in the growth-of-masking function for the shortest delay time in Figure 3.12; the function steepens for the highest signal level. The effect is also apparent, but less clearly so, for the longer time delays of the signal.

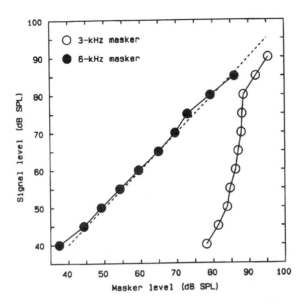

Figure 3.16: Data from Oxenham and Plack (1997) for normally hearing subjects. Thresholds for detecting a 6 kHz signal following a 3 kHz or 6 kHz masker are shown. The signal level was fixed, and the masker level was varied to determine the threshold. Symbols represent the mean thresholds of three normally hearing subjects. The dashed line has a slope of one; linear growth of masking would give data parallel to this line.

For the data shown in Figure 3.12, the signal was relatively long; its overall duration was 20 ms. For such a signal, the signal level at threshold is generally below the masker level. It is this *difference* in level that gives rise to the shallow slopes of the growth-of-masking functions. However, if the signal is made very brief, and it is presented immediately after the end of the masker, the signal level at threshold may be close to the masker level. Under these conditions, the growth-of-masking function is predicted to have a slope of 1; each 10 dB change in masker level should lead to a 10 dB change in signal threshold.

Oxenham and Plack (1997) performed just such an experiment. They measured forward masking for a 6 kHz sinusoidal masker and a signal of the same frequency. They used a very brief signal and a very short time delay between the masker and signal. The level of the signal at threshold was found to be approximately equal to the masker level, and the growth-of-masking function had a slope of 1; each 10 dB increase in masker level was accompanied by a 10 dB increase in signal level. This is illustrated in Figure 3.16 (filled symbols) and it is consistent with the explanation offered above.

In another condition, they used a masker frequency well *below* the signal frequency. The masker frequency was 3 kHz instead of 6 kHz. In this condition, the growth-of-masking function had a slope much *greater* than 1;

a 10 dB increase in masker level was accompanied by a 40 dB increase in signal level, as shown by the open symbols in Figure 3.16. This can be explained in the following way: the signal threshold depends on the response evoked by the masker at the CF corresponding to the signal frequency. The growth of response on the BM for sinusoids with frequencies well below the CF is linear. Thus, the signal is subject to compression while the masker is not (essentially the opposite of the situation illustrated in Figure 3.15). This gives rise to the steep growth-of-masking function.

The ratio of the slopes of the growth-of-masking functions for the 6 kHz masker and the 3 kHz masker reflects the difference in slope of the BM input-output function for a tone at the CF (6 kHz) and a tone well below CF (3 kHz). The slopes actually differ by a factor of about four. Assuming that the response to the 3 kHz tone is linear (at the place with CF = 6 kHz), this implies that the input-output function for the 6 kHz tone has a slope of about 0.25 for mid-range sound levels. This is consistent with direct estimates of the slopes of BM input-output functions, as described in Chapter 1.

The audibility of partials in complex tones

A complex tone is a sound that contains many sinusoidal components and that evokes a subjective sensation of *pitch* (see Chapter 6 for a definition of pitch). The sounds produced by musical instruments are nearly always complex tones. When the waveform of a sound repeats regularly as a function of time, the sound is said to be *periodic*. For such sounds, the sinusoidal components have frequencies that are integer multiples of a common *fundamental frequency*. The components are referred to as *harmonics*. The harmonics are numbered, the first harmonic being the fundamental component. For example, the note 'A' played on an oboe would have a fundamental frequency (first harmonic) of 440 Hz, a second harmonic of 880 Hz, a third harmonic of 1320 Hz, and so on. Some sounds contain frequency components whose frequencies are not integer multiples of a common fundamental. However, they may still evoke a pitch. Examples are the tones produced by bells and gongs. Such sounds are called inharmonic complex tones. The term *partial* is used to refer to any frequency component in a complex tone, whether it is a harmonic or not.

To a limited extent, human listeners are able to hear pitches corresponding to the individual partials in complex tones. This is not the usual way that complex tones are perceived; rather, it is common to hear a single pitch corresponding to the fundamental frequency; see Chapter 6. However, it is possible to 'hear out' some individual partials if attention is directed in an appropriate way. One very effective method is to remove a single partial and then re-introduce it. That partial then seems to 'pop out' and is heard as a separate tone.

Plomp (1964a) and Plomp and Mimpen (1968) investigated the limits of the ability to hear out partials in complex tones. They used tones with twelve sinusoidal components. The listeners had a three-position switch that they could use to hear either the complex tone or one of two comparison sinusoidal tones. One of the comparison tones had the same frequency as a partial in the complex; the other lay halfway between that frequency and the frequency of the adjacent higher or lower partial. The listener had to judge which of these two comparison tones was a component of the complex. Plomp and Mimpen used two types of complex tone: a harmonic complex tone containing harmonics 1 to 12, where the frequencies of the components were integer multiples of that of the fundamental, and an inharmonic complex tone, where the frequencies of the components were mistuned from simple frequency ratios. Figure 3.17 shows their results, plotted in terms of the frequency separation between a given partial and neighbouring partials necessary for that partial be heard out with 75% accuracy.

Plomp and Mimpen's data are consistent with the hypothesis that a partial can just be heard out from neighbouring partials when it is separated from those partials by 1.25 times the ERB of the auditory filter. The solid line in Fig. 3.17 shows the ERB of the auditory filter, estimated

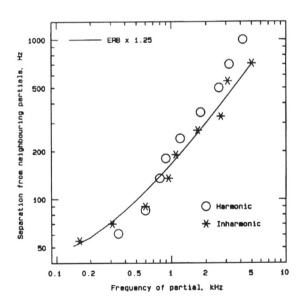

Figure 3.17: Data from Plomp (1964a) and Plomp and Mimpen (1968) on the audibility of partials in complex tones. The symbols show the frequency separation of a partial from neighbouring partials necessary for that partial to be heard out with 75% accuracy, plotted as a function of the frequency of the partial. The solid curve shows the ERB multiplied by 1.25, plotted as a function of frequency.

using the notched-noise method described earlier in this chapter, multiplied by 1.25. This line fits the data rather well. The data of Moore and Ohgushi (1993) on the audibility of partials in inharmonic complex tones are also consistent with the idea that partials can be heard out with about 75% accuracy when the partials are separated by about 1.25 ERBs. Separations greater than 2 ERBs are sufficient to give near-perfect scores, whereas separations less than 1 ERB lead to very low scores. Partials that can be heard out are often described as *resolved,* while partials that cannot be heard out are described as *unresolved.*

For harmonic complex tones, the lower harmonics are separated by more than 1.25 ERBs. For example, for the note 'A' mentioned above, the separation between the second and third harmonics (880 Hz and 1320 Hz) corresponds to about 3 ERBs. However, the higher harmonics are separated by less than 1.25 ERBs. For example, the separation between the ninth and tenth harmonics (3960 Hz and 4400 Hz) corresponds to only 0.9 ERBs. Generally, about the first to the fifth harmonics in a complex tone can be heard out reasonably well. Harmonics above the eighth are very difficult to hear out. Between the fifth and eighth harmonics there is a transition region, where the harmonics can be heard out to some extent; they are partially resolved. These results have important implications for theories of the pitch perception of complex tones, as described in Chapter 6.

I am not aware of any studies of the ability of people with cochlear hearing loss to hear out partials from complex sounds. However, it seems very likely that the reduced frequency selectivity commonly associated with cochlear hearing loss (which is described in more detail below) would have adverse effects on this ability. This is discussed further in Chapter 6.

Effects of cochlear damage on frequency selectivity in simultaneous masking

Complicating factors

Comparisons of frequency selectivity in normal and hearing-impaired people are complicated by several factors. One factor is the sound level of the stimuli used. As mentioned above, the auditory filters of normally hearing subjects broaden on the low-frequency side with increasing level. This effect probably depends on the active mechanism in the cochlea. At low sound levels, this mechanism strongly enhances the tuning on the low-frequency side of the auditory filter. However, as the sound level increases, the contribution of the active mechanism is progressively reduced, and the low-frequency side of the auditory filter broadens.

The active mechanism is usually damaged or completely non-functioning in ears with cochlear damage. Hence, changes in frequency selectivity with level are absent or much less pronounced (Moore, Laurence and Wright, 1985; Stelmachowicz, Lewis, Larson et al., 1987; Nelson and Schroder, 1997). As a result, the differences between normal and hearing-impaired subjects tend to decrease at high sound levels.

A second complicating factor is off-frequency listening. Some measures of frequency selectivity, especially PTCs, can be strongly influenced by off-frequency listening. More importantly, the role of off-frequency listening may vary markedly depending on the sensation level of the stimuli and the frequency selectivity of the subject. For example, if PTCs are measured for a normally hearing subject using a signal at 70 dB SPL, there is a strong potential for off-frequency listening in some conditions. On the other hand, if a hearing-impaired subject with an absolute threshold of 60 dB SPL is tested with a 70 dB SPL signal, the potential for off-frequency listening is much reduced. In practice, the extent to which off-frequency listening affects masked thresholds for hearing-impaired persons depends on the way that absolute thresholds vary with frequency. Although these problems can be reduced by presenting a notched noise with the variable masker, as described earlier, this has not usually been done in studies with hearing-impaired subjects. Hence, in what follows, studies of PTCs will be described only briefly, while measures controlling off-frequency listening will be described in more detail. For a more detailed review of the results of PTC measurements, see Tyler (1986).

Psychophysical tuning curves

There have been many studies comparing PTCs in normal subjects and subjects with cochlear hearing loss (Leshowitz, Linstrom and Zurek, 1975; Hoekstra and Ritsma, 1977; Zwicker and Schorn, 1978; Bonding, 1979b; Florentine, Buus, Scharf et al., 1980; Tyler, Wood and Fernandes, 1982; Carney and Nelson, 1983; Festen and Plomp, 1983; Stelmachowicz, Jesteadt, Gorga et al., 1985; Nelson, 1991). Although the studies differ in detail, their results are in general agreement that PTCs are broader than normal in the impaired subjects; an example was given in Figure 3.1. However, it is difficult to quantify the differences from normal, owing to the problems discussed above. Most studies have found that the sharpness of tuning of PTCs decreases with increasing absolute threshold, although the correlation between threshold and sharpness of tuning varies markedly across studies. No systematic differences in PTCs have been reported between cochlear losses of different origin, such as noise-induced, Ménière's disease, ageing, and hereditary losses. In some cases, PTCs have been found that are W-shaped rather than V-shaped (Hoekstra and Ritsma, 1977). These may be a psychoacoustical analogue of the W-shaped neural tuning curves that are sometimes found in animals with cochlear damage (see Figure 1.20).

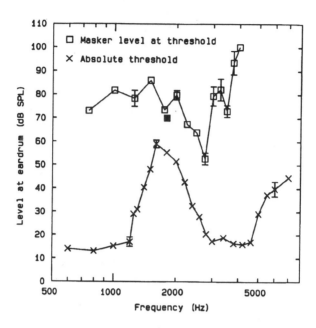

Figure 3.18: Data obtained from a subject with a presumed mid-frequency dead region. The crosses indicate the absolute thresholds. The open squares show a PTC obtained using a sinusoidal signal and a narrowband noise masker. The signal had a frequency of 1800 Hz, and it was presented at 15 dB SL (solid square).

Sometimes, PTCs have been found whose tips are shifted well away from the signal frequency (Thornton and Abbas, 1980; Florentine and Houtsma, 1983; Turner, Burns and Nelson, 1983). This can happen when the signal frequency falls in a dead region. The most-studied situation of this type is when there is a low-frequency dead region, i.e. when there is severe damage to the IHCs at the apical end of the cochlea (see Chapter 2). The detection of low-frequency tones is then mediated by neurones with high CFs. If the signal to be detected has a frequency corresponding to the dead region, the tip of the tuning curve lies well above the signal frequency. In other words, a masker centred well above the signal in frequency is more effective than a masker centred close to the signal frequency. This happens because the higher frequency masker lies closer to the CFs of the neurones mediating detection of the signal.

An example of a PTC obtained from a subject with a presumed mid-frequency dead region is shown in Figure 3.18 (data gathered by Joseph Alcántara in my laboratory). The absolute thresholds, specified as the sound pressure level at the eardrum, are shown as crosses. Absolute thresholds for frequencies from 600 to 1200 Hz, and from 3000 to 5000 Hz are nearly normal, but there is a distinct mid-frequency elevation between 1300 and 2800 Hz. Probably, absolute thresholds for frequencies in the range 1300 to 2800 Hz were determined by excitation spreading to lower CFs (for frequencies from 1300 to 1600 Hz) or higher CFs (for frequencies from 1800 to 2800 Hz). For determination of the PTC (open squares), the signal had a frequency of 1800 Hz and it was presented at a level 15 dB above the absolute threshold, as indicated by the filled square. The tip of the PTC falls well above the signal frequency. In fact, the tip falls at 3000 Hz, which is the frequency at which absolute threshold has returned to a nearly normal value.

Auditory filter shapes measured with notched noise

Auditory filter shapes of subjects with cochlear impairments have been estimated in several studies using notched-noise maskers (Tyler, Hall, Glasberg et al., 1984; Glasberg and Moore, 1986; Dubno and Dirks, 1989; Laroche, Hétu, Quoc et al., 1992; Peters and Moore, 1992; Stone, Glasberg and Moore, 1992; Leek and Summers, 1993; Sommers and Humes, 1993; Leeuw and Dreschler, 1994). The results generally agree in showing that auditory filters are broader than normal in hearing-impaired subjects and that, on average, the degree of broadening increases with increasing hearing loss.

Consider, as an example, the study of Glasberg and Moore (1986). They measured auditory filter shapes in subjects with unilateral and bilateral cochlear impairments; in the former case differences between the normal and impaired ears cannot be attributed to extraneous factors such as age or ability to concentrate. The same noise spectrum level (50 dB, corresponding to an overall level of 79 dB SPL at 1 kHz) was used for the normal and impaired ears. Results for six subjects at a centre frequency of 1 kHz are shown in Figure 3.19.

The filter shapes for the normal ears (top panel) are similar to one another, and all show a high degree of frequency selectivity. The filter shapes for the impaired ears vary greatly in shape across subjects, but they are all broader than those for the normal ears on at least one side. The most common feature is a marked broadening on the low-frequency side. This indicates an increased susceptibility to masking by low-frequency sounds, such as car noise and air-conditioning noise.

Figure 3.20 summarises values of the ERB of the auditory filter obtained from subjects with cochlear hearing loss in my laboratory and in the laboratory of Robert Peters. The summary was prepared by Michael Stone. The upper panel shows ERB values plotted relative to the value for young normally hearing subjects at moderate sound levels, as given by equation 3.1. The lower panel shows ERB values plotted relative to the value for young normal subjects tested at the same sound pressure level as the impaired subjects, assuming that the ERB for normal subjects varies with level as described by Glasberg and Moore (1990). In both cases, the ERB values are plotted as a function of the absolute threshold (dB HL) at the test frequency. There is a clear trend

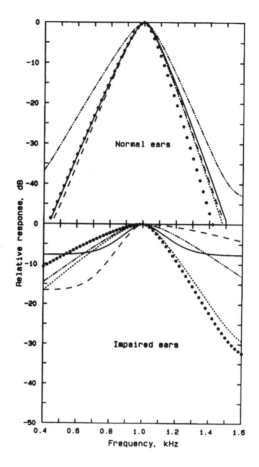

Figure 3.19: Auditory filter shapes at a centre frequency of 1 kHz for the normal (top) and impaired (bottom) ears of six subjects with unilateral cochlear impairments.

for the ERB to increase with increasing absolute threshold. The increase is less in the lower panel as the auditory filters for normal subjects broaden with increasing level of the test stimuli. However, the trend is still quite clear. There is also considerable scatter in the data, indicating that the ERB of the auditory filter cannot be predicted reliably from the absolute threshold.

The scatter in the data shown in Figure 3.20 may reflect different ways in which cochlear damage can occur, as described in Chapter 1 (Liberman and Dodds, 1984; Liberman, Dodds and Learson, 1986). In one common case, the damage is primarily to the OHCs and the IHCs are intact. This results in reduced effectiveness of the active mechanism, but a relatively normal mechanism for transducing BM movement into neural responses. In this case, the degree of auditory-filter broadening is correlated with the loss of sensitivity (elevated absolute threshold), and

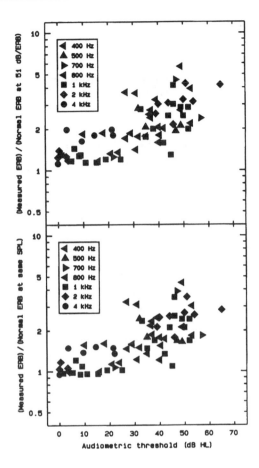

Figure 3.20: Values of the ERB of the auditory filter for subjects with cochlear hearing loss, plotted as a function of absolute threshold (dB HL) at the test frequency. The ERB values are plotted either relative to the values given by Eq. 3.1, or relative to the ERBs for young normally hearing subjects tested at the same sound level.

the broadening of the auditory filter can occur on both sides or mainly on the low-frequency side.

In a second case, both the OHCs and IHCs are damaged. Both the active mechanism and the transducer mechanism are adversely affected. This results in a considerable elevation of absolute threshold and the filter is normally broadened on both sides. In a final (rare) case, the damage is mainly to the IHCs, with minimal damage to the OHCs. The transducer mechanism is severely affected in this case, but the active mechanism still functions, albeit with reduced effectiveness because of the high sound level needed to evoke a neural response. In this case, the absolute threshold is elevated, but the sharpness of tuning is only slightly worse than normal.

In summary, all methods of estimating frequency selectivity suggest that it decreases with increasing hearing loss. However, for a given elevation in absolute threshold, there can be considerable scatter both in the degree of broadening and in the asymmetry of the auditory filter. This large variability may arise from different patterns of hair cell loss within the cochlea.

Effects of cochlear damage on forward masking and suppression

Several workers have compared results from simultaneous and forward masking in an attempt to measure suppression effects in hearing-impaired subjects. Usually, the signal level has been fixed, and the masker has been varied to determine a masked threshold. Essentially, it is assumed that threshold is reached when the masker produces a fixed output from the auditory filter centred at the signal frequency.

Wightman, McGee and Kramer (1977) compared PTCs in simultaneous and forward masking for subjects with high-frequency hearing losses. They found that, when both the signal and the masker were in regions of normal sensitivity, the PTCs obtained in forward masking were sharper than those found in simultaneous masking. However, when the signal was in the frequency region of reduced sensitivity, or just below it, the differences were much reduced. They also attempted to measure suppression more directly, using the two-tone unmasking paradigm described earlier. Unmasking was observed when the 'suppressor' tone fell in frequency regions of normal sensitivity, but not when it fell in the region of the hearing loss. Wightman et al. concluded that the suppression mechanism was rendered ineffective by the hearing loss. They took their results to support the hypothesis that, in normally hearing subjects, suppression is responsible for the differences between PTCs in simultaneous and forward masking. Penner (1980b) and Mills and Schmeidt (1983) studied two-tone unmasking in subjects with noise-induced hearing loss, and obtained similar results to those of Wightman et al.

Moore and Glasberg (1986b) measured PTCs in simultaneous and forward masking separately for each ear of subjects with unilateral moderate cochlear losses. A notched noise was presented with the narrow-band variable masker to restrict off-frequency listening, to provide a consistent detection cue in forward masking, and to equate the levels of the PTCs around their tips for the normal and impaired ears. For the normal ears, they found, as expected, that the PTCs were usually sharper in forward masking than in simultaneous masking. The PTCs were broader for the impaired ears, and the differences between simultaneous and forward masking were reduced or absent. An example of their results is given in Figure 3.21. These results are consistent with

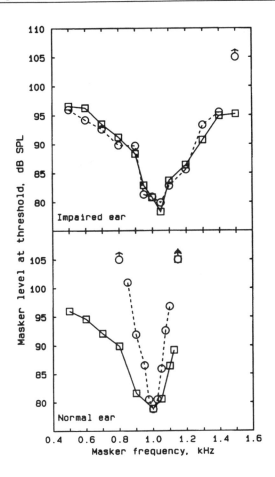

Figure 3.21: PTCs determined for the normal (bottom) and impaired (top) ears of a subject with a unilateral cochlear impairment, for simultaneous masking (squares) and forward masking (circles). Up-pointing arrows indicate that the masker level required for threshold was greater than 105 dB SPL. Data from Moore and Glasberg (1986b).

the idea that suppression is reduced or absent in people with cochlear hearing loss.

In another experiment using five subjects with unilateral cochlear hearing loss, Moore and Glasberg (1986b) used notched noise as a simultaneous and a forward masker. The signal level was fixed and the masker level was varied to determine threshold for each notch width used. For the normal ears, the rate of change of masker level at threshold with notch width was greater in forward masking than in simultaneous masking, indicating a higher effective degree of frequency selectivity in forward masking. For the impaired ears, the differences between simultaneous and forward masking were smaller, although they were completely absent for only one subject. These results suggest that the suppression mechanism was reduced in effectiveness in the impaired ears, but was not completely inoperative, except in one case.

In summary, the results of the various experiments are in agreement in showing that:

- Two-tone unmasking in forward masking is small or absent when the stimuli fall in a frequency region where there is cochlear hearing loss.
- Differences in frequency selectivity between simultaneous and forward masking are much smaller than normal in hearing-impaired subjects.

Taken together, these findings strongly support the idea that suppression is reduced or absent in people with cochlear hearing loss.

Effects of cochlear hearing loss on BM input-output functions

It was argued above that the slopes of growth-of-masking functions in forward masking for normally hearing subjects depend strongly on the

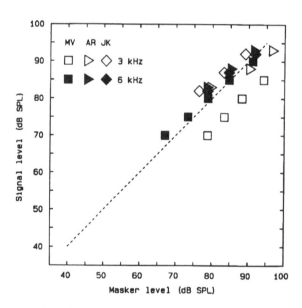

Figure 3.22: Data from Oxenham and Plack (1997) for three subjects with cochlear hearing loss. Individual data from subjects MV, AR and JK are plotted. Thresholds for detecting a 6 kHz signal following a 3 kHz or 6 kHz masker are shown. The signal level was fixed, and the masker level was varied to determine the threshold. The dashed line has a slope of one; linear growth of masking would give data parallel to this line.

compression that occurs on the BM. The shallow slopes that are typically observed (see Figure 3.12) are a consequence of the fact that the masker typically falls in a range of levels where the BM input-output function is highly compressive (has a shallow slope) whereas the signal typically falls in a range of levels where the function is more linear (the slope is steeper). If the compression on the BM is lost as a consequence of cochlear hearing loss, then the growth-of-masking functions in forward masking (in dB per dB) should have slopes close to unity, except when the signal is very close to its absolute threshold. Furthermore, the slope should remain close to unity, regardless of the relative frequencies of the masker and signal, as all frequencies should be processed linearly. Empirical data have confirmed these predictions (Oxenham and Moore, 1995, 1997; Oxenham and Plack, 1997). This is illustrated in Figure 3.22, which shows individual data from three subjects with moderate cochlear hearing loss in the same conditions as those used for the normally hearing subjects in Figure 3.16. In contrast to Figure 3.16, all three hearing-impaired subjects in Figure 3.22 show linear growth-of-masking functions for both the 6 kHz and the 3 kHz masker. This is consistent with the view that cochlear damage results in a loss of BM compression.

Perceptual consequences of reduced frequency selectivity, loss of suppression and steeper BM input-output functions

Frequency selectivity plays an important role in many aspects of auditory perception. Hence, when frequency selectivity is reduced in people with cochlear hearing loss, these aspects of perception can be expected to alter. Some of these aspects - specifically, loudness perception, frequency discrimination, pitch perception and speech perception - are discussed in more detail in later chapters of this book. The steeper BM input-output functions produced by cochlear damage also affect many aspects of auditory perception (Moore and Oxenham, 1998); again, several of these are discussed later in this book. This section will consider some of the aspects of perception that are directly affected by reduced frequency selectivity.

Susceptibility to masking

It is obvious from the studies discussed earlier that masking effects are often more pronounced in hearing-impaired subjects than in normal subjects. However, the size of the difference depends greatly on the spectral characteristics of the signal and masker. When the signal and masker overlap spectrally (for example, when the signal is a sinusoid and the masker is a broad-band noise without distinct spectral peaks), masked thresholds are usually only slightly greater for hearing-impaired listeners than for normal listeners. However, when the signal and masker differ in spectrum, masking may be considerably greater in the hearing-impaired. There are two situations where this might apply. One is when the average spectrum of a masking sound differs from that of a signal. For example, the signal may be a high-frequency warning siren, and the masker may be primarily low-frequency noise from air-conditioning or machinery. The second is when the signal and the masker differ in their short-term spectra. For example, the signal might be a vowel sound for an attended talker and the masker might be a different vowel sound from an interfering talker. A hearing-impaired person with reduced frequency selectivity will be less able than normal to take advantage of the spectral differences between the two vowels. This issue is examined in more detail in Chapter 8.

Timbre perception

Timbre is often defined as 'that attribute of auditory sensation in terms of which a listener can judge that two sounds having the same loudness and pitch are dissimilar'. Differences in timbre allow us to distinguish between the same note played on, say, the piano or the flute. Timbre depends on both spectral and temporal aspects of sounds. Changing either the long-term spectral shape of a sound or its temporal envelope may lead to a change in perceived timbre (see Handel, 1995, for a review).

The aspects of timbre perception that are affected by spectral shape almost certainly depend on the frequency selectivity of the ear. The spectral shape of a sound is represented in the excitation pattern evoked by the sound, and the timbre is related to the shape of the excitation pattern (Plomp, 1976). In an ear with cochlear damage, frequency selectivity is usually reduced. Hence, the excitation pattern contains less detail about the spectrum than would be the case for a normal ear. This would be expected to lead to a reduced ability to distinguish sounds on the basis of their spectral shape. Also, the internal representation of spectral shape may be influenced by suppression. Suppression in a normal ear may enhance the contrast between the peaks and dips in the excitation pattern evoked by a complex sound (Tyler and Lindblom, 1982; Moore and Glasberg, 1983b). This may make it easier to pick out spectral features, such as formants in vowel sounds. The loss of suppression associated with cochlear damage would thus lead to greater difficulty in picking out such features.

For many sounds, such as different musical instruments (for example, xylophone versus harpsichord), the differences in spectral shape are so large that even very poor frequency selectivity allows discrimination between them. However, it may be more difficult for a person with reduced frequency selectivity to distinguish sounds that differ in spectrum in more subtle ways. There has been little study of the ability of hearing-impaired people to distinguish musical instruments. However, different steady-state vowels are primarily distinguished by their spectral shapes, and studies of vowel perception suggest that reduced frequency selectivity can, indeed, lead to difficulties in the discrimination and identification of vowels. These studies are reviewed in Chapter 8.

Chapter 4
Loudness Perception and Intensity Resolution

Introduction

Loudness corresponds to the subjective impression of the magnitude of a sound. The formal definition of loudness is: that attribute of auditory sensation in terms of which sounds can be ordered on a scale extending from quiet to loud. As loudness is subjective it is very difficult to measure in a quantitative way. Estimates of loudness can be strongly affected by bias and context effects of various kinds (Gabriel, Kollmeier and Mellert, 1997; Laming, 1997). For example, the impression of loudness of a sound with a moderate level (say, 60 dB SPL) can be affected by presenting a high-level sound (say, 100 dB SPL) before the moderate level sound. This chapter starts by describing some of the ways in which loudness perception has been studied in normally hearing people. It then goes on to consider changes in loudness perception associated with cochlear hearing loss.

Loudness perception in normally hearing people

Equal-loudness contours and loudness level

It is often useful to be able to compare the loudness of sounds with that of a standard, reference sound. The most common reference sound is a 1000 Hz sinusoid. The *loudness level* of a sound is defined as the level of a 1000 Hz sinusoid that is equal in loudness to the sound. The unit of loudness level is the *phon*. Thus, the loudness level of any sound in phons is the level (in dB SPL) of the 1000 Hz sinusoid to which it sounds equal in loudness. For example, if a sound appears to be as loud as a 1000 Hz sinusoid with a level of 45 dB SPL, then the sound has a loudness level of 45 phons. To determine the loudness level of a given sound, the subject is asked to adjust the level of a 1000 Hz sinusoid until it appears to have the same loudness as that sound. The 1000 Hz sinusoid and the test sound are presented alternately rather than simultaneously.

In a variation of this procedure, the 1000 Hz sinusoid is fixed in level and the test sound is adjusted to give a loudness match. If this is repeated for various different frequencies of a sinusoidal test sound, an *equal-loudness contour* is generated (Fletcher and Munson, 1933). For example, if the 1000 Hz sinusoid is fixed in level at 40 dB SPL, then the 40 phon equal-loudness contour is generated. The exact shapes of equal-loudness contours vary markedly across studies (Gabriel, Kollmeier and Mellert, 1997), and there is currently no agreement as to the 'correct' values. Some examples are shown in Figure 4.1; the curves are actually predictions based on a model of loudness (Moore, Glasberg and Baer, 1997; loudness models are described later in this chapter), but they are similar in form to empirically obtained equal-loudness contours for young normally hearing people. The figure shows equal-loudness contours for binaural listening for loudness levels from 10 phons to 110 phons, and it also includes the absolute threshold (MAF) curve. The listening conditions were assumed to be similar to those for determining the MAF curve, namely that the sound came from a frontal direction in a free field (i.e. in a situation where there is no reflected sound from walls, floor or ceiling). The equal-loudness contours are of similar shape to the MAF curve, but tend to become flatter at high loudness levels.

Note that the subjective loudness of a sound is not directly proportional to its loudness level in phons. For example, a sound with a loudness level of 80 phons sounds much more than twice as loud as a sound with a loudness level of 40 phons.

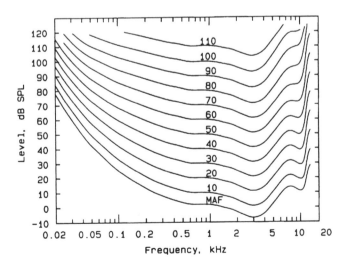

Figure 4.1: Equal-loudness contours for various loudness levels. The lowest curve is the absolute threshold (MAF) curve. The curves are based on a loudness model (Moore, Glasberg and Baer, 1997).

The scaling of loudness

Several methods have been developed that attempt to measure 'directly' the relationship between the physical magnitude of sound and perceived loudness (Stevens, 1957). In one, called *magnitude estimation,* sounds with various different levels are presented, and the subject is asked to assign a number to each one according to its perceived loudness. In a second method, called *magnitude production,* the subject is asked to adjust the level of a sound until it has a loudness corresponding to a specified number.

On the basis of results from these two methods, Stevens suggested that loudness, *L,* was a *power function* of physical intensity, *I:*

$$L = kI^{0.3}$$

(4.1)

where *k* is a constant depending on the subject and the units used. In other words, the loudness of a given sound is proportional to its intensity raised to the power 0.3. Note that this implies that loudness is *not* linearly related to intensity; rather, it is a *compressive* function of intensity. An approximation to equation 4.1 is that the loudness doubles when the intensity is increased by a factor of 10; the latter corresponds to a 10 dB increase in level. In practice, equation 4.1 only holds for sound levels above about 40 dB SPL. For lower levels than this, the loudness changes with intensity more rapidly than predicted by equation 4.1.

The unit of loudness is the *sone.* One sone is defined arbitrarily as the loudness of a 1000 Hz sinusoid at 40 dB SPL, presented binaurally from a frontal direction in a free field. Figure 4.2 shows the relationship between loudness level in phons and loudness in sones. For a 1000 Hz sinusoid, presented under the conditions specified above, the loudness level is equal to the physical level in dB SPL. Figure 4.2, like Figure 4.1, is based on predictions of a loudness model (Moore, Glasberg and Baer, 1997), but it is consistent with empirical data obtained using scaling methods (Hellman and Zwislocki, 1961). Since the loudness in sones is plotted on a logarithmic scale, and the decibel scale is itself logarithmic, the curve shown in Figure 4.2 approximates a straight line for loudness levels above 40 phon, the range for which equation 4.1 holds.

Another method of relating loudness sensations to physical intensity involves categorical judgements of loudness. This method has been used extensively to assess loudness perception in hearing-impaired persons. The subject is presented with a test sound and is asked to judge its loudness by using one of several verbal categories (Pascoe, 1978; Hellbrück and Moser, 1985; Kiessling, Steffens and Wagner, 1993; Cox, Alexander, Taylor et al., 1997). An example is the Loudness Growth in

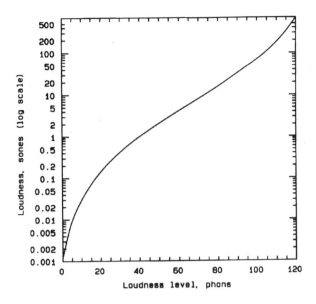

Figure 4.2: Loudness in sones (log scale), plotted as a function of loudness level in phons. The curve is based on a loudness model (Moore, Glasberg and Baer, 1997).

Half-Octave Bands (LGOB) Test described by Allen and Jeng (1990) and adapted by Pluvinage (1989) and by Moore, Johnson, Clark and Pluvinage (1992). The stimuli are half-octave wide bands of noise centred at 500, 1000, 2000 and 4000 Hz. In an initial phase of the test, each centre frequency is tested separately. On each trial, the noise band is presented as a series of three bursts, and the subject is required to indicate the loudness of the bursts by pressing one of seven buttons labelled 'cannot hear', 'very soft', 'soft', 'comfortable', 'loud', 'very loud', and 'too loud'. The sound level is varied randomly from trial to trial over the range from 30 to 110 dB SPL.

In the second phase, all stimuli consistently eliciting responses of 'can't hear' or 'too loud' are eliminated, and a series of trials is presented in which both the centre frequency and level of the noise bands are randomised. The results of the second phase are used to construct functions relating perceived loudness to level at each centre frequency. Sometimes, the verbal categories are transformed to a numerical scale, for example, ranging from 0 to 50.

Estimates of loudness obtained by numerical ratings or categorical ratings can be strongly influenced by factors such as the range of stimuli used and the instructions given (Heller, 1991; Hellbrück, 1993; Hohmann, 1993). Often, listeners distribute their responses across the range of available categories whatever range of stimulus levels is used (Garner, 1954). For example, if the stimuli range in level from 30 to

90 dB SPL, then (for normally hearing listeners) the 30 dB stimulus might be judged as 'very soft' and the 90 dB stimulus might be judged as 'too loud'. If the stimuli range in level from 20 dB to 110 dB SPL, then the 20 dB stimulus might be judged as 'very soft' and the 110 dB stimulus might be judged as 'too loud'. However, there is no easy way of determining what is the 'correct' range to use. Hence, caution is needed in interpreting results obtained using these methods, especially when comparing across studies using different methods and different stimulus ranges.

The detection of intensity changes

The normal auditory system is remarkable both in terms of its absolute sensitivity and in terms of the range of sound intensities to which it can respond. The most intense sound that can be heard without immediately damaging the ears has a level about 120 dB above that of the faintest sound that can be detected. This corresponds to a ratio of intensities of 1 000 000 000 000:1. Over this whole range, relatively small changes in sound intensity can be detected.

The smallest detectable change in intensity has been measured for many different types of stimuli by a variety of methods. The three main methods are:

- Modulation detection. The stimulus is amplitude modulated (made to vary in amplitude) at a slow regular rate and the listener is required to detect the modulation. Usually, the modulation is sinusoidal. For an example of the waveform of such a sound, see the upper-right panel of Figure 6.5.
- Increment detection. A continuous background stimulus is presented, and the subject is required to detect an increment in the level of the background.
- Intensity discrimination of gated or pulsed stimuli. Two (or more) separate pulses of sound are presented successively, one being more intense than the other(s), and the subject is required to indicate which pulse was the most intense.

In all of these tasks, the subjective impression of the listener is that a change in loudness is being detected. For example, in modulation detection the modulation is heard as a fluctuation in loudness. In increment detection the increment is heard as a brief increase in loudness of the background, or sometimes as an extra sound superimposed on the background. In intensity discrimination of gated or pulsed stimuli, the most intense pulse appears louder than the other(s). Although there are some minor discrepancies in the experimental results for the different types of method, the general trend is similar. For wide-band noise, or for bandpass filtered noise, the smallest detectable intensity change is approximately a constant fraction of the intensity of the stimulus. If I is the intensity of a noise band, and ΔI is the smallest detectable change in intensity (both in linear units), then $\Delta I/I$ is roughly constant. This is an example of *Weber's Law*, which states that the smallest detectable change in a stimulus is proportional to the magnitude of that stimulus. The value of $\Delta I/I$ is called the *Weber fraction*. If the smallest detectable change in level is expressed in decibels, i.e. as $\Delta L = 10\log_{10}\{(I+\Delta I)/I\}$, then this, too, is constant. For wide-band noise, ΔL has a value of about 0.5 to 1 dB. This holds from about 20 dB above threshold to 100 dB above threshold (Miller, 1947). The value of ΔL increases for sounds that are close to the absolute threshold.

For sinusoids, Weber's Law does not hold (Riesz, 1928; Harris, 1963; Viemeister, 1972; Jesteadt, Wier and Green, 1977b). Instead it is found that $\Delta I/I$ decreases somewhat with increasing I. This has been called the 'near miss' to Weber's Law. The data of Riesz for modulation detection show a value of ΔL of 1.5 dB at 20 dB SL, 0.7 dB at 40 dB SL, and 0.3 dB at 80 dB SL (all at 1000 Hz). The change in ΔL with level is somewhat less for pulsed tones (intensity discrimination of gated or pulsed stimuli) than for modulated tones (modulation detection).

Effects of cochlear hearing loss on loudness perception

Most, if not all, people with cochlear hearing loss show a phenomenon called *loudness recruitment* (Fowler, 1936; Steinberg and Gardner, 1937). This may be described as follows. The absolute threshold is higher than normal. When a sound is increased in level above the elevated absolute threshold, the rate of growth of loudness level with increasing sound level is greater than normal. When the level is sufficiently high, usually around 90 to 100 dB SPL, the loudness reaches its 'normal' value; the sound appears as loud to the person with impaired hearing as it would to a normally hearing person. With further increases in sound level above 90-100 dB SPL, the loudness grows in an almost normal manner.

A complementary way of describing the same effect is in terms of dynamic range. This refers to the range of sound levels between the absolute threshold and the level at which sounds become uncomfortably loud. For example, for a person with normal hearing, the threshold for detecting a mid-frequency sound might be around 0 dB SPL, whereas the sound might become uncomfortably loud at a level of around 100 dB SPL. The dynamic range would then be 100 dB. Typically, in people with cochlear hearing loss, the absolute threshold is elevated, but the level at which sounds become uncomfortably loud is about the same as normal (except in cases of severe or profound loss). Hence the

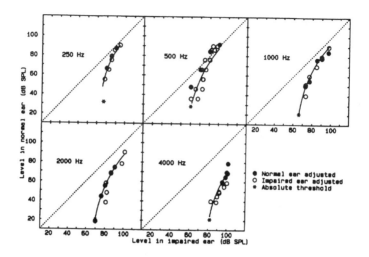

Figure 4.3: Loudness-matching functions for a subject with a unilateral cochlear hearing loss. Asterisks show the absolute threshold for each ear. Each panel shows results for a different signal frequency. The curves are predictions of the model described in the text. The diagonal dotted lines indicate equal levels in the two ears.

dynamic range is reduced compared to normal. Sometimes, especially in cases of severe hearing loss, the loudness does not reach its 'normal' value at high sound levels, but remains somewhat below that which would occur in normal hearing. This is called 'under recruitment' or 'partial recruitment'. The opposite case also sometimes occurs, where high-level sounds appear louder to a hearing-impaired person than to a normally hearing person. This is called 'over recruitment'. However, the most common pattern is that of complete recruitment, where for sounds at high levels the loudness is about the same for normally hearing and hearing-impaired persons.

Loudness recruitment is most easily demonstrated in people who have a unilateral cochlear hearing impairment. It is then possible to obtain loudness matches between the two ears. Usually, a tone is presented alternately to the two ears. The level is fixed in one ear, and the level is adjusted in the other ear until the loudness is judged to be the same at the two ears. The clinical version of this method is known as the alternating binaural loudness balance (ABLB) test. Figure 4.3 shows an example of measurements of this type obtained by Moore and Glasberg (1997). Results were obtained at five different centre frequencies, using sinusoidal tone bursts as stimuli. The exact experimental method is described in Moore, Wojtczak and Vickers (1996). The level of the tone in the normal ear that matches the loudness of the tone in the impaired ear is plotted as a function of the level in the impaired ear. At each frequency tested there is clear evidence of loudness recruitment; the slopes of the curves (in dB/dB) are greater than unity. For some of

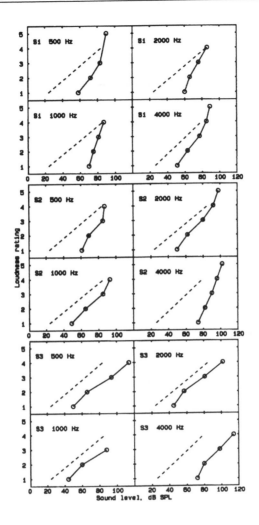

Figure 4.4: Results of three subjects for a categorical loudness scaling procedure (circles). The dashed lines show typical results for normally hearing subjects. The centre frequency of the half-octave wide band of noise used is indicated in each panel. A loudness rating of 1 corresponds to 'very soft' and a rating of 5 corresponds to 'very loud'.

the frequencies tested (250 and 500 Hz), the level required for equal loudness in the normal ear approaches the level in the impaired ear at high levels, i.e. complete loudness recruitment occurs. For other frequencies (2000 and 4000 Hz), only partial recruitment occurs, at least up to the highest level tested. The solid lines are predictions of a model that is described below.

Loudness recruitment can also be demonstrated in people with bilateral cochlear hearing loss. One method of doing this involves the use of the categorical loudness scaling procedure described earlier. Some examples of growth-of-loudness curves obtained using the LGOB method (Allen and Jeng, 1990) are given in Figure 4.4 (data from Moore, Johnson, Clark and Pluvinage, 1992). The numbers 1-5 correspond to the five categories of loudness from 'very soft' to 'very loud'. In each panel, the dashed line indicates typical results for subjects with normal hearing. The four panels at the top show results for a subject with marked loudness recruitment; all of the curves have steep slopes, and at high levels the loudness reaches or even exceeds that which would occur in a normal ear. The bottom four panels show results for a subject with little or no loudness recruitment. The curves are shifted down vertically relative to those for normally hearing subjects, but the slopes are almost normal. This pattern of results is common in cases of conductive hearing loss, but rare in cases of cochlear damage. Most subjects with cochlear hearing loss give results between these two extremes, a typical example being shown in the middle four panels.

A third way of measuring loudness recruitment is to use magnitude estimation or magnitude production, as described earlier for normally hearing subjects (Stevens, 1957). These techniques give a similar pattern of results to the categorical loudness scaling procedures; almost all subjects with cochlear damage show some degree of loudness recruitment, as indicated by the fact that the rate of growth of loudness with increasing sound level is greater than normal (Hellman and Meiselman, 1990, 1993).

On average, the steepness of loudness growth curves increases with increasing absolute threshold at the test frequency (Miskolczy-Fodor, 1960; Glasberg and Moore, 1989; Hellman and Meiselman, 1990, 1993; Kiessling, Steffens and Wagner, 1993). This is consistent with the idea that threshold elevation and loudness recruitment are both linked to the loss of the active mechanism in the cochlea. However, there can be considerable individual differences in the rate of loudness growth for a given degree of hearing loss; examples are given later in this chapter (see Figure 4.10). These individual differences probably arise largely from differing relative amounts of OHC and IHC damage, as will be explained.

When the absolute threshold is high, the dynamic range can be very small indeed. For example, for subject S2 in Figure 4.4, a 75 dB tone at 4000 Hz was judged 'very soft', whereas a 100 dB tone was judged 'very loud', indicating a dynamic range of only about 25 dB. In some cases, the dynamic range can be as small as 10 dB.

The measures of loudness recruitment described above were all obtained with bursts of sound whose amplitude envelope was constant during their presentation time. However, loudness recruitment also influences the perception of sounds whose amplitude fluctuates from moment to moment. Examples of such sounds include speech and music. For speech, the most prominent fluctuations occur at rates from about 0.5 Hz up to 32 Hz (Steeneken and Houtgast, 1980). For sounds that are amplitude modulated at rates up to 32 Hz, recruitment results in a magnification of the perceived amount of fluctuation (Moore, Wojtczak and Vickers, 1996); the sound appears to 'wobble' more than it would for a normally hearing person. The magnification of the perceived fluctuation is roughly independent of the modulation rate over the range 4 to 32 Hz. The fact that the magnification does not decrease with increasing modulation frequency is consistent with the idea that recruitment results mainly from the loss of fast-acting compression on the BM. This idea is elaborated later in this chapter.

A model of normal loudness perception

To understand how loudness recruitment occurs, it is helpful to consider models of loudness perception. Most models of loudness are based on concepts proposed by Fletcher and Munson (1937) and by Zwicker (1958; Zwicker and Scharf, 1965). Figure 4.5 shows a block diagram of a model of loudness perception developed by Moore and Glasberg (1996), but based on these earlier models. The first two stages are fixed filters to account for the transmission of sound through the outer and middle ear (see Chapter 1, Figures 1.3 and 1.4). The next stage is the calculation of an excitation pattern for the sound under consideration; the concept of the excitation pattern was described in Chapter 3. This pattern can be thought of as representing the distribution of excitation at different points along the BM. The excitation patterns are calculated from auditory filter shapes, as described in Chapter 3. The frequency scale of the excitation pattern is translated to a scale that is related to how the sound is represented in the auditory system. This is the ERB scale described in Chapter 3; each ERB corresponds roughly to a constant distance of about 0.89 mm along the BM. Panel A of Figure 4.6 shows excitation patterns for a 1000 Hz sinusoid with a level ranging from 20 to 100 dB SPL in 10 dB steps. The patterns are plotted on an ERB scale. The corresponding frequency is shown at the top.

The next stage is a transformation from excitation level to *specific loudness, N,* which is the loudness per ERB. The specific loudness is a

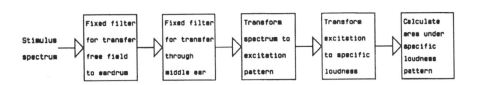

Figure 4.5: A block diagram of the loudness model developed by Moore and Glasberg (1996).

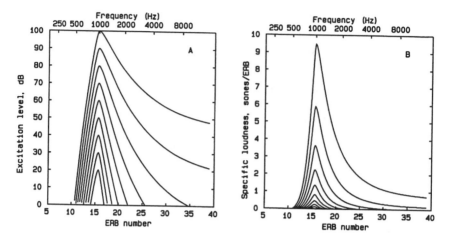

Figure 4.6: Panel A shows excitation patterns for a 1000 Hz sinusoid with a level ranging from 20 to 100 dB SPL in 10-dB steps. The patterns are plotted on an ERB scale. The corresponding frequency is shown at the top. Panel B shows the corresponding specific loudness patterns, calculated using the model of Moore and Glasberg (1996).

kind of loudness density. It represents the loudness that would be evoked by the excitation within a 0.89 mm range on the BM if it were possible to present that excitation alone (without any excitation at adjacent regions on the BM). The relationship between excitation and N is specified with the excitation expressed in linear power units, E, rather than excitation level in dB, L_E. The relationship between E and L_E is:

$$L_E = 10\log_{10}(E/E_0)$$

(4.2)

where E_0 is the peak excitation produced by a sound at 0 dB SPL. The specific loudness is related to the excitation at a given centre frequency by the following equations:

$$N = C[(E_{SIG}/E_0)^\alpha - (E_{THRQ}/E_0)^\alpha] \text{ for } E_{SIG} > E_{THRQ}$$

(4.3)

$$N = 0 \text{ for } E_{SIG} < E_{THRQ}$$

(4.4)

where E_{SIG} is the excitation produced by the stimulus, E_{THRQ} is the excitation at absolute threshold at that centre frequency, and C and α are constants. The value of α is less than one (α is approximately equal to

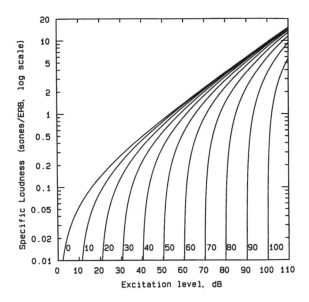

Figure 4.7: Functions showing the transformation from excitation level to specific loudness, N, for a series of values of the excitation level at absolute threshold, L_{ETHRQ}; the value for each curve (in decibels) is plotted next to that curve. The value of N is plotted on a log scale as a function of excitation level in decibels (also a log scale).

0.2), so equation 4.3 defines a *compressive* relationship between excitation and specific loudness. For example, when E_{SIG} is much greater than the threshold value, if E_{SIG} is increased by a factor of 10, N increases by a factor of only 1.58. However, the function becomes steeper when E_{SIG} approaches E_{THRQ}. When E_{SIG} is less than E_{THRQ}, the specific loudness is zero, as indicated by equation 4.4.

The function defined by equation 4.3 is plotted in Figure 4.7 for a series of values of the excitation level at absolute threshold $\{L_{ETHRQ} = 10\log_{10}(E_{THRQ}/E_0)\}$. For normally hearing people, the values of L_{ETHRQ} are always small, except at very low frequencies. However, for hearing-impaired people, the values of L_{ETHRQ} may be higher, as described in the next section. In Figure 4.7, the value of N is plotted on a logarithmic scale as a function of excitation level in decibels (also a log scale). At high excitation levels, the curves show an asymptotic slope corresponding to the value of the constant α. However, the steepness of the initial part of the curves depends on the value of L_{ETHRQ}; the higher L_{ETHRQ}, the steeper are the curves.

The compressive non-linearity in the model can be thought of as representing the overall effects of the transformation from the physical stimulus to neural activity. At least two non-linearities contribute to this overall effect: the compressive nonlinearity of the BM input-output function, and the non-linear transformation from BM velocity or amplitude to neural activity (Yates, 1990); see Figure 1.15.

The model is unrealistic in the sense that the filtering on the BM and the non-linear input-output function on the BM are not two separate processes; it is almost certainly incorrect to represent them as two sequential stages in the model. Nevertheless, the end result in the model is probably similar to what would be obtained in a more realistic model of BM responses, such as proposed by Giguère and Woodland (1994).

If the specific loudness is plotted as a function of frequency or number of ERBs, the resulting pattern is called a *specific loudness pattern*. Specific loudness patterns for a 1000 Hz sinusoid with a level ranging from 20 to 100 dB SPL are shown in panel B of Figure 4.6. The overall loudness of a given sound, in sones, is assumed to be equal to the sum of the loudness in each ERB. This is equal to the total area under the specific loudness pattern plotted as N versus ERB. Thus, the loudness of any sound, including a single sinusoid, is assumed to depend partly on the spread of excitation along the BM.

A model of loudness perception applied to cochlear hearing loss

Introduction

The perception of loudness may be affected by at least four changes that occur with cochlear hearing loss:

- The elevation in absolute threshold, which may be caused by OHC damage, IHC damage, or a combination of the two (Ryan and Dallos, 1975); see Chapters 1 and 2.
- A reduction in or loss of the compressive nonlinearity in the input-output function of the BM, which is mainly associated with OHC damage; see Chapters 1 and 3.
- Loss of frequency selectivity, which results in broader excitation patterns, which is again associated mainly with OHC damage; see Chapters 1 and 3.
- Complete loss of IHCs or functional neurones at certain places within the cochlea (dead regions); see Chapters 2 and 3.

Individual differences in loudness-growth functions may reflect differences in any or all of these factors. Moore and Glasberg (1997) considered the possible influence of each of these factors and how they could be incorporated into a modified loudness model. Florentine and Zwicker (1979), Leijon (1990), Humes, Jesteadt and Lee (1992) and Florentine, Buus and Hellman (1997) have also described loudness models to account for loudness perception in cases of cochlear hearing loss. However, unlike the model presented below, their models did not attempt to account separately for the effects of OHC and IHC damage. The model of Moore and Glasberg (1997) is described below.

Elevation of absolute threshold

As described in Chapter 2, elevation of absolute threshold due to cochlear damage can occur in two main ways. Firstly, damage to the OHCs can result in reduced BM vibration for a given low sound level. Hence, the sound level has to be increased to give a just-detectable amount of vibration. Secondly, IHC damage can result in reduced efficiency of transduction, so the amount of BM vibration needed to reach threshold is higher than normal. In principle, it is possible to partition the overall hearing loss at a given frequency into a component due to OHC damage and a component due to IHC (and neural) damage:

$$HL_{OHC} + HL_{IHC} = HL_{TOTAL}$$

(4.5)

For example, if the total hearing loss at a given frequency is 60 dB, 40 dB of that loss might be due to OHC damage and 20 dB to IHC damage. The maximum gain of the active mechanism is usually estimated to be about 65 dB at high frequencies and somewhat less at low frequencies (Yates, 1995). In the model, it is assumed that HL_{OHC} cannot be greater than 65 dB for CFs of 2 kHz and above and 55 dB for CFs below that. Any loss greater than this must reflect a mixture of OHC loss and IHC loss. Hearing losses less than this may also reflect a mixture of OHC loss and IHC loss.

The value of HL_{TOTAL} at a given frequency can be measured directly (it simply corresponds to the audiometric threshold in dB HL). In the model, it is specified at the standard audiometric frequencies of 125, 250, 500, 1000, 2000, 4000, 6000 and 8000 Hz. Linear interpolation is used to calculate values at intermediate frequencies. However, the values of HL_{OHC} and HL_{IHC} can only be estimated indirectly. Of course, once HL_{OHC} is estimated, then HL_{IHC} can also be estimated using equation 4.5. Moore and Glasberg (1997) estimated the values of HL_{OHC} at each audiometric frequency from measurements of the rate of growth of loudness with sound level. More details are given below.

Reduced compressive non-linearity

As described earlier, the function relating specific loudness to excitation automatically steepens as the value of the excitation level at absolute threshold (L_{ETHRQ}) increases (see Figure 4.7). Increasing L_{ETHRQ} may be an appropriate way to model the consequences of pure OHC loss, as OHC loss is accompanied both by reduced sensitivity and by steeper input-output functions on the BM, and the two are closely coupled. In an ear where the damage is confined largely to the OHCs, with IHCs intact, the transformation from BM velocity or amplitude to neural activity probably remains largely normal.

In an ear with 'pure' IHC damage (which is probably rare), the steepness of the input-output functions on the BM may be nearly normal. In such a case, it would be inappropriate to model the loss simply by an increase in the absolute threshold as this would lead to a steepening of the function relating specific loudness to excitation. The loss due to IHC damage is modelled, following Launer (1995; Launer, Hohmann and Kollmeier, 1997), by a simple attenuation of the excitation level at the frequency in question. For example, if the value of HL_{IHC} is 30 dB, then the excitation level is reduced by 30 dB. The loss due to OHC damage is modelled by raising the excitation level required to reach absolute threshold, L_{ETHRQ}. The value of L_{ETHRQ} is set to be greater than the normal value by the amount HL_{OHC}. For example, if HL_{OHC} is 40 dB, then L_{ETHRQ} is set to a value 40 dB greater than normal. Thus, the component of the loss associated with OHC damage automatically leads to a steepening of the function relating specific loudness to excitation.

Reduced frequency selectivity

Frequency selectivity is usually reduced in cases of cochlear hearing loss; see Chapter 3. For a sinusoidal stimulus, this leads to an excitation pattern, which is broader in an impaired ear than in a normal ear. Moore and Glasberg (1997) developed a series of equations that described empirically how the sharpness of the auditory filters varied with sound level and with hearing loss. The degree of broadening with hearing loss was assumed to depend specifically on HL_{OHC} rather than on HL_{TOTAL}. Figure 4.8 shows excitation patterns calculated from filter shapes based on these equations, for flat hearing losses of 40 dB and 60 dB. For the purpose of calculating these curves, the values of HL_{OHC} were assumed to be 32 and 48 dB, respectively, i.e. the value of HL_{OHC} was assumed to be 80% of HL_{TOTAL}. The patterns were calculated for 1 kHz tones with levels from 20 to 100 dB SPL and they are plotted on an ERB scale, with the corresponding frequency shown at the top. Notice that the patterns become broader with increasing hearing loss, but also the patterns change less in shape with increasing hearing loss. The dashed lines indicate the peak excitation levels that would be produced by tones at absolute threshold. Excitation falling below these lines would be inaudible. The curves below the dashed lines have been plotted only to show more clearly the changes in shape with level.

Estimating the values of HL_{OHC}

The rate of growth of loudness with increasing sound level for a sinusoid with a specific frequency depends mainly on two factors: the steepness of the function relating specific loudness to excitation level at that centre frequency (see Figure 4.7), and the broadness of the excitation pattern evoked by the sound (see Figure 4.8). Both of the factors are assumed to be linked to the value of HL_{OHC} at that frequency; as HL_{OHC} becomes larger, specific loudness grows more steeply with excitation level, and excitation patterns become broader. Hence, the steepness of the loudness-growth function should be closely related to the value of HL_{OHC}; the greater the value of HL_{OHC}, the steeper should be the loudness-growth function. The value of HL_{OHC} at a given frequency can be estimated from the steepness of the loudness-growth function at that frequency.

Figure 4.9 illustrates the effect of varying the parameter HL_{OHC} for a hypothetical person with a flat hearing loss of 60 dB at all frequencies in one ear, the other ear having completely normal audiometric thresholds. The figure shows the predicted sound levels required to match the loudness of a 1 kHz sinusoid between the two ears. To generate these predictions, the loudness was calculated as a function of level for each ear separately, and the loudness functions were used to calculate the levels giving equal loudness in the two ears.

The slopes of the functions vary with HL_{OHC}. They are steep and have a downward curvature for large values of HL_{OHC}, but are shallower and become almost straight for moderate values of HL_{OHC}, and even have a slight upward curvature for very small values of HL_{OHC}. Measured loudness growth functions can vary markedly in slope and in curvature across subjects, even for subjects with similar absolute thresholds (Hellman and Meiselman, 1990; 1993; Kiessling, Steffens and Wagner, 1993; Launer, 1995); some examples are given later in this chapter. The model can account for the range of measured loudness growth functions by varying the parameter HL_{OHC}.

Complete loss of functioning IHCs or neurones (dead regions)

As described in Chapters 2 and 3, sometimes a person with cochlear hearing loss may have a region of the cochlea where there are no functioning IHCs and/or neurones. Evidence for such dead regions can be obtained in several ways:

• From masking experiments, as described in Chapter 3; see Figure 3.14.
• From the values of absolute thresholds. When the absolute threshold is high (greater than about 80 dB HL) at a given frequency, but lower at adjacent frequencies, there is a reasonable probability of a dead region corresponding to that frequency. This is especially true when

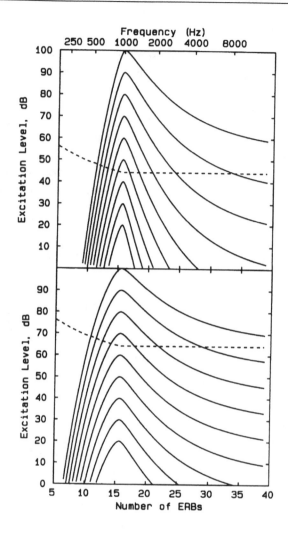

Figure 4.8: Excitation patterns calculated for hypothetical hearing-impaired people with flat losses of 40 dB (upper panel) or 60 dB (lower panel). The value of HL_{OHC} was assumed to be 32 dB for the former and 48 dB for the latter. Patterns are shown for 1-kHz tones with levels ranging from 20 to 100 dB SPL. The dashed lines indicate the peak excitation levels that would be produced by tones at absolute threshold. Excitation falling below these lines would be inaudible.

the absolute threshold changes rather abruptly (by about 30 dB or more) between two adjacent (half-octave spaced) audiometric frequencies (Hellman, 1994; Florentine, Buus and Hellman, 1997).

- From subjective reports. When there are no high-frequency IHCs or neurones, high-frequency tones are reported to sound noise-like (Moore, Laurence and Wright, 1985; Murray and Byrne, 1986) or distorted (Villchur, 1973).

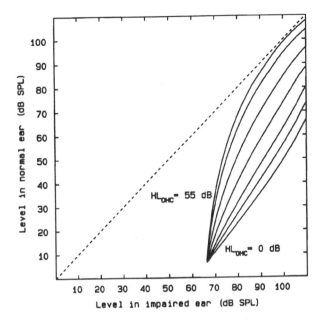

Figure 4.9: The effect on predicted loudness-matching functions of changing the value of the parameter HL_{OHC} for a hypothetical subject with a flat hearing loss of 60 dB in one ear and normal hearing in the other ear. The value of HL_{OHC} was 0, 10, 20, 30, 40, 50 or 55 dB. The diagonal dotted line indicates equal levels in the two ears.

The effects of a dead region are included in the loudness model by setting the excitation to a very low value (effectively zero) over the frequency range corresponding to the region assumed to be dead. This has the effect that the specific loudness evoked from that region is zero.

Using the model to account for loudness recruitment

The model can be used to evaluate the relative importance of the factors described above. Indeed, it is possible within the model to include or remove each factor; for example, frequency selectivity can be set to 'normal' values instead of having the values appropriate for the hearing loss. Analyses of this type indicate that *the main cause of loudness recruitment is the steeper input-output function on the BM.* Reduced frequency selectivity (greater spread of excitation) also plays some role, as suggested by Kiang, Moxon and Levine (1970) and by Evans (1975), but that role is not very great. The minor role of greater-than-normal spread of excitation in producing loudness recruitment is also suggested by experimental studies in which noise was used to mask the excitation at CFs remote from the signal frequency (Hellman, 1978; Moore, Glasberg, Hess et al., 1985; Hellman and Meiselman, 1986; Zeng and

Turner, 1991); the noise had little effect on the rate of loudness growth measured for hearing-impaired subjects.

The solid lines in Figure 4.3, which was presented earlier in this chapter, show predictions of the model. The data were obtained using a subject with a hearing loss of 71 dB at 4000 Hz and 100 dB at 8000 Hz. Masking data suggested that she had a dead region at high frequencies, and to model her data it was assumed that the dead region extended from 4000 to 20 000 Hz. Thus, for a signal at 4000 Hz, the growth of loudness with increasing level in the impaired ear was predicted to depend mainly on the downward spread of excitation. In that case, the broadening of the auditory filters plays a significant role. Note that the predicted growth of loudness would be steeper if no dead region were assumed (a similar point was made by Florentine, Buus and Hellman, 1997). Generally, the model fits the data rather well. It can account for the near-complete recruitment at 250 and 500 Hz, and for the partial recruitment at 2000 and 4000 Hz.

The circles in Figure 4.10 show the loudness matching data presented by Miskolczy-Fodor (1960). He placed subjects into four groups, according to their hearing loss at the test frequency; 40, 50, 60 or 80 dB loss. All subjects were classified as having cochlear hearing loss. There is considerable scatter across subjects with the same hearing loss, and the scatter is larger for the greater hearing losses. Probably, a large part of the individual variability can be explained in terms of differing patterns and degrees of OHC and IHC damage. To predict the results using the model it was assumed that the hearing losses were 'flat' and that there were no dead regions. A 1 kHz sinusoid was used as the input to the model, although the data were actually obtained for several different signal frequencies. Unfortunately, Miskolczy-Fodor does not provide any information that would allow the results to be analysed separately for different frequencies. The solid lines in Figure 4.10 show the predictions of the model assuming that the value of HL_{OHC} was 70% of HL_{TOTAL}, up to the maximum possible values of HL_{OHC} (55 dB at low frequencies and 65 dB at high frequencies). These lines lie well within the range of the data points for hearing losses of 50, 60 and 80 dB, but tend to lie towards the low end of the range of data points for hearing losses of 40 dB.

The dotted lines show predictions based on the assumption that HL_{OHC} was 80% of HL_{TOTAL}, again up to the maximum possible values. The dotted line fits the data slightly better for hearing losses of 40 dB, but fits slightly less well for losses of 50 dB and 60 dB. The prediction for losses of 80 dB is almost the same for the two cases, since HL_{OHC} was limited to 55 dB for frequencies up to 1 kHz.

The upper dashed line shows the predictions of the model assuming that HL_{OHC} had the maximum possible values at all frequencies. Except for the group of subjects with 80 dB loss, very few of the observed data

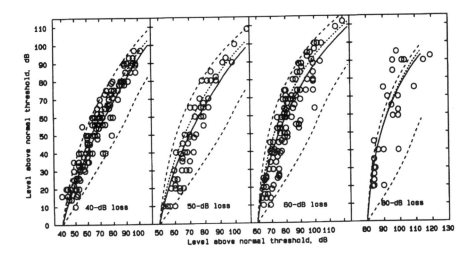

Figure 4.10: The circles show loudness-matching data of Miskolczy-Fodor (1960), for 300 subjects categorised according to the degree of hearing loss in their impaired ears. The solid curves are predictions of the model assuming that the hearing losses were flat, and that $HL_{OHC} = 0.7HL_{TOTAL}$, while the dotted curves are predictions assuming that $HL_{OHC} = 0.8HL_{TOTAL}$. The upper dashed lines are predictions assuming that HL_{OHC} had the maximum possible values, while the lower dashed lines are predictions assuming that HL_{OHC} was zero.

points lie above the dashed line, indicating that the model is able to predict the steepest observed loudness matching functions. The lower dashed line shows the loudness matching functions predicted assuming that HL_{OHC} was zero. Few of the points come close to this line, suggesting that it is rare to have a hearing loss due to IHC damage without some associated OHC damage.

The great majority of data points lie within the range bounded by the two dashed curves, indicating that the model has the flexibility to deal with the range of individual differences encountered. The only exception is for the group with 80 dB losses. However, it should be remembered that the data include results for signal frequencies above 1 kHz, while the predictions were generated using a 1 kHz signal. The use of a higher signal frequency as input to the model would allow steeper loudness-matching functions to be predicted, as HL_{OHC} is permitted to be greater at frequencies of 2 kHz and above. It appears that 'typical' loudness matching functions can be predicted assuming that HL_{OHC} is 80% of HL_{TOTAL} for mild (40 dB) losses, and 70% of HL_{TOTAL} for moderate to severe (50-80 dB) losses.

In summary, the loudness model developed by Moore and Glasberg (1997) can account for the rapid growth of loudness typically associated with cochlear hearing loss. By varying the parameter HL_{OHC}, and taking into account dead regions, the model can also account for individual variability in loudness growth functions. According to the model, the main cause of loudness recruitment is reduced compressive non-linearity of the input-output function on the BM, although reduced frequency selectivity (broader excitation patterns) also plays some role.

Effects of bandwidth on loudness

Normal hearing

In normally hearing subjects, if the bandwidth of a sound is varied keeping the *overall* intensity fixed, the loudness remains constant as long as the bandwidth is less than a certain value, called the critical bandwidth (CB) for loudness. If the bandwidth is increased beyond the CB, the loudness increases (Zwicker, Flottorp and Stevens, 1957). In other words, for a fixed overall intensity, a sound appears louder when its spectrum covers a wide frequency range than when its spectrum covers a narrow frequency range. The reason for this effect can be understood by considering how specific loudness patterns change with bandwidth. With increasing bandwidth, up to the CB, the specific loudness patterns become lower at their tips, but broader; the decrease in area around the tip is almost exactly cancelled by the increase on the skirts, so that the total area remains almost constant (Moore and Glasberg, 1986d; Moore, Glasberg and Baer, 1997). When the bandwidth is increased beyond the CB, the increase on the skirts is greater than the decrease around the tip, and the total area, and hence the predicted loudness, increases. Since the increase depends on the summation of specific loudness at different CFs, the increase in loudness is often described as *loudness summation*.

Impaired hearing

Several studies have shown that loudness summation is reduced in people with cochlear hearing loss; the increase in loudness with increasing bandwidth is less than occurs in normally hearing people (Scharf and Hellman, 1966; Bonding, 1979a; Florentine and Zwicker, 1979; Bonding and Elberling, 1980). Often, the experiments have involved comparisons of loudness between narrow-band noises and broad-band noises. Typically, one sound, the reference sound, is fixed in level, and the other sound, the comparison sound, is adjusted in level to achieve equal loudness. The two sounds are alternated. For normally hearing subjects, the level of the sound with the greater bandwidth is usually lower than that of the sound with the narrower bandwidth, at the point of equal loudness. The extent of this level difference, ΔL, varies with overall level, being greatest at moderate sound levels (Zwicker,

Flottorp and Stevens, 1957; Zwicker and Scharf, 1965; Bonding, 1979a; Bonding and Elberling, 1980; Zwicker and Fastl, 1990). For hearing-impaired subjects, the value of ΔL is usually markedly smaller than normal.

Figure 4.11 shows an example of results of this type, obtained by Florentine and Zwicker (1979). They measured the value of ΔL needed for equal loudness of a 709 Hz wide noise and a 5909 Hz wide noise, both geometrically centred at 4000 Hz, using normally hearing subjects and subjects with noise-induced hearing loss. The absolute thresholds of the latter were about 45 dB higher than normal at 4000 Hz. The value of ΔL is plotted as a function of the level of the narrower band of noise. The difference varies somewhat with level, and is larger for the normally hearing subjects (squares) than for the hearing-impaired subjects (circles). Error bars indicate inter-quartile ranges.

To predict the results using the loudness model, the value of HL_{OHC} was assumed to be either 50% or 80% of HL_{TOTAL}. The predictions for the normal subjects (solid line) have the right form, but slightly underestimate the values of ΔL for sound levels in the range 40-70 dB SPL, and

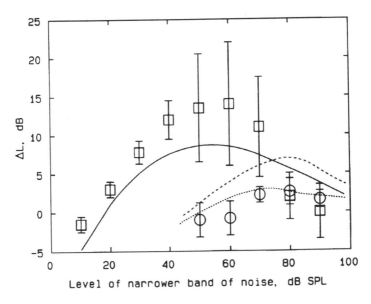

Figure 4.11: The symbols show data of Florentine and Zwicker (1979), showing differences in overall level, ΔL, between a 709 Hz wide noise and a 5909 Hz wide noise required for equal loudness. Both noises were geometrically centred at 4000 Hz. Results are shown for normally hearing subjects (squares), and subjects with noise-induced hearing losses of about 45 dB at 4 kHz (circles). Error bars indicate inter-quartile ranges. Predictions of the model are shown for normally hearing subjects (solid line), and hearing-impaired subjects with $HL_{OHC} = 0.8HL_{TOTAL}$ (dashed line) and $HL_{OHC} = 0.5HL_{TOTAL}$ (dotted line).

overestimate the values of ΔL at 80 and 90 dB. The predictions of the model are in line with other data in the literature, which show slightly less loudness summation than in Figure 4.11 at medium levels and slightly more at higher levels (Zwicker, Flottorp and Stevens, 1957; Zwicker and Fastl, 1990). The predictions for the hearing-impaired subjects with HL_{OHC} equal to 80% of HL_{TOTAL} (dashed line) fall above the obtained values of ΔL, while the predictions for HL_{OHC} equal to 50% of HL_{TOTAL} (dotted line) are accurate both in absolute value and in the form of the results.

At low sensation levels, the values of ΔL are slightly negative for both normally hearing and hearing-impaired subjects. This effect is correctly predicted by the model. It can be described by saying that when the bandwidth of a low-level noise is increased, keeping the overall level constant, the loudness decreases. It occurs for the following reason. At low SLs, specific loudness decreases very rapidly with decreasing excitation level (see Figure 4.7). As the bandwidth is increased, keeping overall intensity constant, the excitation spreads over a wider range of CFs, but the excitation in the central part of the excitation pattern decreases. This leads to a large decrease in specific loudness; indeed the excitation may fall below the threshold value at some CFs, giving zero specific loudness. The decrease in the central part of the specific loudness pattern more than offsets the increase at the edges, so overall loudness decreases.

In summary, loudness summation is typically reduced in people with cochlear hearing loss. In contrast to what happens with normally hearing people, the loudness of a sound of fixed intensity does not usually increase markedly with increasing bandwidth beyond the CB. It is likely that the reduced loudness summation observed in people with cochlear hearing loss depends both on loss of the compressive non-linearity on the BM (which is the main cause of loudness recruitment) and on reduced frequency selectivity.

Effect of cochlear hearing loss on intensity resolution

As described earlier, the ability to detect changes in intensity, or to compare the intensity of two separate sounds, is usually assumed to be based on the loudness sensations evoked by the sounds. In persons with cochlear hearing loss, a given change in intensity usually results in a larger-than-normal change in loudness. Hence, it might be expected that intensity discrimination would be better than normal. However, this expectation is based on the assumption that the just-detectable change in loudness is unaffected by the cochlear damage, and this assumption may not be valid.

Following early evidence that loudness recruitment was specific to cochlear damage (Dix, Hallpike and Hood, 1948), there were many studies exploring the possibility that better-than-normal intensity discrimination could be used as an indirect measure of loudness recruitment and hence as an indicator of cochlear hearing loss (Lüscher and Zwislocki, 1949). These studies led to the Short Increment Sensitivity Index (SISI) test (Jerger, Shedd and Harford, 1959; Jerger, 1962), reviewed by Buus, Florentine and Redden (1982a; 1982b). This test measures the ability to detect brief (200 ms) 1 dB increments in level of a continuous tone presented at 20 dB SL. Typically, cochlear hearing loss leads to an *improvement* in the ability to detect the changes in level.

However, intensity resolution is not always better than normal in persons with cochlear hearing loss. The results depend on the level of testing and on the pattern of hearing loss of the subject. Typically, people with cochlear hearing loss show better intensity discrimination than normal when the comparison is made at equal, low, sensation levels, e.g. 10 or 20 dB SL. However, intensity discrimination is usually about the same as normal (but is sometimes worse than normal) when the comparison is made at equal, high, sound pressure levels. This is true for increment detection (Buus, Florentine and Redden, 1982a; 1982b), modulation detection (Glasberg and Moore, 1989; Turner, Zwislocki and Filion, 1989) and pulsed-tones intensity discrimination (Glasberg and Moore, 1989; Turner, Zwislocki and Filion, 1989; Schroder, Viemeister and Nelson, 1994).

It is not entirely clear why loudness recruitment only leads to better-than-normal intensity discrimination at low SLs. It is possible that the variability in the loudness sensation increases with increases in the slope of the loudness growth function. A steeper loudness growth function in an ear with recruitment leads to a larger change in average loudness for a given change in intensity, but this does not necessarily lead to improved intensity discrimination because the variability of the loudness sensation increases by about the same factor (Zwislocki and Jordan, 1986).

Perceptual consequences of altered loudness perception

Consequences of loudness recruitment and reduced dynamic range

The most prominent change in loudness perception associated with cochlear hearing loss is loudness recruitment and reduced dynamic range. For sounds with inherent amplitude fluctuations, such as speech or music, this results in an exaggeration of the perceived dynamic qualities. The sound appears to fluctuate more in loudness than it would for a normally hearing person. When listening to speech, the loudness differences between consonants and vowels may be greater than normal. When listening to music, the *forte* passages may be perceived at almost normal loudness, but the *piano* passages may be inaudible. Simulations of these effects may be found on the compact disc 'Audio demonstrations to accompany perceptual consequences of cochlear damage' (Moore, 1997a). One might regard the normal auditory system as containing a built-in fast-acting automatic gain control system; this system is lacking or reduced in effectiveness in people with cochlear hearing loss. The perception of exaggerated loudness changes can play a role in several other aspects of auditory perception. The role in temporal processing is reviewed in Chapter 5, and the role in speech perception is reviewed in Chapter 8.

The reduction in dynamic range has practical implications for the design and use of hearing aids. Many hearing aids act primarily as linear amplifiers, except that they have some form of output limiting or clipping to prevent the user from being exposed to excessively loud sounds. The limiting/clipping is usually associated with unpleasant sounding distortion (Crain and van Tasell, 1994; see also Chapter 1, Figure 1.1) so, in practice, users set the volume control so as to avoid limiting/clipping in most everyday situations. Thus, the aid acts as a linear amplifier most of the time; the amplification is independent of the input sound level.

When linear amplification is used, and the volume control is set so that the more intense sounds are at a comfortable loudness, then some weak sounds will be inaudible, owing to the reduced dynamic range. If the volume control is set to make the weak sounds audible, then intense sounds will be unpleasantly loud (or will sound distorted because of limiting/clipping). In practice, the amount of amplification selected for use in everyday life is often rather small (Leijon, 1989), meaning that many weak environmental and speech sounds would be inaudible. Users of linear hearing aids probably select low gains for use in everyday life partly to be sure of avoiding unpleasantly loud sounds, and partly to avoid the distorted sound associated with limiting/clipping.

These problems can be largely overcome by the use of hearing aids incorporating *automatic volume control* or *compression;* such aids are described in more detail in Chapter 9.

Perceptual consequences of reduced loudness summation

As described earlier, a narrow-band sound and a broad-band sound with the same intensity usually differ considerably in loudness for normally hearing people (the broadband sound being louder), but differ less or not at all in loudness for people with cochlear hearing loss. This means that the relative loudness of complex sounds may differ for normally hearing and hearing-impaired people; sound A might be judged louder than sound B by a normally hearing person, but might be judged as less loud than sound B by a hearing-impaired person. This complicates the fitting of hearing aids, especially hearing aids with multi-band compression (see Chapter 9 for details of such aids).

Perceptual consequences of altered intensity discrimination

As reviewed above, intensity discrimination by people with cochlear hearing loss can be better than normal when the comparison is made at equal SL. However, intensity discrimination is not better than normal and can be worse than normal when the comparison is made at equal SPL. However, even when intensity discrimination is worse than normal, this does not appear to lead to marked problems, since it is rare in everyday life for critical information to be carried by small changes in intensity. Although intensity contrasts can convey information in speech, the contrasts involve rather large changes in intensity, changes that are well above the threshold of detection for both normally hearing and hearing-impaired persons.

Potential problems can arise when hearing aids incorporating fast-acting compression are used; details are given in Chapter 9. Such hearing aids reduce differences in level between sounds. If a large amount of compression is used, then information-bearing intensity contrasts may be reduced to the point where they are difficult for the hearing-impaired person to discriminate. This can lead to impaired speech perception (Plomp, 1994). However, moderate amounts of compression do not seem to have such deleterious effects, and even have beneficial effects by restoring audibility of weak sounds. These issues are discussed further in Chapter 9.

Chapter 5
Temporal Resolution and Temporal Integration

Introduction

All sounds are characterised by pressure variations over time. However, if the intensity of a sound remains constant over time and if its frequency content is also constant over time, the sound is said to be steady; it is heard as an unchanging sound. An example is a sustained tone produced by a musical instrument such as the oboe. A sound such as a broadband white noise (which contains equal energy at all frequencies) is also heard as a steady sound, even though its waveform is not regular but fluctuates rapidly from moment to moment. In the case of the noise, the fluctuations are mostly too rapid to be heard distinctly. Temporal resolution refers to the ability to detect changes over time. Often, it involves detection of changes in the envelope of a sound - for example, the detection of a brief gap in a sound or detection of amplitude modulation of a sound. Forward and backward masking may also be regarded as situations involving temporal resolution (Moore, Glasberg, Plack et al., 1988). If a brief signal is presented close in time to a masker, then temporal resolution may be insufficient to separate the signal and masker, and masking will occur. One way to conceptualise this process is to assume that the representation of sounds at higher levels in the auditory system takes some time to build up and decay. For example, one might explain forward masking by assuming that, when the masker is turned off, the internal representation of the masker takes some time to decay. If a brief signal is presented during this decay time, then forward masking may occur.

It is important to distinguish between temporal resolution (or acuity) and temporal integration (or summation). The latter refers to the ability of the auditory system to add up information over time to enhance the detection or discrimination of stimuli; generally, the longer a sound is, the better it is detected and discriminated. Temporal integration is described in the last part of this chapter.

Many studies have shown that temporal resolution can be adversely affected by cochlear hearing loss. To understand why temporal resolution is affected, it is helpful to use a model of temporal processing in the normal auditory system and to consider how the different stages of the model may be altered by cochlear pathology. That is the approach taken in this chapter.

In characterising temporal resolution in the auditory system, it is important to take account of the filtering that takes place in the peripheral auditory system. The different frequency components in complex sounds are partly resolved on the BM. One can regard the auditory system as having frequency-selective 'channels', each channel being responsive to a limited range of frequencies. Temporal resolution depends on two main processes: analysis of the time pattern occurring within each frequency channel; and comparison of the time patterns across channels. This chapter concentrates on within-channel processes, since there have been few studies of across-channel processing in hearing-impaired subjects.

Modelling within-channel temporal resolution in normal hearing

An example of a model of temporal resolution is illustrated in Figure 5.1. Each stage of the model is discussed below.

Bandpass filtering

There is an initial stage of bandpass filtering, reflecting the action of the auditory filters. For simplicity, only one filter is shown; in reality there is an array of parallel channels, each like that shown in the figure. When a brief signal is passed through a bandpass filter, the filter responds over a longer duration than that of the input signal. Generally, the narrower the filter, the more the output is stretched in time relative to the input. This is illustrated in Figure 5.2, which shows the response of a simulated auditory filter to a brief impulse. The filter was centred at 1000 Hz. The narrowest filter had a bandwidth of 150 Hz (which is slightly greater than the average normal auditory filter bandwidth for a centre frequency

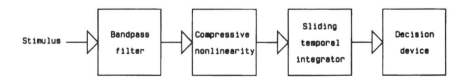

Figure 5.1: A block diagram showing the stages of a model of temporal resolution.

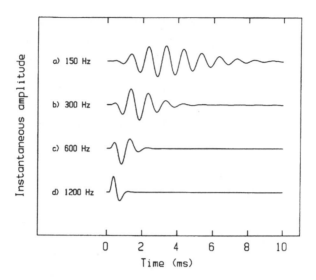

Figure 5.2: The response to a brief impulse of a simulated auditory filter, with a bandwidth of 150 Hz, and filters with bandwidths two times, four times or eight times greater than that value. All filters are centred at 1 kHz. The responses are not drawn to scale. The peak amplitude of the response actually increases as the filter bandwidth increases.

of 1000 Hz) and the other filters had bandwidths two, four and eight times that value. The response, called the impulse response, clearly shortens in time as the filter becomes broader. The auditory filters have bandwidths that decrease progressively with decreasing centre frequency (Glasberg and Moore, 1990) - see Chapter 3. One might expect, therefore, that the auditory filters would play some role in limiting temporal resolution, this effect being greater at low centre frequencies. The evidence relating to this question will be presented later.

Non-linearity

Each filter is followed by a non-linear device. This non-linear device is meant to reflect the operation of several processes that occur in the peripheral auditory system. For example, nerve spikes tend to occur at a specific phase of the stimulating waveform on the BM. An effect resembling this can be achieved by a non-linear process called half-wave rectification; in this process, only the parts of the waveform with a specific polarity (for example, the positive parts) are passed, whereas the parts of the waveform with opposite polarity are set to zero. Another significant non-linearity is the compressive input-output function of the BM - see Chapter 1 and Figure 1.10. In recent models of temporal resolution, the non-linear device includes these two processes, i.e. rectification and a compressive non-linearity, resembling the compressive input-output function on the BM (Oxenham and Moore, 1994, 1997; Moore, Peters and Glasberg, 1996). As noted in Chapters 3 and 4, it is unrealistic to treat the filtering on the BM and the compressive non-linearity as separate stages, but this probably does not seriously undermine the usefulness of the model. A method for determining the characteristics of the non-linearity is described later in this chapter.

The sliding temporal integrator

The output of the non-linear device is fed to a 'smoothing' device, which can be implemented either as a lowpass filter (Viemeister, 1979) or a sliding temporal integrator (Moore, Glasberg, Plack et al., 1988; Plack and Moore, 1990). Usually, the smoothing device is thought of as occurring after the auditory nerve; it is assumed to reflect a relatively central process. The device determines a kind of weighted average of the output of the compressive non-linearity over a certain time interval or 'window'. An example of a weighting function is shown in Figure 5.3. This function is sometimes called the 'shape' of the temporal window. Most weight is given to the output of the non-linear device at times close to the temporal centre of the window, and progressively less weight is given to the output at times farther from the centre. The window itself is assumed to slide in time, so that the output of the temporal integrator is like a weighted running average of the input. This has the effect of smoothing rapid fluctuations while preserving slower ones. When a sound is turned on abruptly, the output of the temporal integrator takes some time to build up. Similarly, when a sound is turned off, the output of the integrator takes some time to decay.

It is often assumed that backward and forward masking depend on the process of build-up and decay. For example, if a brief signal is rapidly followed by a masker (backward masking) the response to the signal may still be building up when the masker occurs. If the masker is sufficiently intense, then its internal effects may 'swamp' those of the signal. Similarly, if a brief signal follows soon after a masker (forward masking), the decaying response to the masker may swamp the response to the signal.

The operation of the sliding temporal integrator is illustrated in Figure 5.4. The panels on the left-hand side show several different signals applied to the input of the integrator. These signals can be thought of as corresponding to the envelopes of audio signals, not the waveforms themselves. The output of the sliding temporal integrator is shown on the right. In response to a brief pulse (panel a), the output builds up and then decays. The build up is more rapid than the decay, because the window shape is asymmetric in time. In fact, the impulse

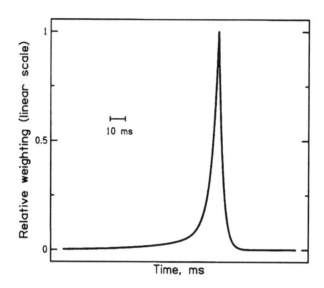

Figure 5.3: The 'shape' of the temporal window. This is a weighting function applied to the output of the non-linear device. It performs a weighted running average of the output of the non-linear device. The shape is plotted with a linear ordinate as a function of time.

response shown in the right-hand part of panel a is simply the window shape played backwards in time. The asymmetry assumed for the window shape makes it possible to account for an asymmetry between forward and backward masking; when the time interval between the masker and the signal is increased, backward masking decreases more rapidly than forward masking (Oxenham and Moore, 1994). In response to an input with a rectangular envelope (panel b), the output builds up, stays at a steady value for some time, and then decays. In response to an input with a temporal gap (panel c), the output shows a build up, a steady part, a dip, another steady part, and then a decay. The dip corresponds to the gap, but it is like a partially filled-in representation of the gap. In response to an input with a slow sinusoidal fluctuation, such as might be produced by an amplitude modulated tone (panel d), the output also shows a sinusoidal modulation; slow fluctuations are preserved at the output of the sliding temporal integrator. In response to an input with a fast sinusoidal fluctuation (panel e), the output shows a much reduced amount of fluctuation; fast fluctuations are attenuated at the output of the sliding temporal integrator.

The decision device

The output of the sliding temporal integrator is fed to a decision device. The decision device may use different 'rules' depending on the task

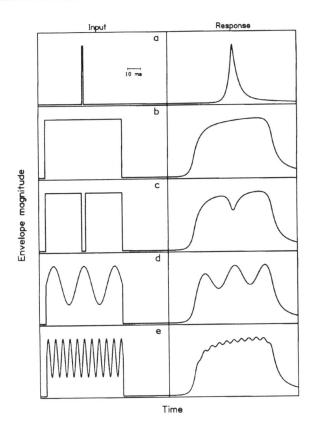

Figure 5.4: Examples of the influence of the sliding temporal integrator on the envelopes of sounds. The panels on the left show inputs to the sliding temporal integrator. The panels on the right show the corresponding outputs.

required. For example, if the task is to detect a brief temporal gap in a signal, the decision device might look for a 'dip' in the output of the temporal integrator (Moore, 1997b). If the task is to detect amplitude modulation of a sound, the device might assess the amount of modulation at the output of the sliding temporal integrator (Viemeister, 1979).

Characterising the non-linear device and the sliding temporal integrator

In the model, the characteristics of the auditory filters are based on auditory filter shapes derived from masking experiments, as described in Chapter 3. However, it is also necessary to define the characteristics of the non-linearity and the sliding temporal integrator. An approach to this problem was described by Oxenham and Moore (1994). They performed an experiment in which they used a noise masker and a brief 6 kHz signal. In one set of conditions the signal was presented after the masker (forward masking). In another set it was presented before the masker (backward masking). In a third set of conditions, the signal was presented between two bursts of the masker; this involves a combination of forward and backward masking. As described earlier, forward and backward masking can be accounted for in terms of the build up and decay processes at the output of the sliding temporal integrator.

An interesting effect is observed in cases when a forward and backward masker are combined. It might be thought that, if two different maskers are equally effective (i.e. each produces the same amount of masking) then the combination of the two maskers would result in a doubling of the signal energy required for threshold (Green and Swets, 1974); this corresponds to an increase in the signal level at threshold of 3 dB. In fact, the signal threshold often increases by more than this. The amount by which signal threshold exceeds the prediction is referred to as 'excess masking'. Combining two equally effective non-simultaneous maskers (one forward and one backward) *consistently* results in excess masking, usually of 7-12 dB at moderate sound levels (Wilson and Carhart, 1971; Cokely and Humes, 1993).

This excess masking can be explained if it is assumed that each stimulus (the forward masker, signal and backward masker) is subjected to a compressive non-linearity before the effects of the stimuli are combined in a linear temporal integrator (Penner, 1980a; Penner and Shiffrin, 1980), as assumed in the model of temporal resolution shown in Figure 5.1. To understand how the compressive non-linearity accounts for excess masking, consider the following. Imagine that two equally effective non-simultaneous maskers (one forward and one backward) are presented together. At the output of the temporal integrator, the decay of response to the forward masker is summed with the build up of response to the backward masker. It is assumed that, at the time when the brief signal produces its own maximum response at the output of the temporal integrator, the effects of the forward and backward masker are equal (as they are equally effective maskers). The integrator itself is a linear device, and so the internal effect evoked by the two maskers is simply double the effect evoked by either alone. Thus, in order to reach threshold, the level of the signal has to be increased relative to the level required for a single masker. In fact, to reach the signal threshold, the *internal* effect of the signal must also be doubled. This requires more than a 3 dB increase in signal threshold because the signal itself is independently compressed.

Oxenham and Moore (1994) showed that their results could be used to separate the effects of the temporal integrator and the compressive non-linearity prior to the integrator. A good fit to their forward and backward masking data was obtained when the stimulus intensity at the output of the simulated auditory filter was raised to a power between 0.25 and 0.35. If, for example, the intensity is raised to the power 0.3, then a tenfold increase in power (corresponding to 10 dB) would be needed to double the internal effect of the signal. Thus, for two equally effective maskers, one forward and one backward, excess masking of 7 dB is predicted.

Oxenham and Moore (1994) also used their data to derive the weighting characteristic or 'shape' of the temporal window (see the schematic illustration in Figure 5.3), following an approach proposed by Moore, Glasberg, Plack and Biswas (1988). However, the derivation is rather complex, and is beyond the scope of this book. The reader is referred to the original publications for details. In fact, the weighting function shown in Figure 5.3 corresponds to that derived by Oxenham and Moore.

In the next section, data on temporal resolution in normally hearing people are presented and interpreted in terms of the model. Then, data on temporal resolution in hearing-impaired people are described and evaluated.

Temporal resolution in normal hearing

The effect of centre frequency on gap detection

As mentioned above, if the auditory filter plays a role in limiting temporal resolution, one would expect temporal resolution to improve with increasing frequency. Several researchers have measured thresholds for detecting a gap in narrow-band sounds (tones or bands of noise) as a function of centre frequency; the duration of the gap is adjusted to find the point where it is just detectable. When a narrow-band sound is turned off and on abruptly to introduce a temporal gap, energy 'splatter' occurs outside the nominal frequency range of the sound; this may be heard as a click or a thud. People can use the click or thud as a cue for detecting the gap. However, it is usually argued that this reflects the use of spectral information rather than temporal information; it depends upon frequency selectivity rather than upon temporal resolution *per se*. Two methods have been used to prevent the splatter being detected. In one, the narrow-band sound is presented in a background sound, usually a broad-band noise, designed to mask the splatter. In the other, the gap is introduced by turning the sound off and on again gradually; this reduces spectral splatter but it prevents the use of very brief gaps.

The pattern of results found for the detection of gaps in bands of noise depends on the bandwidth of the noise, and on how that bandwidth varies with centre frequency. If the *relative* bandwidth is held constant (i.e. the bandwidth is a constant proportion of the centre frequency) then gap thresholds decrease monotonically with increasing centre frequency (Fitzgibbons and Wightman, 1982; Fitzgibbons, 1983;

Shailer and Moore, 1983). This is the effect that would be expected if the auditory filters played a role in limiting gap detection. However, if the absolute bandwidth is held constant, gap thresholds do not vary markedly with centre frequency (Shailer and Moore, 1985; De Filippo and Snell, 1986; Eddins, Hall and Grose, 1992). On the other hand, if the bandwidth is varied keeping either the centre frequency or the upper spectral edge fixed, gap thresholds increase with decreasing noise bandwidth (Shailer and Moore, 1983; 1985; Eddins, Hall and Grose, 1992; Glasberg and Moore, 1992; Snell, Ison and Frisina, 1994; Eddins and Green, 1995).

To understand this pattern of results it is necessary to take account of the fact that noise bands fluctuate randomly in amplitude from moment to moment. The rapidity of these fluctuations increases with increasing bandwidth. The slow fluctuations are easy to hear as changes in loudness from moment to moment. More rapid fluctuations are heard as a kind of 'roughness'. Gap thresholds for noise bands are probably partly limited by the inherent fluctuations in the noise (Shailer and Moore, 1983, 1985; Green, 1985; Eddins and Green, 1995). Randomly occurring dips in the noise are 'confused' with the gap to be detected. The confusion is maximal for dips comparable in duration to the gap. In practice, this means that noise with a narrow bandwidth, and hence slow fluctuations, creates the greatest confusion and gives the largest gap thresholds. The data are consistent with this view.

In summary, gap thresholds measured using bands of noise do not provide clear evidence of an improvement in temporal resolution with centre frequency. However, the gap thresholds are influenced by the inherent fluctuations in the noise. The slow fluctuations associated with small bandwidths lead to large gap thresholds.

Shailer and Moore (1987) studied the ability of subjects to detect a temporal gap in a sinusoid, which has no inherent fluctuations. To mask spectral splatter associated with the introduction of the gap, the sinusoid was presented in a continuous noise with a spectral notch at the frequency of the sinusoid. In one of their conditions, called 'preserved phase', the sinusoid was turned off at a positive-going zero crossing (as the waveform was about to change from negative to positive values) and it started (at the end of the gap) at the phase it would have started at if it had continued without interruption. Thus, it was as if the gap had been 'cut out' from a continuous sinusoid.

Shailer and Moore (1987) found that the gap threshold was roughly constant at about 5 ms for centre frequencies of 400, 1000 and 2000 Hz. Recently, Moore, Peters and Glasberg (1993) measured gap thresholds for centre frequencies of 100, 200, 400, 800, 1000 and 2000 Hz, using a condition similar to the preserved-phase condition of Shailer and Moore. The gap thresholds were almost constant, at 6-8 ms over the frequency range 400-2000 Hz, but increased somewhat at 200 Hz, and

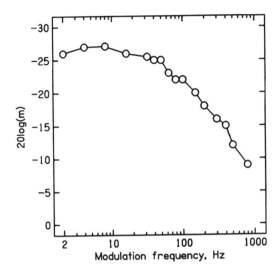

Figure 5.5: A temporal modulation transfer function (TMTF). A broadband white noise was sinusoidally amplitude modulated, and the threshold amount of modulation required for detection was plotted as a function of modulation rate. The amount of modulation is specified as $20\log(m)$, where m is the modulation index (m can vary between 0 and 1; a value of 1 corresponds to 100% modulation). The higher the sensitivity to modulation, the more negative is $20\log(m)$. Adapted from Bacon and Viemeister (1985).

increased markedly, to about 18 ms, at 100 Hz. Individual variability also increased markedly at 100 Hz.

Overall, the results of experiments using narrowband stimuli indicate that temporal resolution does not vary markedly with frequency, except at very low frequencies (200 Hz and below). This suggests in turn that the smoothing produced by the auditory filters does not play a major role, except perhaps at very low frequencies.

Temporal modulation transfer functions

Gap detection experiments give a single number - the gap threshold - to describe temporal resolution. A more general approach is to measure the threshold for detecting changes in the amplitude of a sound as a function of the rapidity of the changes. In the simplest case, white noise is sinusoidally amplitude modulated, and the amount of modulation required to detect the modulation is determined as a function of modulation rate. The function relating the threshold amount of modulation to modulation rate is known as a *temporal modulation transfer function (TMTF)*. Modulation of white noise does not change its long-term magnitude spectrum. An example of the results is shown in Figure 5.5, adapted from Bacon and Viemeister (1985). For low modulation rates, performance is limited by the amplitude resolution of the ear, rather than by temporal resolution. Thus, the threshold is independent of modulation rate for rates up to about 16 Hz. As the rate increases beyond 16 Hz, temporal resolution starts to have an effect; the threshold increases, and for rates above about 1000 Hz the modulation is difficult to detect at all. Thus, sensitivity to amplitude modulation decreases progressively as the rate of modulation increases. The shapes of TMTFs do not vary much with overall sound level, but the ability to detect the modulation does worsen at low sound levels.

The rate of recovery from forward masking

As described in Chapter 3, the threshold for detecting a signal in forward masking decreases progressively with increasing time delay of the signal relative to the end of the masker (see Figure 3.12). As described earlier, the rate of recovery from forward masking is often considered as a measure of temporal resolution; the more rapidly the threshold drops as the time interval between the masker and signal increases, the better is temporal resolution. However, the rate of decrease of threshold (often described as the decay of masking), depends on the masker level; the decay is more rapid for higher masker levels. This effect can be understood by considering the form of the input-output function on the BM, as illustrated schematically in Figure 1.11 (Oxenham and Moore, 1997). To understand this, consider an example based on the following assumptions:

- The threshold for detecting a brief signal is measured for two different times following the end of the masker, t_1 and t_2, where $t_1 < t_2$.
- The internal effect of the masker, E_M, as reflected in the output of the sliding temporal integrator, decays by a factor X over this time; this decay is determined by the shape of the temporal 'window', as illustrated in Figure 5.3.
- X is independent of the overall masker level. This is equivalent to assuming that the temporal integrator is linear.
- The threshold for detecting the brief signal is reached when the peak internal effect evoked by the signal, E_S, is a constant proportion of the internal effect of the masker at the times t_1 and t_2.

To take a specific example, assume that $X = 0.1$; the internal effect of the masker at time t_1 is 10 times the effect at t_2. In order to reach threshold at the two different delay times, the internal effect of the signal, E_S, has to be a factor of 10 greater at time t_1 than at time t_2. Consider now how much the signal intensity has to be changed in order to give a change in its internal effect by a factor of 10. If the masker is intense, then the signal thresholds will be relatively high; the signal levels at threshold might fall in the range 40 to 80 dB SPL, where the input-output function on the BM is highly compressive. Assuming a typical amount of mid-level compression, the signal intensity would have to change by a factor of about 1000 in order to change its internal effect by a factor of 10. This corresponds to a change in signal level of about 30 dB. Thus, when the masker is sufficiently intense to give signal thresholds in the range 40 to 80 dB, the signal threshold would decay by 30 dB when its delay time following the masker was increased from t_1 to t_2.

Consider, now, the situation where the masker is at a lower level, and the signal threshold is correspondingly lower. Say, for example, that thresholds fall in the range 10-30 dB, where the input-output function on the BM approaches linearity. In this case, the intensity of the signal needs to be changed by a factor only a little greater than 10 to change its internal effect by a factor of 10. In other words, the signal threshold would decay by only a little more than 10 dB when its delay time following the masker was increased from t_1 to t_2. Clearly, the decay of masking is much less in this case than in the case where the signal levels were higher.

In practice, the input-output function on the BM becomes progressively more compressive as the input level is increased over the range 15 to about 50 dB. For the masker levels and signal durations typically used in forward masking experiments, signal thresholds fall within this range. Hence, a progressive change in the rate of decay of forward masking would be expected with increasing masker level; that is exactly what is observed (see Figure 3.12). Notice however, that the rate of decay of forward masking is predicted to depend on the *signal* level at short delay times, not the masker level. Of course, higher masker levels usually imply higher signal levels, but a higher signal level at threshold could also be achieved by using a shorter signal, for example.

In summary, the rate of decay of forward masking is greater for higher masker levels. This can be understood by assuming that the sliding temporal integrator is linear, but the non-linearity prior to the temporal integrator is more compressive at medium levels than at low levels; less compression leads to a slower rate of decay of forward masking.

Temporal resolution in people with cochlear damage

Some measures of temporal resolution in subjects with cochlear damage appear to show reduced temporal resolution whereas others do not. Several factors can affect the results, and not all of these are directly connected with temporal processing itself. This section considers several of these factors.

The influence of sound level on gap detection and the rate of decay of forward masking

One important factor influencing measures of temporal resolution is the sound level used. Many measures of temporal resolution show that performance in normally hearing subjects worsens at low sensation levels (SLs) (Plomp, 1964b; Shailer and Moore, 1983; Buus and Florentine, 1985; Fitzgibbons and Gordon-Salant, 1987; Peters, Moore and Glasberg, 1995). This is not unique to temporal resolution; performance on many tasks worsens at low SLs, presumably because less neural information is available, or because of the greater effects of internal noise at low SLs. It is not generally possible to test hearing-impaired subjects at high SLs because they have loudness recruitment; sounds with levels of 90-100 dB SPL appear as loud as they would to a normal listener, as described in Chapter 4. On some measures of temporal resolution, such as the detection of gaps in bands of noise, hearing-impaired subjects appear markedly worse than normal subjects when tested at the same SPLs, but only slightly worse at equal SLs (Fitzgibbons and Wightman, 1982; Tyler, Summerfield, Wood et al., 1982; Glasberg, Moore and Bacon, 1987; Nelson and Thomas, 1997). For example, Nelson and Thomas (1997) measured gap detection thresholds for normally hearing and hearing-impaired listeners using a 650 Hz wide noise centred at about 2850 Hz. At equal SLs, most hearing-impaired listeners showed near-normal performance, especially when the SL was relatively low. However, at equal SPLs, and also when the level was adjusted to give comfortable loudness, the hearing-impaired listeners had markedly larger gap thresholds than normal.

As mentioned earlier, the rate of decay of forward masking is often considered as a measure of temporal resolution; the more rapidly the threshold drops as the time interval between the masker and signal increases, the better is temporal resolution. The effect of overall level for the case of forward masking is illustrated in Figure 5.6, adapted from Glasberg, Moore and Bacon (1987). They tested subjects with cochlear hearing loss in one ear only. The brief sinusoidal signal was presented at various times during and following a noise masker. The masker was presented at a fixed high level to the impaired ear of each subject. In the normal ear it was presented both at the same SPL and at the same SL as for the impaired ear.

It is clear from the figure that the rate of decay of forward masking is much more rapid for the normal ear than for the impaired ear when the comparison is made at equal SPL. However, at equal SL, the difference is much reduced. This effect of level is not unexpected, since the rate of decay of forward masking in normal ears depends strongly on sound level, as described in Chapter 3 and earlier in this chapter. The slow rate of decay of forward masking found in normally hearing people at low sound levels was explained above in terms of the reduced compressive

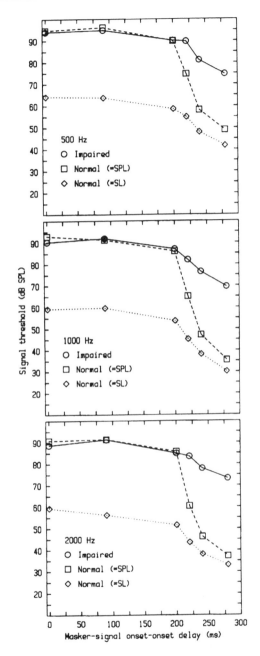

Figure 5.6: The threshold for detection of a brief sinusoidal signal presented at various times during and following a noise masker. The temporal position of the signal is plotted relative to the onset of the masker; times greater than 200 ms correspond to forward masking. Mean results are shown for the normal and impaired ears of five subjects with unilateral cochlear damage. Each panel shows results for a different signal frequency. The masker was presented at a single high level to the impaired ear (84 dB SPL). The masker was presented to the normal ear either at the same SPL or the same SL.

non-linearity of the BM input-output function at low levels. Similarly, the slow rate of decay of forward masking that is commonly found in people with cochlear hearing loss probably depends partly on the loss of compressive non-linearity on the BM. A prediction derived from this explanation is that the rate of decay of forward masking in people with cochlear hearing loss should vary less with level than is the case for normally hearing subjects. Indeed, if the input-output function on the BM is completely linear, then the rate of decay of forward masking should not vary at all with level. Experimental results are consistent with this prediction. In subjects with moderate-to-severe cochlear hearing loss, the rate of decay of forward masking is almost invariant with level (Oxenham and Moore, 1995; 1997).

In summary, two common measures of temporal resolution - gap detection and the rate of decay of forward masking - both show deleterious effects of cochlear hearing loss when the normal and impaired ears are compared at equal SPLs. At equal SLs the discrepancy between normal and impaired hearing is less. Unfortunately, people with cochlear hearing loss usually listen at low SLs, since loudness recruitment makes it impossible to present sounds at high SLs without discomfort occurring. Hence, in practice, cochlear hearing loss leads to poorer temporal resolution than normal.

The influence of audible bandwidth on TMTFs and gap detection

Another important consideration is the bandwidth available to the listeners. This can be clearly seen by consideration of studies measuring the temporal modulation transfer function (TMTF). Several studies measuring TMTFs for broad-band noise carriers showed that hearing-impaired listeners were generally less sensitive to high rates of modulation than normal listeners (Formby, 1982; Lamore, Verweij and Brocaar, 1984; Bacon and Viemeister, 1985). However, this may have been largely a consequence of the fact that high frequencies were inaudible to the impaired listeners (Bacon and Viemeister, 1985); most of the subjects used had greater hearing losses at high frequencies than at low, as is typical in cases of noise-induced hearing loss. When the broad-band noise is lowpass filtered, to simulate the effects of threshold elevation at high frequencies, normally hearing subjects also show a reduced ability to detect modulation at high rates (Bacon and Viemeister, 1985).

Bacon and Gleitman (1992) measured TMTFs for broad-band noise using subjects with relatively flat hearing losses. They found that at equal (high) SPLs performance was similar for hearing-impaired and normally hearing subjects. At equal (low) SLs, the hearing-impaired subjects tended to perform better than the normally hearing subjects. Moore, Shailer and Schooneveldt (1992) controlled for the effects of listening bandwidth by measuring TMTFs for an octave-wide noise band centred at 2 kHz, using subjects with unilateral and bilateral cochlear hearing loss. Over the frequency range covered by the noise, the subjects had reasonably constant thresholds as a function of frequency, both in their normal and their impaired ears. This ensured that there were no differences between subjects or ears in terms of the range of audible frequencies in the noise. To ensure that subjects were not making use of information from frequencies outside the nominal passband of the noise, the modulated carrier was presented in an unmodulated broadband noise background. The results for the subjects with unilateral impairments are shown in Figure 5.7. It can be seen that performance is similar for the normal and impaired ears, both at equal SPL and equal SL, although there is a slight trend for the impaired ears to perform better at equal SL.

Studies of gap detection also show clear effects of the audible frequency range of the stimuli. Thresholds for detecting gaps in broadband noise become progressively larger as the audible frequency range of the stimuli is reduced by increasing high-frequency hearing loss

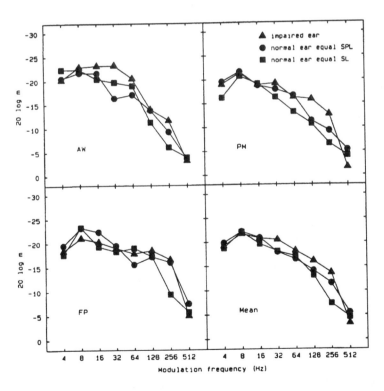

Figure 5.7: Temporal modulation transfer functions (TMTFs) obtained using a bandpass noise carrier for the normal and impaired ears of three subjects with unilateral cochlear hearing loss. Mean results for the three subjects are shown in the bottom right panel.

(Florentine and Buus, 1984; Buus and Florentine, 1985; Salvi and Arehole, 1985).

To summarise the results so far, people with cochlear hearing loss often show reduced temporal resolution as a result of the low SL of the stimuli and/or the reduced audible bandwidth of the stimuli. When these factors are controlled for, hearing-impaired subjects often perform as well as, or even better than normal.

The influence of changes in the compressive non-linearity

For certain types of sounds, the temporal resolution of subjects with cochlear hearing loss seems to be worse than normal, even when the stimuli are well above threshold and when all of the components of the stimuli fall within the audible range. This happens mainly for stimuli that contain slow random fluctuations in amplitude, such as narrow bands of noise. For such stimuli, subjects with cochlear damage often show larger gap detection thresholds than normal (Fitzgibbons and Wightman, 1982; Florentine and Buus, 1984; Buus and Florentine, 1985; Glasberg, Moore and Bacon, 1987). However, gap detection is not usually worse than normal when the stimuli are sinusoids, which do not have inherent amplitude fluctuations (Moore and Glasberg, 1988b; Moore, Glasberg, Donaldson et al., 1989). Glasberg, Moore and Bacon (1987) and Moore and Glasberg (1988b) suggested that the poor gap detection for narrowband noise stimuli might be a consequence of loudness recruitment, the abnormally rapid growth of loudness with increasing intensity that occurs commonly in cases of cochlear hearing loss - see Chapter 4. For a person with recruitment, the inherent amplitude fluctuations in a narrow-band noise would result in larger-than-normal loudness fluctuations from moment to moment (Moore, Wojtczak and Vickers, 1996), so that inherent dips in the noise might be more confusable with the gap to be detected.

This idea can also be expressed in terms of the model of temporal resolution. It seems likely that loudness recruitment is caused primarily by a reduction in the compressive non-linearity found in the normal cochlea - see Chapter 4. When cochlear damage occurs, the cochlea behaves in a more linear way, and the input-output function of the BM becomes less compressive, having a slope closer to unity (on log-log coordinates); see Figure 1.19.

To assess the idea that steeper input-output functions lead to impaired gap detection for stimuli with fluctuating envelopes, Glasberg and Moore (1992) processed the envelopes of narrow bands of noise so as to modify the envelope fluctuations. The envelope was processed by raising it to a power, N. If N is greater than unity, this has the effect of magnifying fluctuations in the envelope, thus simulating the effects of recruitment; higher powers correspond to greater degrees of simulated recruitment. If N is less than unity, fluctuations in the envelope are reduced. This represents a type of signal processing that might be used to compensate for recruitment; it resembles the operation of a fast-acting compressor or automatic gain control (AGC) system; see Chapter 9.

Values of N used were 0.5, 0.66, 1.0, 1.5 and 2. For $N = 1$, the stimuli were the same as unprocessed noise. A value of $N = 2$ simulates the type of recruitment typically found in cases of moderate to severe cochlear damage, where, for example, a 50 dB range of stimulus levels gives the same range of loudness as a 100 dB range of stimulus levels in a normal ear. Several different bandwidths of the noise were used.

Some examples of the envelopes of unprocessed and processed stimuli are shown in Figure 5.8. The envelopes are plotted on a logarithmic (dB) scale, as this seems more relevant to loudness perception than a linear amplitude scale. The bottom panel shows the envelope of a 'normal' noise band ($N = 1$) with a bandwidth of 10 Hz. The top panel shows the effect of squaring the envelope ($N = 2$), whereas the middle panel shows the result of raising the envelope to the power 0.5. The envelope fluctuations are obviously greatest in the top panel and smallest in the middle panel.

To prevent the detection of spectral splatter associated with the gap or with the envelope processing, the stimuli were presented in a

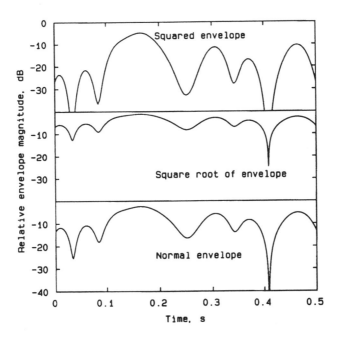

Figure 5.8: Examples of the envelopes of noise bands with $N = 1$ (unprocessed, bottom panel), $N = 0.5$ (middle panel) and $N = 2$ (top panel). The noise bandwidth was 10 Hz. The envelope magnitudes are plotted on a decibel scale.

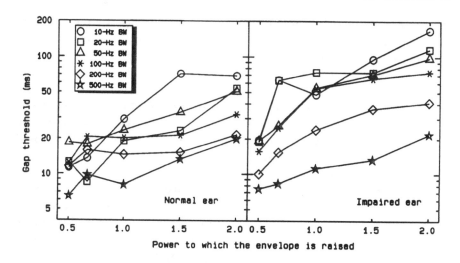

Figure 5.9: Thresholds for detecting a gap in a noise band whose envelope had been processed to enhance or reduce fluctuations. Gap thresholds are plotted as a function of the power to which the envelope was raised, with noise bandwidth as parameter; the higher the power, the greater the fluctuations. Results are shown for each ear of a subject with unilateral cochlear hearing loss.

continuous background noise. The spectrum of the noise was chosen so that it would be as effective as possible in masking the splatter while minimising its overall loudness.

Figure 5.9 shows an example of results obtained using a subject with unilateral hearing loss of cochlear origin. The stimuli were presented at 85 dB SPL, a level which was well above the absolute threshold for both the normal and impaired ears (although the SL was lower in the impaired ear). The results for the normal ear were very similar to those of three normally hearing subjects who were also tested. Gap thresholds increased significantly with decreasing noise bandwidth. This is as expected, since the inherent fluctuations in the noise are slower, and more confusable with the gap to be detected, when the bandwidth is narrow.

For all noise bandwidths, gap thresholds increased as N increased. This effect was particularly marked for the smaller noise bandwidths. There was a significant interaction between bandwidth and N, reflecting the fact that changes in gap threshold with N were greater for small bandwidths. This supports the idea that fluctuations in the noise adversely affect gap detection; greater fluctuations lead to worse performance, especially when the fluctuations are slow.

Gap thresholds were larger for the impaired than for the normal ear. The overall geometric mean gap threshold was 12.8 ms for the normal ear and 27.2 ms for the impaired ear. Performance for the normal ear with $N = 2$ was roughly similar to performance for the impaired ear with unprocessed noise bands ($N = 1$); geometric mean gap thresholds were

26.9 ms for the former and 26.5 ms for the latter. Thus, the simulation of recruitment in the normal ear was sufficient to produce impaired gap detection, comparable to that actually found in the impaired ear.

For both normal-hearing and hearing-impaired subjects, the effects of changing N decreased with increasing noise bandwidth. One reason for this is that slow fluctuations can be followed by the auditory system, whereas rapid fluctuations are smoothed to some extent by the central temporal integration process described earlier. The rapid fluctuations of the wider noise bands are smoothed in this way, thus reducing their influence on gap detection.

The results suggest that, for most subjects with cochlear hearing loss, recruitment, or equivalently, a reduction in the compressive non-linearity on the BM, may provide a sufficient explanation for increased gap thresholds. Thus, it is not usually necessary to assume any abnormality in temporal processing occurring after the cochlea. However, a few subjects show impairments in temporal resolution even using non-fluctuating stimuli (Jesteadt, Bilger, Green et al., 1976; Moore and Glasberg, 1988b; Moore, Glasberg, Donaldson et al., 1989; Plack and Moore, 1991) or noise stimuli with a fairly large bandwidth (Nelson and Thomas, 1997), especially subjects with large hearing losses. It is possible that the subjects showing this impaired resolution had damage to both OHCs (affecting the active process and the compressive non-linearity) and IHCs (reducing the amount of information conveyed in the auditory nerve), or that they had a retrocochlear component to their hearing loss.

For deterministic stimuli that have no inherent random fluctuations, hearing-impaired subjects can actually perform a little better than normally hearing subjects when tested at equal SLs. This applies, for example, to the detection of gaps in sinusoids (Moore and Glasberg, 1988b; Moore, Glasberg, Donaldson et al., 1989).

Temporal integration at threshold

Temporal integration in normally hearing people

It has been known for many years (Exner, 1876) that the absolute threshold for detecting a sound depends upon the duration of the sound. For durations up to a few hundred milliseconds, the intensity required for threshold decreases as the duration increases. For durations exceeding about 500 ms, the sound intensity at threshold is roughly independent of duration. Many workers have investigated the relation between threshold and duration for tone pulses, over a wide range of frequencies and durations. The early work of Hughes (1946) and Garner and Miller (1947) indicated that, over a reasonable range of durations, the ear appears to integrate the intensity of the stimulus over time in the detection of short duration tone bursts. This is often called *temporal integration.* In other words, the threshold corresponds to a constant *energy* rather than a constant intensity. For durations up to about 500 ms, the following formula is approximately true:

$$I \times t = \text{constant}$$

$$(5.1)$$

where I is the threshold intensity for a tone pulse of duration t.

Thresholds as a function of duration are often plotted on dB versus log-duration co-ordinates. When plotted in this way, energy integration is indicated by the data falling on a straight line with a slope of -3 dB per doubling of duration; each time the duration is doubled, the intensity at threshold is halved, corresponding to a 3 dB decrease in level. Although the average data for a group of subjects typically give a slope close to this value, the slopes for individual subjects can differ significantly from -3 dB per doubling. This suggests that it would be unwise to ascribe too much significance to the average slope. It seems very unlikely that the auditory system would actually integrate stimulus energy; it is almost certainly neural activity that is integrated (Zwislocki, 1960; Penner, 1972). It may also be the case that the auditory system does not actually perform an operation analogous to integration. Rather, it may be that the threshold intensity decreases with increasing, duration partly because a longer stimulus provides more chances to detect the stimulus through repeated sampling. This idea is sometimes called 'multiple looks' (Viemeister and Wakefield, 1991).

Temporal integration in people with cochlear hearing loss

For people with cochlear hearing loss, the change in threshold intensity with signal duration is often smaller than it is for normally hearing people. If the thresholds are plotted on dB versus log-duration co-ordinates, the slopes are usually much less in absolute value than the typical value of -3 dB/doubling found for normally hearing people. This is often described as reduced temporal integration (Gengel and Watson, 1971; Pedersen and Elberling, 1973; Elliott, 1975; Chung, 1981; Hall and Fernandes, 1983; Carlyon, Buus and Florentine, 1990). There is a trend for higher absolute thresholds to be associated with flatter slopes. In other words, the greater the hearing loss, the more reduced is the temporal integration.

Explanations for reduced temporal integration in people with cochlear hearing loss

A number of explanations have been advanced to account for reduced temporal integration in people with cochlear hearing loss (Florentine,

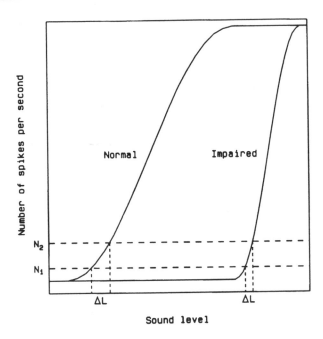

Figure 5.10: Schematic illustration of rate-versus-level functions in single neurones of the auditory nerve for a normal ear (left curve) and an impaired ear (right curve). The horizontal dashed lines indicate the mean firing rate needed for threshold for a long-duration sound (lower line, rate N_1) and a short-duration sound (upper line, rate N_2) on the assumption that threshold corresponds to a fixed total number of spikes.

Fastl and Buus, 1988). One of the most plausible is that it results from a reduction or complete loss of the compressive non-linearity on the BM. This leads to steeper input-output functions on the BM and to steeper rate-versus-level functions in the auditory nerve - see Chapter 1. According to the models of temporal integration proposed by Zwislocki (1960) and by Penner (1972) this will automatically lead to reduced temporal integration. Figure 5.10 illustrates schematically two rate-versus-level functions: the left-hand curve shows a typical function for a low-threshold neurone in a normal auditory system; the right-hand curve shows a typical function for a neurone in an auditory system with OHC damage. The curve is shifted to the right, reflecting a loss of sensitivity, and is steeper, reflecting loss of the compressive non-linearity on the BM. It is assumed that there is some residual compression on the normal BM at levels close to threshold; although the input-output function steepens at low levels (as illustrated in Figure 1.10), it does not become completely linear.

Consider now how steeper rate-versus-level functions can lead to reduced temporal integration. Assume that, to a first approximation, the threshold for detecting a sound requires a fixed number of neural spikes to be evoked by that sound. Assume also, for the sake of simplicity, that the neurones involved in detection at absolute threshold are relatively homogeneous in terms of their rate-versus-level functions. The lower dashed horizontal line in Figure 5.10 indicates the number of neural spikes per second, N_1, needed to achieve absolute threshold for a long-duration sound; in practice of course, the absolute threshold depends upon the activity of many neurones, but if they are all similar, then the argument can be illustrated by considering just one. Notice that N_1 is the spike rate; the total number of spikes evoked by a sound of duration D would be $N_1 \times D$. If the duration of the sound is decreased by a factor R, then the level has to be increased to restore the total number of spikes evoked by the sound. Assume that the higher spike rate needed for the shorter-duration sound is N_2, where $N_2 = R \times N_1$. For example, if the duration is halved, the spike rate has to be increased by a factor of two to achieve the same total spike count. The increase in level, ΔL, needed to achieve this increased rate is greater for the normal than for the impaired ear, because the rate-versus-level function is steeper for the impaired ear, and this explains the reduced temporal integration.

Temporal integration at suprathreshold levels

A phenomenon similar to temporal integration at threshold is found for the perception of the loudness of sounds that are above the detection threshold. For normally hearing subjects, if the intensity of a sound is held constant, and the duration is varied, the loudness increases with duration for durations up to 100-200 ms. If a sound of a particular duration is chosen as a reference sound, and a sound of shorter duration is adjusted so that it appears equally loud to the reference sound, then the shorter duration sound is adjusted to a higher intensity. As a very rough summary of the data, it may be stated that, for durations up to about 80 ms, constant energy leads to constant loudness; each time the duration is halved the intensity has to be doubled to maintain constant loudness. This is equivalent to saying that the level must be increased by 3 dB for each halving of duration. However, considerable variability occurs across studies. For reviews see Zwislocki (1969), Scharf (1978) and Buus, Florentine and Poulsen (1997).

The amount of temporal integration for loudness is sometimes quantified by estimating the difference in level between equally loud short and long tones. For example, if the difference in level required for equal loudness of a 100 ms tone and a 10 ms tone is 10 dB, it may be stated that the amount of temporal integration is 10 dB. Buus, Florentine and Poulsen (1997) found that, for normally hearing listeners, the amount of temporal integration for 5 kHz sinusoidal tone bursts, varied with sound level, being greatest for medium sound levels. They explained this in terms of the function relating loudness to sound level, pointing out that this function was shallower for medium sound levels than for very low or very high sound levels - see Chapter 4, Figure 4.2. The explanation is similar, in principle, to that given in the previous section to explain differences in temporal integration at threshold between normally hearing and hearing-impaired people.

To understand how temporal integration for loudness might be related to the slopes of loudness-growth functions, consider the following example. Assume that the duration and level of a reference sound are fixed, and the duration of a test sound is decreased, keeping the level fixed, until the loudness is half of the loudness of the reference sound. Assume also that the duration at which the loudness is halved is similar for all values of the reference level. To measure the amount of temporal integration, the level of the shorter sound has to be increased by an amount sufficient to double its loudness. If the function relating loudness to level is relatively steep, as it is at very low and very high sound levels, then only a small increase in sound level, say 6 dB, will be needed to double the loudness. If the function relating loudness to level is relatively shallow, as it is at medium sound levels, then a larger increase in sound level, say 12 dB, will be needed to double the loudness. This can explain why temporal integration is greater at medium levels than at very low or very high levels.

As described in Chapter 4, the functions relating loudness to sound level are typically steeper for people with cochlear hearing loss than for normally hearing people. According to the arguments given above, this should lead to reduced temporal integration for loudness. I am aware of only one study of the effect of duration on loudness for hearing-impaired persons (Pedersen and Poulsen, 1973). That study found that temporal integration for loudness was *not* reduced by hearing loss. However, Pedersen and Poulsen only tested people with hearing impairment caused by presbyacusis, and these people had mild hearing losses (30 to 40 dB) at the test frequency of 1000 Hz. Therefore, temporal integration for loudness might be reduced in cases of cochlear hearing losses that were more severe, or had other causes. Further experimental data are needed to clarify this issue.

Perceptual consequences of abnormal temporal processing in people with cochlear hearing loss

Consequences of abnormal temporal resolution

It has been argued above that the sliding temporal integrator in the model of temporal resolution is probably normal in most people with cochlear hearing loss. However, the non-linearity preceding the integrator is less compressive in impaired ears than in normal ears. For stimuli with inherent slow amplitude fluctuations (such as narrow bands of noise) this can lead to poorer temporal resolution, since the inherent fluctuations become more confusable with the temporal feature to be detected. However, for deterministic stimuli (such as sinusoids) or for broad-band noise stimuli, performance is similar for normal and impaired ears, when the comparison is made at equal SLs. Unfortunately, most sounds in everyday life are characterised by unpredictable fluctuations in amplitude from moment to moment. For such sounds, people with cochlear damage will have more difficulty than normal in following the temporal structure of the sounds. In addition, temporal resolution may be poor because the sounds are at low SLs and/or because the audible bandwidth of the stimuli is restricted. All of these factors can lead to problems in understanding speech and in discriminating and identifying music and environmental sounds. For example, it may be difficult for a person with cochlear hearing loss to detect a weak consonant sound following soon after a relatively intense vowel sound.

Consequences of reduced temporal integration

One consequence of reduced temporal integration is that the hearing loss, as measured by the change in absolute threshold relative to 'normal' values, varies according to the duration of the test sounds; the hearing loss is not as great for short sounds as it is for long sounds. Consider, as an example, two sounds with durations of 400 ms and 10 ms. For a normally hearing person the level required for detection of these two sounds might be, for example, 4 dB SPL and 20 dB SPL, respectively; the shorter sound has to be about 16 dB higher in level to reach the absolute threshold. For a person with moderate cochlear hearing loss, the threshold for detecting the longer sound, might be 54 dB SPL, i.e. 50 dB higher than normal. However, the threshold for detecting the shorter sound might be 60 dB SPL, which is only 40 dB higher than normal. Thus the 'loss' relative to normal hearing is 10 dB less for the shorter sound than for the longer sound.

It is not obvious what is the 'correct' duration at which to measure absolute thresholds. Clinically, audiometric thresholds are usually measured using tones lasting several hundred milliseconds, and many prescriptive formulae for fitting hearing aids (see Chapter 9) are based on such measurements. However, it would seem just as valid to measure thresholds for brief sounds and to specify hearing loss in that way. Many hearing-impaired persons have difficulty in detecting weak consonants, and those consonants are often of short duration - e.g. p, t or k.

As described above, I am aware of only one study of temporal integration for loudness in hearing-impaired people, and that study used listeners with mild hearing losses at the test frequency. It is not known whether temporal integration for loudness differs for normally hearing and for hearing-impaired people with moderate-to-severe hearing losses. If it does, this would complicate the design of hearing aids that attempt to restore loudness to 'normal' (Kollmeier and Hohmann, 1995) - see Chapter 9 for further discussion of these. The amplification appropriate for long-duration sounds may be inappropriate for short duration sounds.

Chapter 6
Pitch Perception and
Frequency Discrimination

Introduction

Pitch is a subjective attribute of sound defined in terms of what is *heard*. It is related to the physical repetition rate of the waveform of a sound; for a pure tone (a sinusoid) this corresponds to the frequency, and for a periodic complex tone to the *fundamental frequency*. Increasing the repetition rate gives a sensation of increasing pitch. Pitch is defined formally as 'that attribute of auditory sensation in terms of which sounds may be ordered on a musical scale' (American Standards Association, 1960). In other words, variations in pitch give rise to a sense of melody. Variations in pitch are also associated with the intonation of voices, and they provide cues as to whether an utterance is a question or a statement. As pitch is a subjective attribute, it cannot be measured directly. Often, the pitch of a sound is assessed by adjusting the frequency of a sinusoid until the pitch of the sinusoid matches the pitch of the sound in question. The frequency of the sinusoid then gives a measure of the pitch of the sound. Sometimes a periodic complex sound, such as a pulse train, is used as a matching stimulus. In this case, the repetition rate of the pulse train gives a measure of pitch.

The ability to detect changes in frequency over time is called frequency discrimination. Usually, the changes in frequency are heard as changes in pitch. It is important to distinguish between frequency selectivity and frequency discrimination. The former refers to the ability to resolve the frequency components of a complex sound, as described in Chapter 3. If a complex tone with many harmonics is presented, a given harmonic can only be 'heard out' from the complex tone if it is separated from neighbouring harmonics by about 1.25 ERBs (Plomp, 1964a; Moore and Ohgushi, 1993; Moore, 1997b) - see Chapter 3 for a description of the ERB scale and for a description of the ability to hear out harmonics. For example, for a complex tone with a fundamental frequency of 150 Hz, the sixth harmonic (900 Hz) is separated from the neighbouring harmonics (750 Hz and 1050 Hz) by about 1.25 ERBs and it would just be possible to 'hear it out' as a separate tone. Frequency discrimination often involves much smaller frequency differences. For example, a 1000 Hz sinusoid can just be discriminated from a 1003 Hz sinusoid when the two sinusoids are presented successively with a brief silent interval between them.

Theories of pitch perception

For many years there have been two theories of pitch perception. One, the 'place' theory, is based on the fact that different frequencies (or frequency components in a complex sound) excite different places along the BM, and hence neurones with different characteristic frequencies. The place theory assumes that the pitch of a sound is related to the excitation pattern produced by that sound; for a pure tone the pitch is generally assumed to correspond to the position of maximum excitation.

An alternative theory, called the 'temporal' theory, is based on the assumption that the pitch of a sound is related to the time pattern of the neural impulses evoked by that sound. These impulses tend to occur at a particular phase of the waveform on the BM, a phenomenon called phase locking - see Chapter 1. The intervals between successive neural impulses approximate integer multiples of the period of the waveform and these intervals are assumed to determine the perceived pitch. The temporal theory cannot be applicable at very high frequencies, since phase locking does not occur for frequencies above about 5 kHz. However, the tones produced by most musical instruments, the human voice, and most everyday sound sources, have fundamental frequencies well below this range.

Many researchers believe that the perception of pitch involves both place mechanisms and temporal mechanisms. However, one mechanism may be dominant for a specific task or aspect of pitch perception, and the relative role of the two mechanisms almost certainly varies with centre frequency.

The place and temporal theories were originally proposed to account for the perception of the pitch of pure tones. Later, they were extended to account for the perception of complex tones. This chapter follows a similar sequence. It first presents experimental data on the perception of pure tones, and describes the theoretical implications of those data. The effect of cochlear hearing loss on the pitch perception of pure tones is then described. Next, the chapter presents data on the perception of complex tones, which are much more common in everyday life. Finally, the effect of cochlear hearing loss on the pitch perception of complex tones is described.

The perception of the pitch of pure tones by normally hearing people

The frequency discrimination of pure tones

The smallest detectable change in frequency is called the frequency difference limen *(DL)*. There have been two common ways of measuring frequency discrimination. One measure involves the discrimination of two successive steady tones with slightly different frequencies. On each trial, the tones are presented in a random order and the listener is required to indicate whether the first or second tone is higher in frequency. The frequency difference between the two tones is adjusted until the listener achieves a criterion percentage correct, for example 75%. This measure will be called the *DLF* (difference limen for frequency). A second measure uses tones that are frequency modulated. In such tones, the frequency moves up and down in a regular periodic manner about the mean (carrier) frequency. The number of times per second that the frequency goes up and down is called the modulation rate. Typically, the modulation rate is rather low (between 2 and 20 Hz), and the changes in frequency are heard as fluctuations in pitch - a kind of 'warble'. To determine a threshold for detecting frequency modulation, two tones are presented successively; one is modulated in frequency and the other has a steady frequency. The order of the tones on each trial is random. The listener is required to indicate whether the first or the second tone is modulated. The amount of modulation (also called the modulation depth) required to achieve a criterion response (e.g. 75% correct) is determined. This measure will be called the *FMDL* (frequency modulation detection limen).

An example of results obtained with the two methods is given in Figure 6.1 (data from Sek and Moore, 1995). Expressed in Hz, both DLFs and FMDLs are smallest at low frequencies, and increase monotonically with increasing frequency. Expressed as a proportion of centre frequency, as in Figure 6.1, DLFs are smallest for middle frequencies and are larger for very high and very low frequencies. FMDLs vary less with frequency than DLFs. Both DLFs and FMDLs tend to get somewhat smaller as the sound level increases; this is not shown in the figure - but see Wier, Jesteadt and Green (1977) and Nelson, Stanton and Freyman (1983).

Place models of frequency discrimination (Henning, 1967; Siebert, 1970; Zwicker, 1970) predict that frequency discrimination should be related to frequency selectivity; both should depend on the sharpness of tuning on the BM. Zwicker (1970) has attempted to account for frequency discrimination in terms of changes in the excitation pattern evoked by the sound when the frequency is altered. Zwicker inferred the

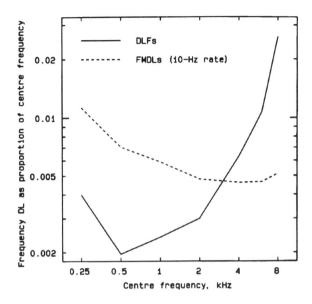

Figure 6.1: Thresholds for detecting differences in frequency between steady pulsed tones (DLFs) and for detecting frequency modulation (FMDLs), plotted as a percentage of the centre frequency and plotted against centre frequency. The modulation rate for the FMDLs was 10 Hz. The data are taken from Sek and Moore (1995).

shapes of the excitation patterns from masking patterns such as those shown in Figure 3.9 (see Chapter 3 for details). In his original formulation of the model, Zwicker intended it to apply only to FMDLs; others (Freyman and Nelson, 1986) have tried to apply the model to account for DLFs.

The model is illustrated in Figure 6.2. The figure shows two excitation patterns corresponding to two tones with slightly different frequencies. A change in frequency results in a sideways shift of the excitation pattern. The change is assumed to be detectable whenever the excitation level at some point on the excitation pattern changes by more than a certain threshold value. Zwicker suggested that this value was about 1 dB. The change in excitation level is greatest on the steeply sloping low-frequency side of the excitation pattern. Thus, in this model, the detection of a change in frequency is functionally equivalent to the detection of a change in level on the low-frequency side of the excitation pattern. The steepness of the low-frequency side is roughly constant when the frequency scale is expressed in units of the ERB of the auditory filter (see Chapter 3) rather than in terms of linear frequency. The slope is about 18 dB per ERB. To achieve a change in excitation level of 1 dB, the frequency has to be changed by one eighteenth of an ERB. Thus, Zwicker's model predicts that

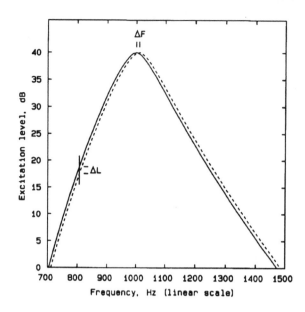

Figure 6.2: Schematic illustration of an excitation-pattern model for frequency discrimination. Excitation patterns are shown for two sinusoidal tones differing slightly in frequency; the two tones have frequencies of 1000 Hz and 1010 Hz. It is assumed that the difference in frequency, ΔF, can be detected if the excitation level changes anywhere by more than a criterion amount. The biggest change in excitation level is on the low-frequency side. The change is indicated by ΔL.

the frequency DL at any given frequency should be about one eighteenth (= 0.056) of the ERB at that frequency. Frequency modulation detection limen do conform fairly well to this prediction of the model, especially when the modulation rate is fairly high (10 Hz or above), as illustrated in Figure 6.3. The dashed line in this figure shows the ratio FMDL/ERB, plotted as a function of centre frequency. The modulation rate was 10 Hz. The ratio is roughly constant, and its value is about 0.05, close to the value predicted by the model. However, DLFs vary more with frequency than predicted by the model (Moore, 1974; Moore and Glasberg, 1986d; 1989; Sek and Moore, 1995). This is illustrated by the solid line in Figure 6.3, which shows the ratio DLF/ERB. The ratio varies markedly with centre frequency. The DLFs for frequencies of 2 kHz and below are smaller than predicted by Zwicker's model, while those for frequencies of 6 and 8 kHz are larger than predicted.

The results for the FMDLs are consistent with the place model, but the results for the DLFs are not. The small DLFs at low frequencies probably reflect the use of temporal information from phase locking. Phase locking becomes less precise at frequencies above 1 kHz, and it is

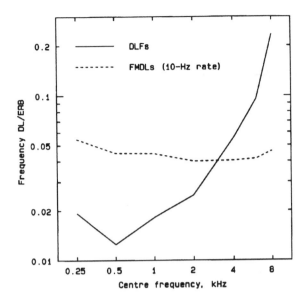

Figure 6.3: DLFs and FMDLs plotted relative to the ERB of the auditory filter at each centre frequency, and plotted as a function of centre frequency. The modulation rate for the FMDLs was 10 Hz. The data are taken from Sek and Moore (1995).

completely lost above 5 kHz. This can account for the marked increase in the DLFs at high frequencies (Goldstein and Srulovicz, 1977).

The ratio FMDL/ERB is not constant across centre frequency when the modulation rate is very low (around 2 Hz), but increases with increasing centre frequency (Moore and Sek, 1995; 1996; Sek and Moore, 1995). For low centre frequencies, FMDLs are smaller for a 2 Hz modulation rate than for a 10 Hz rate, while for high carrier frequencies (above 4 kHz) the reverse is true. For very low modulation rates, frequency modulation may be detected by virtue of the changes in phase locking to the carrier that occur over time. In other words, the frequency is determined over short intervals of time, using phase-locking information, and changes in the estimated frequency over time indicate the presence of frequency modulation. Moore and Sek (1996) suggested that the mechanism for decoding the phase-locking information was 'sluggish'; it had to sample the sound for a certain time in order to estimate its frequency. Hence, it could not follow rapid changes in frequency and it played little role for high modulation rates.

In summary, measures of frequency discrimination are consistent with the idea that DLFs, and FMDLs for very low modulation rates, are determined by temporal information (phase locking) for frequencies up to about 4-5 kHz. The precision of phase locking decreases with increasing frequency above 1-2 kHz, and it is completely absent above about 5 kHz. This can explain why DLFs increase markedly at high frequencies. FMDLs for medium to high modulation rates may be determined by a place mechanism, i.e. by the detection of changes in the excitation pattern. This mechanism may also account for DLFs and for FMDLs for low modulation rates, when the centre frequency is above about 5 kHz.

The perception of musical intervals

Two tones that are separated in frequency by an interval of one *octave* (one has twice the frequency of the other) sound similar. They are judged to have the same name on the musical scale (for example, C3 and C4). This has led several theorists to suggest that there are at least two dimensions to musical pitch. One aspect is related monotonically to frequency (for a pure tone) and is known as 'tone height'. The other is related to pitch class (i.e. the name of the note) and is called 'tone chroma' (Bachem, 1950). For example, two sinusoids with frequencies of 220 and 440 Hz would have the same tone chroma (they would both be called A on the musical scale) but, as they are separated by an octave, they would have different tone heights.

If subjects are presented with a pure tone of a given frequency, f_1, and are asked to adjust the frequency, f_2, of a second tone so that it appears to be an octave higher in pitch, they generally adjust f_2 to be roughly twice f_1. However, when f_1 lies above 2.5 kHz, so that f_2 would lie above 5 kHz, octave matches become very erratic (Ward, 1954). It appears that the musical interval of an octave is only clearly perceived when both tones are below 5 kHz.

Other aspects of the perception of pitch also change above 5 kHz. A sequence of pure tones above 5 kHz does not produce a clear sense of melody (Attneave and Olson, 1971). It is possible to hear that the pitch changes when the frequency is changed, but the musical intervals are not heard clearly. Also, subjects with absolute pitch (the ability to assign names to notes without reference to other notes) are very poor at naming notes above 4-5 kHz (Ohgushi and Hatoh, 1991).

These results are consistent with the idea that the pitch of pure tones is determined by different mechanisms above and below 5 kHz, specifically, by a temporal mechanism at low frequencies and a place mechanism at high frequencies. It appears that the perceptual dimension of tone height persists over the whole audible frequency range, but tone chroma only occurs in the frequency range below 5 kHz. Musical intervals are clearly perceived only when the frequencies of the tones lie in the range where temporal information is available.

The effect of level on pitch

The pitch of a pure tone is primarily determined by its frequency. However, sound level also plays a small role. On average, the pitch of tones below about 2 kHz decreases with increasing level, while the pitch of tones above about 4 kHz increases with increasing sound level. The early data of Stevens (1935) showed rather large effects of sound level on pitch, but more recent data generally show much smaller effects (Verschuure and Van Meeteren, 1975). For tones between 1 and 2 kHz, changes in pitch with level are generally less than 1%. For tones of lower and higher frequencies, the changes can be larger (up to 5%). There are also considerable individual differences both in the size of the pitch shifts with level and in the direction of the shifts (Terhardt, 1974a).

It has sometimes been argued that pitch shifts with level are inconsistent with the temporal theory of pitch; neural interspike intervals are hardly affected by changes in sound level over a wide range. However, changes in pitch with level could be explained by the place theory, if shifts in level were accompanied by shifts in the position of maximum excitation on the BM. On closer examination, these arguments turn out to be rather weak. Although the temporal theory assumes that pitch depends on the temporal pattern of nerve spikes, it also assumes that the temporal information has to be 'decoded' at some level in the auditory system. In other words, the time intervals between neural spikes have to be measured. It is quite possible that the mechanism that does this is affected by which neurones are active and by the spike rates in those neurones; these, in turn, depend on sound level.

The argument favouring the place mechanism is also weak. Chapter 1 described how the peak in the pattern of excitation evoked by a tone shifts towards the base of the cochlea with increasing sound level. The base is tuned to higher frequencies, so the basalward shift should correspond to hearing an increase in pitch. At high sound levels the basalward shift corresponds to a shift in frequency of one-half octave or more. Thus the place theory predicts that the pitch of pure tones should increase with increasing sound level, and the shift should correspond to half an octave or more at high sound levels. In fact, for medium and low-frequency tones, the pitch tends to decrease with increasing sound level. For high-frequency tones, the shift is in the predicted direction, but the shift is always much less than half an octave. If pitch is determined by a place mechanism, then the auditory system must have some way of compensating for changes in excitation patterns with level.

At present there is no generally accepted explanation for the shifts in pitch with level. Given this, the existence of these pitch shifts cannot be used to draw any strong conclusions about theories of pitch. In any case, as already mentioned, the pitch shifts are rather small. In some people with cochlear hearing impairment, shifts in pitch with level can be much larger. Examples are described below.

Frequency discrimination of pure tones by people with cochlear hearing loss

People with cochlear hearing loss usually have auditory filters that are broader than normal - see Chapter 3. Hence, the excitation pattern evoked by a sinusoid is also broader than normal. According to the place theory, this should lead to impaired frequency discrimination. According to the temporal theory, there should not necessarily be a relationship between frequency selectivity and frequency discrimination. However, frequency discrimination could be adversely affected by the reduced precision of phase locking that can occur in cases of cochlear damage - see Chapter 1.

Difference limens for frequency (DLFs)

Several studies have measured DLFs in people with cochlear damage (Gengel, 1973; Tyler, Wood and Fernandes, 1983; Hall and Wood, 1984; Freyman and Nelson, 1986, 1987, 1991; Moore and Glasberg, 1986c; Moore and Peters, 1992; Simon and Yund, 1993). The results have generally shown that frequency discrimination is adversely affected by cochlear hearing loss. However, there is considerable variability across individuals and the size of the DLF has not been found to be strongly correlated with the absolute threshold at the test frequency. Simon and Yund (1993) measured DLFs separately for each ear of subjects with bilateral cochlear damage and found that DLFs could be markedly different for the two ears at frequencies where absolute thresholds were the same. They also found that DLFs could be the same for the two ears when absolute thresholds were different.

Tyler, Wood and Fernandes (1983) compared DLFs and frequency selectivity measured using psychophysical tuning curves (see Chapter 3). They found a low correlation between the two. They concluded that frequency discrimination was not closely related to frequency selectivity, suggesting that place models were not adequate to explain the data. Moore and Peters (1992) measured DLFs for four groups of subjects: young normally hearing, young hearing impaired, elderly with near-normal hearing, and elderly hearing impaired. The auditory filter shapes of the subjects had been estimated in earlier experiments using the notched-noise method (see Chapter 3) for centre frequencies of 100, 200, 400 and 800 Hz. The DLFs for both impaired groups were higher than for the young normal group at all centre frequencies (50-4000 Hz). The DLFs for the elderly group with near-normal hearing were intermediate. The DLFs at a given centre frequency were generally only weakly correlated with the sharpness of the auditory filter at that centre frequency, and some subjects with broad filters at low frequencies had near-normal DLFs at low frequencies. These results suggest a partial dissociation of frequency selectivity and frequency discrimination of pure tones.

Overall, the results of these experiments do not provide strong support for place models of frequency discrimination. This is consistent with the conclusions reached earlier in this chapter, that DLFs for normally hearing people are determined mainly by temporal mechanisms for frequencies up to about 5 kHz. An alternative way of accounting for the fact that cochlear hearing loss results in larger-than-normal DLFs is in terms of loss of neural synchrony (phase locking) in the auditory nerve - see Chapter 1. Goldstein and Srulovicz (1977) described a model for frequency discrimination based on the use of information from the inter-spike intervals in the auditory nerve. This model was able to account for the way that DLFs depend on frequency and duration for normally hearing subjects. Wakefield and Nelson (1985) showed that a simple extension to this model, taking into account the fact that phase locking gets slightly more precise as sound level increases, allowed the model to predict the effects of level on DLFs. They also applied the model to DLFs measured as a function of level in subjects with high-frequency hearing loss, presumably resulting from cochlear damage. They were able to predict the results of the hearing-impaired subjects by assuming that neural synchrony was reduced in neurones with characteristic frequencies corresponding to the region of hearing loss. Of course, this does not prove that loss of synchrony is the cause of the larger DLFs, but it does demonstrate that loss of synchrony is a plausible candidate.

Yet another possibility is that the central mechanisms involved in the analysis of phase-locking information make use of differences in the preferred time of firing of neurones with different characteristic frequencies; these time differences arise from the propagation time of the travelling wave on the BM (Loeb, White and Merzenich, 1983; Shamma, 1985). The propagation time along the BM can be affected by cochlear damage (Ruggero, 1994; Ruggero, Rich, Robles et al., 1996), and this could disrupt the processing of the temporal information by central mechanisms.

Frequency modulation detection limens (FMDLs)

Zurek and Formby (1981) measured FMDLs in ten subjects with sensorineural hearing loss (assumed to be mainly of cochlear origin) using a 3 Hz modulation rate and frequencies between 125 and

4000 Hz. Subjects were tested at a sensation level (SL) of 25 dB, a level above which performance was found (in pilot studies) to be roughly independent of level. The FMDLs tended to increase with increasing hearing loss at a given frequency. For a given degree of hearing loss, the worsening of performance with increasing hearing loss was greater at low frequencies than at high frequencies.

Zurek and Formby suggested two possible explanations for the greater effect at low frequencies. The first is based on the assumption that two mechanisms are involved in coding frequency, a temporal mechanism at low frequencies and a place mechanism at high frequencies. The temporal mechanism may be more disrupted by hearing loss than the place mechanism. An alternative possibility is that absolute thresholds at low frequencies do not provide an accurate indicator of the extent of cochlear damage as these thresholds may be mediated by neurones with characteristic frequencies above the test frequency. For example, if the IHCs at a region of the BM tuned to low frequencies are damaged, then low frequencies may be detected via the 'tails' of the tuning curves of neurones with higher characteristic frequencies. In extreme cases, there may be a dead region at low frequencies; this was described in Chapters 2 and 3 and is discussed in more detail in the following section.

Moore and Glasberg (1986c) measured both FMDLs and thresholds for detecting amplitude modulation (see Chapter 4), using a 4 Hz modulation rate. They used subjects with moderate unilateral and bilateral cochlear impairments. Stimuli were presented at a fixed level of 80 dB SPL, which was at least 10 dB above the absolute threshold. The FMDLs were larger for the impaired than for the normal ears, by an average factor of 3.8 for a frequency of 500 Hz and 1.5 for a frequency of 2000 Hz, although the average hearing loss was similar for these two frequencies. The greater effect at low frequencies is consistent with the results of Zurek and Formby, described above. The amplitude-modulation detection thresholds were not very different for the normal and impaired ears. These thresholds provide an estimate of the smallest detectable change in excitation level. Moore and Glasberg also used the notched-noise method (see Chapter 3) to estimate the slopes of the auditory filters, at each test frequency. The slopes, together with the amplitude-modulation detection thresholds, were used to predict the FMDLs on the basis of Zwicker's excitation-pattern model. The obtained FMDLs were reasonably close to the predicted values. In other words, the results were consistent with the excitation-pattern model.

Grant (1987) measured FMDLs for three normally hearing subjects and three subjects with profound hearing losses. The sinusoidal carrier was modulated in frequency by a triangle function three times per second. Stimuli were presented at 30 dB SL for the normal subjects and at a 'comfortable listening level' (110-135 dB SPL) for the impaired subjects. For all carrier frequencies (100 to 1000 Hz), FMDLs were larger, by an average factor of 9.5, for the hearing-impaired subjects than for the normally hearing subjects. Grant also measured FMDLs when the stimuli were simultaneously amplitude modulated by a noise that was lowpass filtered at 3 Hz. The slow random amplitude fluctuations produced by this amplitude modulation would be expected to impair the use of cues for frequency modulation detection based on changes in excitation level. Consistent with the predictions of the excitation-pattern model, the random amplitude modulation led to increased FMDLs. Interestingly, the increase was much greater for the hearing-impaired than for the normally hearing subjects. When the random amplitude modulation was present, thresholds for the hearing-impaired subjects were about 16 times those for the normally hearing subjects.

As described earlier, it is likely that, for low modulation rates, normally hearing subjects can extract information about frequency modulation both from changes in excitation level and from phase locking (Moore and Sek, 1995; Sek and Moore, 1995). The random amplitude modulation disrupts the use of changes in excitation level but does not markedly affect the use of phase locking cues. The profoundly hearing-impaired subjects of Grant appear to have been relying mainly or exclusively on changes in excitation level. Hence, the random amplitude modulation had severe adverse effects on the FMDLs.

Lacher-Fougère and Demany (1998) measured FMDLs for a 500 Hz carrier, using modulation rates of 2 and 10 Hz. They used five normally hearing subjects and seven subjects with cochlear hearing loss ranging from 30 dB to 75 dB at 500 Hz. Stimuli were presented at a 'comfortable' loudness level. The subjects with losses up to 45 dB had thresholds that were about a factor of two larger than for the normally hearing subjects. The subjects with larger losses had thresholds that were as much as ten times larger than normal. The effect of the hearing loss was similar for the two modulation rates. Lacher-Fougère and Demany suggested that cochlear hearing loss disrupts excitation-pattern (place) cues and phase-locking cues to a roughly equal extent.

In conclusion, FMDLs for hearing-impaired people are generally larger than normal. The larger thresholds may reflect both the broadening of the excitation pattern (reduced frequency selectivity) and disruption of cues based on phase locking.

The perception of pure-tone pitch for frequencies falling in a dead region

In some people with cochlear damage restricted to low-frequency regions of the cochlea, it appears that there are no functioning IHCs with characteristic frequencies corresponding to the frequency region of the loss. In other words, there may be a low-frequency dead region, as described in Chapters 2 and 3. In such cases, the detection of low-frequency tones is mediated by neurones with high characteristic frequencies. One way of demonstrating this is by the measurement of psychophysical tuning curves (PTCs) - see Chapter 3, Figure 3.18. If the signal to be detected has a low frequency, falling within the dead region, the tip of the tuning curve lies well above the signal frequency. In other words, a masker centred well above the signal in frequency is more effective than a masker centred close to the signal frequency (Thornton and Abbas, 1980; Florentine and Houtsma, 1983; Turner, Burns and Nelson, 1983). For example, Florentine and Houtsma (1983) studied a subject with a moderate to severe unilateral low-frequency loss of cochlear origin. For a 1 kHz signal, the tip of the PTC fell between 2.2 and 2.85 kHz, depending on the exact level of the signal.

The perception of pitch in such subjects is of considerable theoretical interest. When there is a low-frequency dead region, a low-frequency pure tone cannot produce maximum neural excitation at the characteristic frequency corresponding to its frequency, since there are no neural responses at that characteristic frequency. The peak in the neural excitation pattern must occur at characteristic frequencies higher than the frequency of the signal. If the place theory is correct, this should lead to marked upward shifts in the pitch of the tone. In fact, this does not happen.

Florentine and Houtsma (1983) obtained pitch matches between the two ears of their unilaterally impaired subject. They presented the stimuli at levels just above absolute threshold, to minimise the spread of excitation along the BM. Pitch shifts between the two ears were small. Turner, Burns and Nelson (1983) studied six subjects with low-frequency cochlear losses. Three of their subjects showed PTCs with tips close to the signal frequency; they presumably had functioning IHCs with characteristic frequencies close to the signal frequency. The other three subjects showed PTCs with tips well above the signal frequency; they presumably had low-frequency dead regions. Pitch perception was studied either by pitch matching between the two ears (for subjects with unilateral losses) or by octave matching (for subjects with bilateral losses, but with some musical ability). The subjects whose PTCs had tips above the signal frequency gave results similar to those of the subjects whose PTCs had tips close to the signal frequency; no distinct pitch anomalies were observed.

These results are hard to explain in terms of the traditional place theory. They show that a pure tone can evoke a low pitch even when there are no functioning IHCs or neurones with characteristic frequencies corresponding to that pitch. The results are more readily explained in terms of the temporal theory; the pitch of the low-frequency tone may be coded in the temporal pattern of neural responses in neurones with characteristic frequencies above the signal frequency.

There have been a few reports of people with hearing losses that increase abruptly at high frequencies who appear to have no functioning IHCs tuned to high frequencies. These subjects report that high-frequency sinusoids do not have a distinct pitch, but sound like noises or buzzes (Villchur, 1973; Moore, Laurence and Wright, 1985; Murray and Byrne, 1986). Presumably, in these cases, neither place coding nor temporal coding mechanisms for pitch can operate effectively. Interestingly, subjects with this type of loss are helped only to a limited extent by hearing aids which attempt to restore audibility of high frequencies; they are helped more by aids which low-pass filter the signal to remove components in the frequency region of high-frequency loss (Villchur, 1973; Moore, Laurence and Wright, 1985; Murray and Byrne, 1986).

Pitch anomalies in the perception of pure tones

Although people with low-frequency hearing loss sometimes perceive the pitch of low-frequency tones in a more or less 'normal' way, cochlear hearing loss at low or high frequencies does sometimes lead to changes in perceived pitch. For people with unilateral cochlear hearing loss, or asymmetrical hearing losses, the same tone presented alternately to the two ears may be perceived as having different pitches in the two ears. This effect is given the name *diplacusis*. Sometimes different pitches are perceived even when the hearing loss is the same in the two ears. The magnitude of the shift can be measured by getting the subject to adjust the frequency of the tone in one ear until its pitch matches that of the tone in the other ear.

According to the place theory, cochlear damage might result in pitch shifts for two reasons. The first applies when the amount of hearing loss varies with frequency and especially when the amount of IHC damage varies with characteristic frequency. When the IHCs are damaged, transduction efficiency is reduced, and so a given amount of BM vibration leads to less neural activity than when the IHCs are intact. When IHC damage varies with characteristic frequency, the peak in the *neural* excitation pattern evoked by a tone will shift away from a region of greater IHC loss. Hence the perceived pitch is predicted to shift away from that region. Early studies of diplacusis (De Mare, 1948; Webster and Schubert, 1954) were generally consistent with this prediction, showing that when a sinusoidal tone is presented in a frequency region of hearing loss, the pitch shifts towards a frequency region where there is less hearing loss. For example, in a person with a high-frequency hearing loss, the pitch was reported to be shifted downwards. However, there are clearly cases where the pitch does not shift as predicted, as described in the previous section.

An alternative way in which pitch shifts might occur is by shifts in the position of the peak excitation on the BM; such shifts can occur even for a flat hearing loss. Chapter 1 described work showing that the tips of tuning curves on the BM and of neural tuning curves were often shifted towards lower frequencies in cases of moderate to severe cochlear damage. This means that the maximum excitation at a given place is produced by a *lower* frequency than normal. Hence, for a given frequency, the peak of the BM response in an impaired cochlea would be shifted towards the base - i.e. towards places normally responding to higher frequencies. This leads to the prediction that the perceived pitch should be shifted upwards. Several studies have found that this is usually the case. For example, Gaeth and Norris (1965) and Schoeny and Carhart (1971) reported that pitch shifts were generally upwards regardless of the configuration of loss. However, it is also clear that individual differences can be substantial and subjects with similar patterns of hearing loss (absolute thresholds as a function of frequency) can show quite different pitch shifts.

Burns and Turner (1986) measured changes in pitch as a function of intensity, by obtaining pitch matches between a tone presented at a fixed level (midway, in dB, between the absolute threshold and 100 dB SPL) and a tone of variable level. The tones were presented alternately to the same ear. As described earlier, normally hearing subjects usually show small shifts in pitch with intensity in this type of task; the shifts are rarely greater than about 3%. The hearing-impaired subjects of Burns and Turner often showed abnormally large pitch-intensity effects, with shifts up to 10%. A common pattern was an abnormally large negative pitch shift with increasing level for low-frequency tones.

Burns and Turner (1986) obtained several other measures from their subjects, including PTCs in forward masking, DLFs, measures of diplacusis, and octave judgements. There was a tendency for increased DLFs and increased pitch-matching variability in frequency regions where the PTCs were broader than normal. The exaggerated pitch-level effects occurred both in frequency regions where PTCs were broader than normal, and (sometimes) in regions where both absolute thresholds and PTCs were normal. The results of the diplacusis measurements and octave matches indicated that the large pitch-intensity effects were mainly a consequence of large increases in pitch at low levels; the pitch returned to more 'normal' values at higher levels.

As pointed out by Burns and Turner, these results are difficult to explain by the place theory. There is no evidence to suggest that peaks in BM responses or in neural excitation patterns of ears with cochlear damage are shifted at low levels but return to 'normal' positions at high levels. Also, even in subjects with similar configurations of hearing loss, the pitch shifts and changes in pitch with level can vary markedly. Furthermore, as pointed out earlier, low-frequency pure tones can evoke low pitches even in people who appear to have no IHCs or neurones tuned to low frequencies.

The results are also problematic for the temporal theory. There is no obvious reason why systematic shifts in pitch should occur as a result of cochlear damage or of changes in level. Unfortunately, there seem to be no physiological data concerning the effects of level on phase locking in ears with cochlear damage. As pointed out earlier, it is possible that the central mechanisms involved in the analysis of phase-locking information make use of the propagation time of the travelling wave on the BM (Loeb, White and Merzenich, 1983; Shamma, 1985). This time can be affected by cochlear damage, and this could disrupt the processing of the temporal information by central mechanisms.

In summary, the perceived pitch of pure tones can be affected by cochlear hearing loss, and changes in pitch with level can be markedly greater than normal. Large individual differences occur, even between subjects with similar absolute thresholds. The mechanisms underlying these effects remain unclear.

The pitch perception of complex tones by normally hearing people

The phenomenon of the missing fundamental

For complex tones the pitch does not, in general, correspond to the position of maximum excitation on the BM. Consider, as an example, a sound consisting of short impulses (clicks) occurring 200 times per second. This sound contains harmonics with frequencies at integer multiples of 200 Hz (200, 400, 600, 800 . . . Hz). The harmonic at 200 Hz is called the *fundamental frequency*. The sound has a low pitch, which is very close to the pitch of its fundamental component (200 Hz), and a sharp timbre (tone quality); it sounds very 'buzzy'. However, if the sound is filtered so as to remove the fundamental component, the pitch does not alter; the only result is a slight change in timbre. This is called the 'phenomenon of the missing fundamental' (Ohm, 1843; Schouten, 1940). Indeed, all except a small group of mid-frequency harmonics can be eliminated, and the low pitch remains the same, although the timbre becomes markedly different.

Schouten (1940, 1970) called the low pitch associated with a group of high harmonics the *residue*. Several other names have been used to describe residue pitch, including *periodicity pitch, virtual pitch,* and *low pitch*. The term residue pitch will be used here. Schouten pointed out that it is possible to hear the change produced by removing the fundamental component and then reintroducing it. Indeed, when the fundamental component is present, it is possible to 'hear it out' as a separate sound. The pitch of that component is almost the same as the pitch of the whole sound. However, the presence or absence of the fundamental component does not markedly affect the pitch of the whole sound.

The perception of a residue pitch does not require activity at the point on the BM that would respond maximally to the fundamental component. Licklider (1956) showed that the low pitch of the residue could be heard when low-frequency noise was present that would mask any component at the fundamental frequency. Even when the fundamental component of a complex tone is present, the pitch of the tone is usually determined by harmonics other than the fundamental. Thus the perception of residue pitch should not be regarded as unusual. Rather, residue pitches are normally heard when listening to complex tones.

The phenomenon of the missing fundamental is not consistent with a simple place model of pitch based on the idea that pitch is determined by the position of the peak excitation on the BM. However, more elaborate place models have been proposed, and these are discussed below.

Discrimination of the repetition rate of complex tones

When the repetition rate of a complex tone changes, all of the components change in frequency by the same ratio, and a change in residue pitch is heard. The ability to detect such changes in pitch is better than the ability to detect changes in a sinusoid at the fundamental frequency (Flanagan and Saslow, 1958) and it can be better than the ability to detect changes in the frequency of any of the individual sinusoidal components in the complex tone (Moore, Glasberg and Shailer, 1984). This indicates that information from the different harmonics is combined or integrated in the determination of residue pitch. This can lead to very fine discrimination; changes in repetition rate of about 0.2% can be detected for fundamental frequencies in the range 100-400 Hz provided that low harmonics are present (e.g. the third, fourth and fifth). The detection of changes in repetition rate is poorer for complex tones that contain only high harmonics (above about the seventh) (Hoekstra and Ritsma, 1977; Moore, Glasberg and Shailer, 1984; Houtsma and Smurzynski, 1990; Carlyon and Shackleton, 1994; Plack and Carlyon, 1995; Carlyon, 1997).

Theories of pitch perception for complex tones

To understand theories of pitch perception for complex tones it is helpful to consider how complex tones are represented in the peripheral auditory system. A simulation of the response of the BM to a complex tone is illustrated in Figure 6.4. In this example, the complex tone is a periodic pulse train, containing many equal-amplitude harmonics. The lower harmonics are partly resolved on the BM, and give rise to distinct peaks in the pattern of activity along the BM. At a place tuned to the frequency of a low harmonic, the waveform on the BM is approximately a sinusoid at the harmonic frequency. For example, at the place with a characteristic frequency of 400 Hz the waveform is a 400 Hz sinusoid. In contrast, the higher harmonics are not resolved, and do not give rise to distinct peaks on the BM. The waveforms at places on the BM responding to higher harmonics are complex, but they all have a repetition rate equal to the fundamental frequency of the sound.

There are two main ways in which the residue pitch of a complex sound might be extracted. Firstly, it might be derived from the frequencies of the lower harmonics that are resolved on the BM. The frequencies of the harmonics might be determined either by place mechanisms (e.g. from the positions of local maxima on the BM) or by temporal mechanisms (from the inter-spike intervals in neurones with characteristic frequencies close to the frequencies of individual harmonics). For example, for the complex tone whose analysis is illustrated in Figure 6.4,

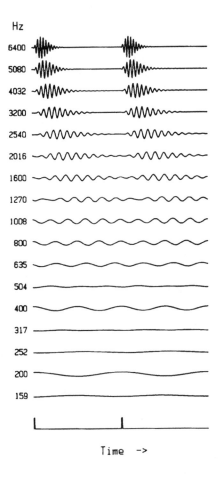

Figure 6.4: A simulation of the responses on the BM to periodic impulses of rate 200 pulses per second. Each number on the left represents the frequency which would maximally excite a given point on the BM. The waveform that would be observed at that point, as a function of time, is plotted opposite that number.

the second harmonic, with a frequency of 400 Hz, would give rise to a local maximum at the place on the BM tuned to 400 Hz. The inter-spike intervals in neurones innervating that place would reflect the frequency of that harmonic; the intervals would cluster around integer multiples of 2.5 ms. Both of these forms of information may allow the auditory system to determine that there is a harmonic at 400 Hz. The auditory system may contain a pattern recogniser that determines the residue pitch of the complex sound from the frequencies of the resolved components (Goldstein, 1973; Terhardt, 1974b). In essence the pattern recogniser tries to find the harmonic series giving the best match to the resolved frequency components; the fundamental frequency of this harmonic series determines the perceived pitch. Say, for example, that the first stage establishes frequencies of 800, 1000 and 1200 Hz to be present. The fundamental frequency whose harmonics would match these frequencies is 200 Hz. The perceived pitch corresponds to this inferred fundamental frequency of 200 Hz. Note that the inferred fundamental frequency is always the highest possible value that fits the frequencies determined in stage one. For example, a fundamental frequency of 100 Hz would also have harmonics at 800, 1000 and 1200 Hz, but a pitch corresponding to 100 Hz is *not* perceived. It is as if the pattern recogniser assumes that the harmonics are successive harmonics, such as the fourth, fifth and sixth, rather than non-successive harmonics like the eighth, tenth and twelfth.

The pitch of a complex tone may also be extracted from the higher unresolved harmonics. As shown in Figure 6.4, the waveforms at places on the BM responding to higher harmonics are complex, but they all have a repetition rate equal to the fundamental frequency of the sound. For the neurones with characteristic frequencies corresponding to the higher harmonics, nerve impulses tend to be evoked by the biggest peaks in the waveform, i.e. by the waveform peaks close to envelope maxima. Hence, the nerve impulses are separated by times corresponding to the period of the sound. For example, in Figure 6.4 the input has a repetition rate of 200 periods per second, so the period is 5 ms. The time intervals between nerve spike would cluster around integer multiples of 5 ms, i.e. 5, 10 15, 20 . . . ms. The pitch may be determined from these time intervals. In this example, the time intervals are integer multiples of 5 ms, so the pitch corresponds to 200 Hz.

Experimental evidence suggests that pitch can be extracted both from the lower harmonics and from the higher harmonics. Usually, the lower, resolved harmonics give a clearer residue pitch, and are more important in determining residue pitch, than the upper unresolved harmonics (Plomp, 1967; Ritsma, 1967; Moore, Glasberg and Peters, 1985). Also, the discrimination of changes in repetition rate of complex tones is better for tones containing only low harmonics than for tones containing only high harmonics (Hoekstra and Ritsma, 1977; Moore,

Glasberg and Shailer, 1984; Houtsma and Smurzynski, 1990; Carlyon and Shackleton, 1994; Plack and Carlyon, 1995; Carlyon, 1997). However, a residue pitch can be heard when only high unresolvable harmonics are present (Ritsma, 1962; 1963; Moore, 1973). Although, this pitch is not as clear as when lower harmonics are present, it is clear enough to allow the recognition of musical intervals and of simple melodies (Moore and Rosen, 1979; Houtsma and Smurzynski, 1990).

Evidence that the time pattern of the waveform evoked on the BM by the higher harmonics plays a role comes from studies of the effect of changing the relative phase of the components in a complex tone. Changes in phase can markedly alter the waveform of a tone. This is illustrated in Figure 6.5, which shows the effect of changing the relative phase of one component in a complex tone containing just three harmonics, the ninth, tenth and eleventh. The left panels show waveforms of the individual sinusoidal components, and the right

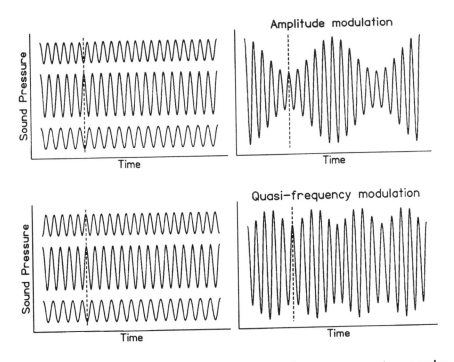

Figure 6.5: The effect of changing the relative phase of one component in a complex tone containing just three harmonics, the ninth, tenth and eleventh. The left panels show waveforms of the individual sinusoidal components, and the right panels show the waveforms of the complex tones produced by adding together the sinusoidal components. For one phase (upper panels), the waveform has an envelope with distinct peaks and dips; this waveform is sometimes called 'amplitude modulated'. For the other phase (lower panels), the envelope is much flatter; this waveform is sometimes called 'quasi-frequency modulated'.

panels show the waveforms of the complex tones produced by adding together the sinusoidal components. For the case illustrated in the top half of the figure, all three components start in 'cosine' phase; this means that the components have their maximum amplitudes at the start of the waveform. Correspondingly, a peak in the envelope of the complex tone occurs at the start of the waveform, and a new peak in the envelope occurs for every ten oscillations in the 'fine structure'. At the point in time marked by the vertical dashed line, a peak in the waveform of the centre component (the tenth harmonic) coincides with minima in the waveforms of the two other harmonics. This gives a minimum in the envelope of the complex tone. Thus, the waveform of the complex tone has an envelope with distinct peaks and dips and is described as 'amplitude modulated'. It might also be described as a 'peaky' waveform.

For the case illustrated in the bottom half of the figure, the phase of the highest component is shifted by 180°; that component starts with a minimum rather than a maximum in its waveform. As a result, the amplitude of the complex tone at the start of the waveform is not as high as for the case when all components started in cosine phase. At the point in time marked by the vertical dashed line, a peak in the waveform of the centre component (the tenth harmonic) coincides with a minimum in the waveform of the eleventh harmonic and a peak in the waveform of the ninth harmonic. The minimum in the envelope of the complex tone is less deep than the minimum when all components started in cosine phase. Thus, the envelope is much flatter, and the envelope actually shows two maxima for each period of the waveform. This waveform is sometimes called 'quasi-frequency modulated', as the time between peaks in the fine structure fluctuates slightly; however this is not easily visible in the figure.

If the harmonics have low harmonic numbers (say the second, third and fourth), they will be resolved on the BM. In this case, the relative phase of the harmonics is of little importance as the envelope on the BM does not change when the relative phases of the components are altered. However, if the harmonics have high harmonic numbers (as in Figure 6.5), then changes in the relative phase of the harmonics can result in changes in the envelope of the waveform on the BM. If this waveform has a peaky envelope, the repetition period will be clearly represented in the intervals between neural impulses. However, if the waveform has a flatter envelope, the repetition period will be less clearly represented.

For tones containing many harmonics, phase has only small effects on the *value* of the pitch heard (Patterson, 1973). This is not surprising, as for such tones temporal information is available from many different points along the BM, and ambiguities in the timing information can be resolved by comparisons across characteristic frequencies; this point is expanded below. Changes in the relative phase of the components can affect the *clarity* of pitch for complex tones with many harmonics

(Lundeen and Small, 1984). For tones containing only a few high harmonics, phase can affect both the pitch value and the clarity of pitch (Moore, 1977; Patterson, 1987a; Shackleton and Carlyon, 1994). These results suggest that the temporal structure of complex sounds does influence pitch perception.

Several researchers have proposed theories in which both place (spectral) and temporal mechanisms play a role; these are referred to as spectro-temporal theories. The theories assume that information from both low harmonics and high harmonics contributes to the determination of pitch. The initial place/spectral analysis in the cochlea is followed by an analysis of the time pattern of the neural spikes evoked at each characteristic frequency (Moore, 1982, 1989; Srulovicz and Goldstein, 1983; Patterson, 1987b; Meddis and Hewitt, 1991; Meddis and O'Mard, 1997). The model proposed by Moore is illustrated in Figure 6.6. The sound is passed through an array of bandpass filters, each corresponding to a specific place on the BM. The time pattern of the neural

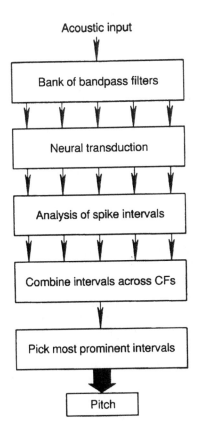

Figure 6.6: A schematic diagram of the spectro-temporal model of pitch perception for complex tones described in Moore (1997b).

impulses at each characteristic frequency is determined by the waveform at the corresponding point on the BM. The inter-spike intervals at each characteristic frequency are determined. Then, a device compares the time intervals present at different characteristic frequencies, and searches for common time intervals. The device may also integrate information over time. In general the time interval which is found most often corresponds to the period of the fundamental component. The perceived pitch corresponds to the reciprocal of this interval. For example, if the most prominent time interval is 5 ms, the perceived pitch corresponds to a frequency of 200 Hz.

As described above, complex tones with low, resolvable harmonics give rise to clear pitches. Changes in repetition rate for such tones are discriminated very well. Tones containing only high, unresolvable harmonics give less clear pitches, and changes in repetition rate are harder to detect. The differences between the two types of tones can be accounted for by spectro-temporal theories (Meddis and Hewitt, 1991; Meddis and O'Mard, 1997). They probably arise because the temporal information conveyed by the resolved harmonics is less ambiguous than the temporal information conveyed by the high harmonics (Moore, 1997b).

Consider two complex tones, one containing three low harmonics, say 800, 1000 and 1200 Hz, and the other containing three high harmonics, say 1800, 2000 and 2200 Hz. For the first tone, the components are largely resolved on the BM. The neurones with characteristic frequencies close to 800 Hz respond as if the input were an 800 Hz sinusoid. The time intervals between successive nerve impulses are multiples of the period of that tone, i.e. 1.25, 2.5, 3.75, 5.0 . . . ms. Similarly, in neurones with characteristic frequencies close to 1000 Hz the intervals between successive nerve spikes are multiples of 1 ms, i.e. 1, 2, 3, 4, 5 . . . ms, and in neurones with characteristic frequencies close to 1200 Hz the intervals are 0.833, 1.67, 2.5, 3.33, 4.17, 5.0 . . . ms. The only interval that is in common across characteristic frequencies is 5 ms, and this unambiguously defines a pitch corresponding to 200 Hz (the missing fundamental).

Consider now the response to the second complex tone, with three high harmonics. These harmonics are not resolved. They give rise to maximum activity at a place on the BM with characteristic frequency close to 2000 Hz. Neurones with characteristic frequencies around 2000 Hz are driven by a complex waveform. The temporal structure of the response is correspondingly complex. Each peak in the fine structure of the waveform is capable of evoking a spike, so many different time intervals occur between spikes. The interval corresponding to the fundamental, 5 ms, is present, but other intervals, such as 4.0, 4.5, 5.5 and 6.0 ms, also occur (Evans, 1978; Javel, 1980). Hence, the pitch is somewhat ambiguous. Increasing the number of harmonics leads to activity across a greater range of places on the BM. The pattern of inter-spike intervals is slightly different for each place, and the only interval that is in common across characteristic frequencies is the one corresponding to the repetition period of the sound. Thus, the pitch becomes less ambiguous as the number of harmonics increases.

In summary, spectro-temporal theories can account for most existing data on the pitch perception of complex tones (Cariani and Delgutte, 1996a; 1996b; Moore, 1997b; Meddis and O'Mard, 1997). The theories assume that both place analysis and temporal analysis are important, and that information about pitch can be extracted both from low harmonics and from high harmonics.

Pitch perception of complex tones by people with cochlear hearing loss

Theoretical considerations

As described in Chapter 3, cochlear hearing loss is usually associated with reduced frequency selectivity; the auditory filters are broader than normal. This makes it more difficult to resolve the harmonics of a complex tone, especially when the harmonics are of moderate harmonic number. For example, for a fundamental frequency (F0) of 200 Hz, the fourth and fifth harmonics would be quite well resolved in a normal auditory system, but would be poorly resolved in an ear where the auditory filters were, say, three times broader than normal. This is illustrated in Figure 6.7, which shows excitation patterns for a complex tone composed of the fourth to tenth harmonics of a 200 Hz fundamental, for a normal auditory system (solid curve), and for an impaired auditory system (dashed curve) in which the auditory filters are three times broader than normal. The former shows distinct ripples corresponding to the lower harmonics, whereas the latter does not.

In the normal auditory system, complex tones with low, resolvable harmonics give rise to clear pitches while tones containing only high, unresolvable harmonics give less clear pitches. As described earlier, the difference between the two types of tones probably arises because the temporal information conveyed by the resolved harmonics is less ambiguous than the temporal information conveyed by the high harmonics. Since cochlear hearing loss is associated with poorer resolution of harmonics, one might expect that this would lead to less clear pitches, and poorer discrimination of pitch than normal. However, for complex tones with many harmonics this effect should be small; spectro-temporal theories assume that information can be combined across different frequency regions to resolve ambiguities.

Spectro-temporal theories also lead to the prediction that the perception of pitch and the discrimination of repetition rate by subjects with broader-than-normal auditory filters might be more affected by the

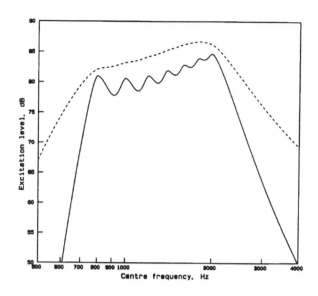

Figure 6.7: Excitation patterns for a harmonic complex tone containing harmonics 4-10 of a 200 Hz fundamental. Each harmonic has a level of 80 dB SPL. Excitation patterns are shown for a normal ear (solid curve), and for an impaired ear (dashed curve) in which the auditory filters are three times as broad as normal.

relative phases of the components than is the case for normally hearing subjects. For subjects with broad auditory filters, even the lower harmonics would interact at the outputs of the auditory filters, giving a potential for strong phase effects.

In addition to producing reduced frequency selectivity, it is possible that cochlear damage leads to abnormalities in phase locking (neural synchrony) - see chapter 1. This could lead to less clear pitches and poorer discrimination of pitch than normal.

Experimental studies

The pitch discrimination of complex tones by hearing-impaired people has been the subject of several studies (Hoekstra and Ritsma, 1977; Rosen, 1987; Moore and Glasberg, 1988c; 1990; Moore and Peters, 1992; Arehart, 1994). Most studies have required subjects to identify which of two successive harmonic complex tones had the higher repetition rate (corresponding to a higher pitch). The threshold determined in such a task will be described as a *DLC* (difference limen for a complex). These studies have revealed the following:

- There was considerable individual variability, both in overall performance and in the effects of harmonic content.

- For some subjects, when F0 was low, DLCs for complex tones containing only low harmonics (1-5) were markedly higher than for complex tones containing higher harmonics, suggesting that pitch was conveyed largely by the higher, unresolved harmonics.
- For some subjects, DLCs were larger for complex tones with lower harmonics (1-12) than for tones without lower harmonics (4-12 and 6-12) for F0s up to 200 Hz. In other words, adding lower harmonics made performance *worse*. This may happen because, when auditory filters are broader than normal, adding lower harmonics can create more complex waveforms at the outputs of the auditory filters. For example, there may be more than one peak in the envelope of the sound during each period, and this can make temporal analysis more difficult (Rosen and Fourcin, 1986; Rosen, 1986).
- The DLCs were mostly only weakly correlated with measures of frequency selectivity. There was a slight trend for large DLCs to be associated with poor frequency selectivity but the relationship was not a close one. Some subjects with very poor frequency selectivity had reasonably small DLCs.
- There can be significant effects of component phase. In several studies, DLCs have been measured with the components of the harmonic complexes added in one of two phase relationships, all cosine phase or alternating cosine and sine phase. The former results in a waveform with prominent peaks and low amplitudes between the peaks (as in the upper right-hand panel of Figure 6.5). The latter results in a waveform with a much flatter envelope (as in the lower right-hand panel of Figure 6.5). The DLCs tended to be larger for complexes with components added in alternating sine/cosine phase than for complexes with components added in cosine phase. However, the opposite effect was sometimes found. The direction of the phase effect varied in an unpredictable way across subjects and across type of harmonic complex. Phase effects tended to be stronger for hearing-impaired than for normally hearing subjects. The variability in the phase effects may arise from variability in the properties of the auditory filters across subjects and across centre frequencies. According to spectro-temporal theories, the time patterns of the waveforms at the outputs of the auditory filters are important for determining pitch. These waveforms are determined by the magnitude and phase response of the auditory filters and these may vary markedly across subjects and centre frequencies depending on the specific pattern of cochlear damage.

Overall, these results suggest that people with cochlear damage depend relatively more on temporal information and less on spectral information than normally hearing people. The results lend support to spectro-temporal theories of pitch perception. The variability in the results across people, even in cases where the audiometric thresholds are similar, may occur partly because of individual differences in the auditory filters and partly because loss of neural synchrony is greater in some people than others. People in whom neural synchrony is well preserved may have good pitch discrimination despite having broader-than-normal auditory filters. People in whom neural synchrony is adversely affected may have poor pitch discrimination regardless of the degree of broadening of their auditory filters.

Perceptual consequences of altered frequency discrimination and pitch perception

Effects on speech perception

The perception of pitch plays an important role in the ability to understand speech. In all languages, the pitch patterns of speech indicate which are the most important words in an utterance, they distinguish a question from a statement and they indicate the structure of sentences in terms of phrases. In 'tone' languages, such as Mandarin Chinese and Thai, pitch can affect word meanings. Pitch also conveys non-linguistic information about the gender, age and emotional state of the speaker. Supplementing lip reading (speechreading) with an auditory signal containing information only about voice pitch can result in a substantial improvement in the ability to understand speech (Risberg, 1974; Rosen, Fourcin and Moore, 1981; Grant, Ardell, Kuhl et al., 1985). The use of a signal that conveys information about the presence or absence of voicing (i.e. about whether a periodic complex sound is present or not) gives less improvement than when pitch is signalled in addition (Rosen, Fourcin and Moore, 1981). It seems likely that reduced ability to discriminate pitch changes, such as occurs in people with cochlear hearing loss, would reduce the ability to use pitch information in this way.

For complex tones, people with cochlear hearing loss are often more affected by the relative phases of the components than are normally hearing people. When a hearing-impaired person is reasonably close to a person speaking and when the room has sound-absorbing surfaces, the waveforms reaching the listener's ears when a voiced sound is produced will typically have one major peak per period. These peaky waveforms may evoke a distinct pitch sensation. On the other hand, when the listener is some distance from the speaker, and when the room is reverberant, the phases of the components become essentially random (Plomp and Steeneken, 1973) with the result that the waveforms are less peaky. In this case, the evoked pitch may be less clear. The ability of hearing-impaired listeners to extract pitch information in everyday situations may be over-estimated by studies using headphones or conducted in rooms with sound-absorbing walls.

For normally hearing listeners, several studies have shown that when two people are talking at once, it is easier to 'hear out' the speech of individual talkers when their voices have different F0s (Brokx and Nooteboom, 1982). This effect probably arises in two main ways (Culling and Darwin, 1993). Firstly, when the F0s of two voices differ, the lower resolved harmonics of the voices have different frequencies and excite different places on the BM. This allows the brain to separate the harmonics of the two voices and to attribute to one voice only those components whose frequencies form a harmonic series. This mechanism would be adversely affected by cochlear hearing loss, since reduced frequency selectivity would lead to poorer resolution of the harmonics. Secondly, the higher harmonics would give rise to complex waveforms on the BM, and these waveforms would differ in repetition rate for the two voices. The brain may be able to use the differences in repetition rate to enhance separation of the two voices. This mechanism might depend on the two voices having different short-term spectra. At any one time, the peaks in the spectrum of one voice would usually fall at different frequencies from the peaks in the spectrum of the other voice. Hence, one voice would dominate the BM vibration patterns at some places, whereas the other voice would dominate at other places. The local temporal patterns could be used to determine the spectral characteristics of each voice. This mechanism would also be impaired by cochlear hearing loss for two reasons. Firstly, reduced frequency selectivity would tend to result in more regions on the BM responding to the harmonics of both voices, rather than being dominated by a single voice. Secondly, abnormalities in temporal coding might lead to less effective representations of the F0s of the two voices.

I am not aware of any experimental studies of the effects of differences in F0 of two talkers on speech perception by hearing-impaired people. However, it is known that people with cochlear hearing loss perform much more poorly than normally hearing people when trying to understand one person when another person is talking (Duquesnoy, 1983; Festen and Plomp, 1990; Hygge, Rönnberg, Larsby et al., 1992; Baer and Moore, 1994; Moore, Glasberg and Vickers, 1995; Peters, Moore and Baer, 1998) - see Chapter 8 for more details. Part of this difficulty may stem from a reduced ability to exploit differences in F0.

Effects on music perception

The existence of pitch anomalies (diplacusis and exaggerated pitch-intensity effects) may affect the enjoyment of music. Changes in pitch with intensity would obviously be very disturbing, especially when listening to a live performance where the range of sound levels can be very large. There have been few, if any, studies of diplacusis for complex sounds but it is likely to occur to some extent. One person studied in our laboratory was a professor of music who had a unilateral cochlear loss. He reported that he typically heard different pitches in his normal ear and impaired ear, and that musical intervals in his impaired ear sounded distorted. Other subjects have reported that some musical notes do not produce a distinct pitch, and that they get no pleasure from listening to music.

Chapter 7
Spatial Hearing and Advantages of Binaural Hearing

Introduction

Two ears are definitely better than one, for several reasons. Firstly, differences in the intensity and time of arrival of sounds at the two ears provide cues that are used to localise sound sources. Secondly, when a desired signal and a background noise come from different locations, comparison of the stimuli reaching the two ears improves the ability to detect and discriminate the signal in the noise. Thirdly, when trying to hear a sound such as speech in the presence of background noise, the speech-to-noise ratio may be much higher at one ear than at the other ear. For example, if the speech comes from the left and the noise from the right, the speech-to-noise ratio will be higher at the left ear than at the right. Under these circumstances, people are able to make use of the ear receiving the higher speech-to-noise ratio. Finally, even when the signals reaching the two ears are identical, the ability to discriminate or identify the signals is often slightly better than when the signals are delivered to one ear only. These advantages of having two ears can be reduced by cochlear hearing loss, but this does not always happen. This chapter reviews several aspects of binaural and spatial hearing, comparing results for normally hearing and hearing-impaired people.

The chapter starts with a review of the ability to localise sounds in space, i.e. to determine the direction that sounds are coming from. It is useful to define some common terms used in studies of sound localisation. The word *binaural* refers to situations where sound reaches both ears. When the stimulus arriving at the two ears is identical, this is referred to as *diotic*. When the sound is different at the two ears, this is called *dichotic*. When earphones are worn, the sound sometimes appears to come from within the head. Judgements of the position within the head (e.g. towards the left ear, towards the right ear, or in the middle of the head) are referred to as *lateralisation* judgements.

The directions of sound sources in space are usually defined relative to the head. For this purpose, three planes are defined, as illustrated in Figure 7.1 (Blauert, 1996). The *horizontal plane* passes through the upper margins of the entrances to the ear canals and the lower margins of the eye sockets. The *frontal plane* lies at right angles to the horizontal plane and intersects the upper margins of the entrances to the ear canals. The *median plane* lies at right angles to the horizontal and frontal planes; points in the median plane are equally distant from the two ears. The point of intersection of all three planes lies roughly at the centre of the head; it defines the origin for a co-ordinate system for specifying the angles of sounds relative to the head. The direction of a sound can be specified by its *azimuth* and its *elevation*. All sounds lying in the median plane have 0° azimuth. All sounds lying in the horizontal plane have 0° elevation. A sound with 0° azimuth and 0° elevation lies directly in front of the head. A sound with 90° azimuth and 0° elevation lies directly opposite the left ear. A sound with 180° azimuth and 0° elevation lies directly behind the head. A sound with 0° azimuth and 90° elevation lies directly above the head, while a sound with 0° azimuth and 270° elevation lies directly below the head. Generally, the azimuth is the angle produced by projection on to the horizontal plane (θ in Figure 7.1), while the elevation is the angle produced by projection on to the median plane (δ in Fig. 7.1).

There are two aspects to performance in localisation of sounds. The first aspect is concerned with how well the perceived direction of a sound source corresponds to its actual direction. For normally hearing people, the perceived direction generally corresponds reasonably well with the actual direction, although for sinusoidal stimuli errors sometimes occur in judging whether a sound is coming from in front or behind, or from above or below the horizontal (Stevens and Newman, 1936); this point is discussed in more detail later on. The second aspect of localisation is concerned with how well subjects can detect a small shift in position of a sound source. This aspect measures the resolution of the auditory system. When resolution is studied using stimuli presented via loudspeakers, the smallest detectable change in angular position, relative to the subject, is referred to as the *minimum audible angle (MAA)*.

The localisation of sinusoids

Cues for localisation

Consider a sinusoidal sound source located to the left side of the head. The sound has to travel further to reach the right ear than to reach the left ear, so the sound is delayed in time in the right ear relative the left. In addition, the sound reaching the right ear is less intense than that reaching the left ear, because the head casts a kind of 'shadow' (see

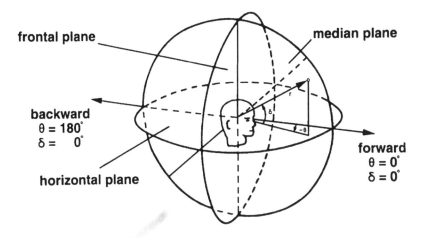

frontal plane

median plane

backward
θ = 180°
δ =   0°

forward
θ = 0°
δ = 0°

horizontal plane

Figure 7.1: Illustration of the co-ordinate system used to define the position of sounds relative to the head. The azimuth is given by the angle θ (positive for leftwards directions and negative for rightwards directions) and the elevation by the angle δ (positive for upward directions and negative for downwards directions). The distance is given by r. Adapted from Blauert (1996).

below for details). There are thus two physical differences in the sound at the two ears, the interaural time difference (ITD) and the interaural intensity difference (IID), which could provide cues as to the location of the sound source. We consider below the magnitudes of these cues and the extent to which they are actually used by the auditory system. Notice that the sounds at the two ears are normally fused and heard as a single sound image. For example, if an IID is present, we do not hear a loud sound towards one side and a softer sound towards the other side; rather a single sound image is heard towards the side receiving the more intense sound. The physical cues of ITD and IID are used by the brain to create a percept at a specific subjective location.

The cues of ITD and IID are not equally effective at all frequencies. Consider first the IID, which is often described as the interaural level difference (ILD), measured in dB. Low-frequency sounds have wavelengths that are long compared with the size of the head, and as a result they bend very well around the head. Thus, little or no 'shadow' is cast by the head. On the other hand, at high frequencies, where the wavelength is short compared with the dimensions of the head, a 'shadow', almost like that produced by a beam of light, occurs. Interaural differences in level are negligible at low frequencies, but may be 20 dB or more at high frequencies. This is illustrated in Figure 7.2, adapted from Feddersen, Sandel, Teas and Jeffress (1957).

Interaural time differences range from 0 (for a sound straight ahead) to about 650 μs for a sound at 90° azimuth (directly opposite one ear).

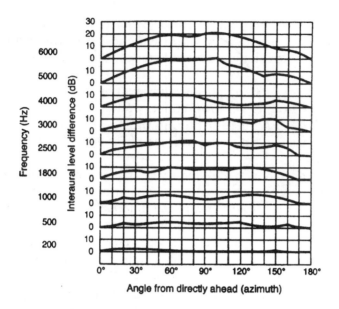

Figure 7.2: Interaural level differences (ILDs) for sinusoidal stimuli plotted as a function of azimuth; each curve is for a different frequency. Adapted from Feddersen et al. (1957).

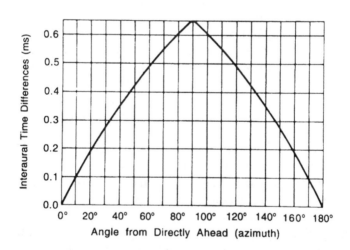

Figure 7.3: Interaural time differences (ITDs) plotted as a function of azimuth. Adapted from Feddersen, Sandel, Teas and Jeffress (1957).

This is illustrated in Figure 7.3, adapted from Feddersen, Sandel, Teas and Jeffress (1957). The ear at which the sound arrives earlier is often called the 'leading' ear; the other ear is called the 'lagging' ear. For a given azimuth, the interaural time difference is roughly independent of the frequency of the sound source. However, the effectiveness of ITDs as a cue for localisation does vary with frequency, as will be explained below. For a sinusoidal tone, a time difference is equivalent to a phase difference between the two ears. For example, if a 500 Hz tone is delayed at one ear by 200 μs, this is equivalent to a phase shift of one-tenth of a period, i.e. 36°. For low-frequency tones, the phase difference provides effective information about the location of the sound. However, for higher-frequency sounds, the phase difference provides an ambiguous cue.

Consider a sinusoid with a frequency of 769 Hz. This has a period of 1.3 ms. If the sinusoid is delayed by 650 μs at one ear relative to the other ear, then the sinusoid has a phase difference of 180° at the two ears. In other words, a peak in the waveform at the left ear coincides with a minimum in the right ear, and vice versa. In this situation, the auditory system has no way of knowing whether the leading ear was the left or the right; the sound at the right ear might be 650 μs ahead of that at the left ear or 650 μs behind. For a high-frequency sinusoid, say around 10 kHz, there may be many cycles of phase difference between the two ears. The auditory system has no way of determining which cycle in the left ear corresponds to a given cycle in the right ear. Thus, the phase difference at the two ears provides unambiguous information for frequencies below 750 Hz but the information becomes increasingly ambiguous at higher frequencies.

The idea that sound localisation is based on interaural time differences at low frequencies and interaural intensity differences at high frequencies has been called the *duplex theory* and it dates back to Lord Rayleigh (1907). It appears to hold for sinusoids but it is not strictly accurate for complex sounds, as will be explained later.

Performance of normally hearing people in localisation and lateralisation

Studies of localisation using sinusoids have usually used tone bursts with gradual onsets and offsets, to minimise cues related to the interaural timing of the envelope; envelope cues are discussed in more detail later in this chapter. Figure 7.4 shows the MAA for sinusoidal signals, plotted as a function of frequency (Mills, 1958; 1972). All stimuli were presented in the horizontal plane, i.e. with an elevation of 0°. Each curve shows results for a different reference azimuth; the task was to detect a shift in azimuth from that direction. The MAA is smallest for a reference azimuth of 0°, i.e. for sounds coming from directly in front of the subject. A shift as small as 1° can be detected for frequencies below 1000 Hz. Performance worsens around 1500 Hz. This is consistent with the duplex theory; at 1500 Hz phase differences between the two ears are ambiguous cues for localisation, and interaural intensity differences

are small. Performance worsens markedly when the reference direction
is moved away from 0° azimuth. Indeed, for reference azimuths of 60°
and 75°, the MAA was so large that it could not be determined when the
frequency was around 1500 Hz.

When resolution is studied using earphones, it is possible to study
the effectiveness of ILDs alone or ITDs alone. The discriminability of
interaural differences is usually measured in a two-alternative forced-
choice task. Two successive binaural stimuli are presented and they
differ in interaural level or time. For example, one stimulus might be
identical at the two ears, while the other stimulus might have an ITD of
ΔT. The task of the subject is to say whether the first stimulus was to the
left or the right of the second stimulus. In other words, the task is to
identify a shift in perceived location associated with a change in interaural amplitude or timing.

Thresholds for detecting changes in ITD are smallest when the reference ITD is zero, corresponding to a sound heard in the centre of the
head (Yost, 1974). In this case, a change in ITD of about 10 μs can be
detected for a frequency of 900 Hz. Such a change would be produced
by moving a sound source through an angle of about 1° relative to the
subject; this corresponds well with the MAA value described above. The
smallest detectable ITD increases somewhat at lower frequencies,
although the threshold is roughly constant at about 3° when it is
expressed as the smallest detectable change in relative phase at the two
ears. Above 900 Hz, the threshold ITD increases markedly, and above
1500 Hz changes in ITD are essentially undetectable. The threshold ITD

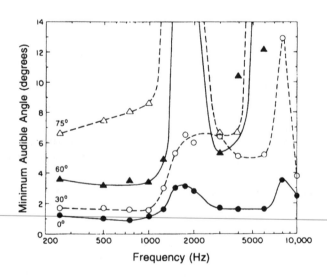

Figure 7.4: The minimum audible angle (MAA) for sinusoidal signals, plotted as a
function of frequency; each curve shows results for a different reference direction.
Data from Mills (1958; 1972).

increases for all frequencies when the reference ITD is greater than zero, i.e. when the reference sound is heard towards one side of the head.

Thresholds for detecting changes in ILD are also smallest when the reference ILD is zero, corresponding to an identical sound at the two ears. In this case, changes in ILD of about 1 dB can be detected across a wide range of frequencies, although performance worsens slightly for frequencies around 1000 Hz (Mills, 1960; Yost and Dye, 1988). When the reference ILD is 15 dB, as would occur for a high-frequency sound well to one side of the head, the threshold change in ILD varies between 1.3 dB (at low and high frequencies) and 2.5 dB (around 1000 Hz).

In summary, the resolution of the binaural system, which determines the ability to detect changes in the position of a sound source, is best for sounds that come from directly ahead (0° azimuth). Resolution at low frequencies is based on the use of ITDs. Changes in ITD cannot be detected for frequencies above 1500 Hz. Changes in ILD can be detected over the whole audible frequency range, but, in practice, ILDs sufficiently large to provide useful cues to sound location occur only at high frequencies.

Performance of hearing-impaired people in localisation and lateralisation

There have been few studies of localisation and lateralisation of sinusoids by hearing-impaired subjects; most studies have used complex stimuli (see below). Nordlund (1964) measured free-field localisation of sinusoids with frequencies 500, 2000 and 4000 Hz. He reported both the mean error (a measure of systematic errors or biases), and the standard deviation (a measure of resolution). For subjects with cochlear losses in both ears, only one out of 13 showed any abnormal results (based on a 99.9% confidence interval). For subjects with unilateral or highly asymmetric cochlear losses, seven out of nine showed at least one abnormal result. However, even for these subjects, the majority of results were within the normal range.

Häusler, Colburn and Marr (1983) reported limited measurements on subjects with unilateral cochlear losses (mainly Ménière's syndrome). Stimuli were presented via earphones. Thresholds for detecting changes in ITD were sometimes very large, but few specific details were given.

Hall, Tyler and Fernandes (1984) measured thresholds for detecting a change in ITD of a 500 Hz sinusoid at a level of 70 dB SPL. They tested six normally hearing subjects and ten subjects with mild-to-moderate symmetrical cochlear hearing losses. The ITD thresholds were markedly larger for the impaired subjects (mean 176 μs) than for the normally hearing subjects (mean 65 μs). The ITD thresholds tended to increase with increasing absolute threshold at 500 Hz, and three subjects with absolute thresholds less than 40 dB SPL had near-normal ITD thresholds.

The poor performance of the subjects with higher absolute thresholds could have been partly due to the low sensation level (SL) of the stimuli.

Smoski and Trahiotis (1986) measured thresholds for detecting changes in ITD using 500 Hz sinusoids delivered by earphones. They used four subjects with mainly high-frequency cochlear losses caused by noise exposure or viral infections. At equal sound pressure level (80 dB SPL), the hearing-impaired subjects had higher ITD thresholds than the two normally hearing subjects tested. However, at an equal SL of 25 dB, ITD thresholds did not differ greatly for the normal and hearing-impaired subjects.

In summary, the limited data available on the localisation and lateralisation of sinusoids suggest that bilateral symmetric cochlear damage does not lead to marked abnormalities, except when the stimuli are at low SLs. Asymmetrical or unilateral damage more often leads to abnormalities. In most studies, abnormalities in localisation were not closely related to audiometric thresholds, although sometimes absolute thresholds and ITD thresholds have been found to be correlated. Sometimes abnormal localisation is found in frequency regions where absolute thresholds are normal.

The localisation of complex sounds

The role of transients and across-frequency comparisons

All sounds which occur in nature have onsets and offsets, and many also change their intensity or their spectral structure as a function of time. Interaural differences in the time of arrival of these transients provide cues for localisation which are not subject to the phase ambiguities which occur for steady sinusoidal tones. For sounds that cover a reasonable frequency range, phase ambiguities can also be resolved by comparisons across frequency; the ITD that is common across all frequencies must be the 'true' ITD (Grantham, 1995; Stern and Trahiotis, 1995).

Performance of normally hearing people

Klump and Eady (1956) measured thresholds for discriminating changes in ITD using stimuli delivered via headphones. They compared three types of stimuli: band-limited noise (containing frequencies in the range 150-1700 Hz); 1000 Hz pure tones with gradual rise and fall times; and clicks of duration 1 ms. For a reference ITD of 0°, the threshold ITDs were 9 μs, 11 μs and 28 μs, respectively. Thus the greatest acuity occurred for the noise stimulus. The single click gave rise to the poorest performance. However, threshold ITDs for click trains can be as small as 10 μs (Dye and Hafter, 1984) when the click rate is reasonably low (200 clicks per second or less). For bursts of noise (lowpass filtered at 5000 Hz), the ability to detect changes in ITD improves with duration of the bursts for durations up to about 700 ms, when the threshold change in ITD reaches an asymptotic value of about 6 μs (Tobias and Zerlin, 1959).

Yost, Wightman and Green (1971) investigated what frequencies were most important for the discrimination of changes in ITD of click trains. They did this by filtering the click trains, and by adding filtered noise to mask the energy in certain frequency regions. They found that discrimination deteriorated for clicks which were highpass filtered, so that only energy above 1500 Hz was present. However, discrimination was largely unaffected by lowpass filtering. Masking with a lowpass noise produced a marked disruption whereas a highpass noise had little effect. Thus discrimination of lateral position on the basis of time delays between the two ears depends largely on the low-frequency content of the clicks, although somewhat poorer discrimination is possible with only high-frequency components.

Henning (1974) investigated the lateralisation of high-frequency sinusoids, which were amplitude modulated; for an example of the waveform of an amplitude-modulated sound, see the upper-right panel of Figure 6.5. He found that the detectability of changes in ITD in the envelope of a 3900 Hz carrier modulated at a frequency of 300 Hz was about as good as the detectability of changes in ITD of a 300 Hz sinusoid. However, there were considerable differences among individual observers; the threshold ITDs had values of 20, 50 and 65 μs for three different subjects (all stimuli had 250 ms durations and 50 ms rise-fall times). Henning found that time delay of the envelope rather than time delay of the 'fine structure' (associated with the carrier frequency) within the envelope determines the lateralisation. The signals could be lateralised on the basis of time delays in the envelope even when the carrier frequencies were different in the two ears. Thus it seems that for complex signals containing only high-frequency components, listeners extract the envelopes of the signals and compare the relative timing of the envelopes at the two ears. However, lateralisation performance is best when the carrier frequencies are identical, and poor lateralisation results when the complex waveforms at each ear have no frequency component in common.

Overall, these results lead to some revision of the basic principles of the duplex theory. Complex sounds containing only high frequencies (above 1500 Hz) can be localised on the basis of ITDs, but this is done by comparing the timing of the *envelope* at the two ears.

Performance of people with cochlear hearing loss

A survey of studies of localisation and lateralisation in hearing-impaired people, for studies up to 1981, has been given by Durlach, Thompson and Colburn (1981). A wide variety of stimuli were used in the studies, but the majority used either wideband noise or filtered noise. Durlach et al. concluded that many of the studies were hard to interpret because they did not distinguish between systematic errors in localisation and poor resolution. Nevertheless, there was a clear trend for poor localisation and lateralisation to occur in people with unilateral or asymmetrical cochlear damage. Subjects with symmetrical cochlear losses often showed near-normal performance, especially when tested at reasonably high sound levels.

Häusler, Colburn and Marr (1983) studied sound localisation and lateralisation in hearing-impaired subjects using broadband noise as a stimulus. They measured MAAs for stimuli presented in free field at various azimuths, and ITDs and ILDs for stimuli presented via earphones. Stimuli were presented at levels ranging from 85 to 100 dB SPL. Some subjects with bilateral sensorineural losses (presumably cochlear in origin) showed MAAs within the normal range, both for stimuli at 0° azimuth, and for stimuli to one side. These subjects nearly always had good speech discrimination scores. Other subjects with bilateral losses showed somewhat larger MAAs than normal, especially for stimuli located to the side. These subjects usually had poor speech discrimination scores. Subjects with unilateral or asymmetric losses (mainly Ménière's syndrome) tended to have larger MAAs than normal, especially for sounds towards the side of the impaired ear, but a few subjects showed performance within the normal range.

Subjects with bilateral sensorineural losses usually showed thresholds for the detection of changes in ITD and ILD that were within the normal range, although a few showed larger ITDs than normal. Subjects with unilateral or asymmetric sensorineural losses (Ménière's) showed threshold ITDs that were normal or slightly larger than normal. However, threshold ILDs were mostly larger than normal.

Hawkins and Wightman (1980) measured thresholds for detecting changes in ITD and ILD for narrow bands of noise centred at 500 and 4000 Hz, using eight subjects with moderate cochlear losses, six of whom had symmetrical losses. The remaining two had unilateral losses caused by Ménière's syndrome. The stimuli were presented at 85 dB SPL and were delivered by earphones. For most subjects, ITD thresholds were much higher than normal at 4000 Hz (greater than $250\,\mu s$ as compared to $40\text{-}80\,\mu s$ for normally hearing subjects). At 500 Hz, ITD thresholds were more variable, with two subjects showing performance within the normal range ($12\text{-}29\,\mu s$) and the remainder showing thresholds in the range $33\,\mu s$ to unmeasurable. The ILD thresholds were often close to normal, except for the subjects with unilateral losses. Abnormally large ITD thresholds were sometimes found when both ILDs and absolute thresholds were normal.

Smoski and Trahiotis (1986) measured thresholds for detecting a change in ITD using narrow-band noises centred at 500 and 4000 Hz and an amplitude modulated 4000 Hz sinusoidal carrier. Stimuli were delivered by earphones. They used four subjects with mainly high-frequency cochlear losses caused by noise exposure or viral infections. At equal sound pressure level (80 dB SPL), the hearing-impaired subjects had higher ITD thresholds than the two normally hearing subjects tested. The difference was small for the 500 Hz stimulus, but was large for the 4000 Hz stimuli. For example, for the 4000 Hz amplitude-modulated stimulus, the threshold ITD averaged 25 μs for the normally hearing subjects, and about 250 μs for the hearing-impaired subjects. However, at an equal sensation level (SL) of 25 dB, ITD thresholds were much larger (200-600 μs), but did not differ greatly for the normal and hearing-impaired subjects.

Kinkel, Kollmeier and Holube (1991) measured thresholds for detecting changes in ITD and ILD of narrow bands of noise presented via earphones at centre frequencies of 500 Hz and 4000 Hz. They used 15 normally hearing subjects and 49 subjects with hearing loss, presumed to be mainly of cochlear origin. Stimuli were presented at 75 dB SPL or at the 'most comfortable level', whichever was the higher. The ITD thresholds were, on average, much larger for the hearing-impaired than for the normally hearing subjects, both at 500 Hz (210 μs versus 38 μs) and at 4000 Hz (530 μs versus 81 μs), although some hearing-impaired subjects had ITDs within the normal range. The average ILD thresholds were also larger for the hearing-impaired than for the normally hearing subjects, both at 500 Hz (4.7 dB versus 2.6 dB) and at 4000 Hz (5.1 dB versus 2.2 dB). However, many hearing-impaired subjects had ILD thresholds within the normal range.

Gabriel, Koehnke and Colburn (1992) measured thresholds for detecting changes in ITD and ILD for narrowband noise stimuli presented via earphones at about 30 dB SL. The centre frequency of the noise was varied from 250 to 4000 Hz in one-octave steps. They used three subjects with symmetrical cochlear losses. Both ITDs and ILDs were generally larger than normal, although results varied markedly across subjects. One subject with a flat loss showed essentially no sensitivity to changes in ITD, except at 500 Hz, where the threshold was 100 μs. That subject also had unusually large ILD thresholds (3-8 dB as compared to about 1 dB for normally hearing subjects). Even for two subjects with similar audiograms and similar causes of hearing loss (noise induced), performance differed markedly both in the values of the thresholds and in their pattern across frequency.

It is clear from these studies that binaural performance can vary markedly across subjects. Subjects with unilateral or asymmetric losses tend to show larger than normal thresholds for detecting changes in ITD and ILD. Subjects with symmetrical losses sometimes show normal or near-normal performance for broad-band noise stimuli. However, they often show impaired performance for narrowband stimuli. It is possible, as pointed out by Colburn and Trahiotis (1992), that good performance

for a restricted frequency range may be enough to ensure good performance for broadband stimuli.

Reasons for large ITD and ILD thresholds in people with cochlear hearing loss

The poor discrimination of ITDs, when it occurs, may be the result of
several factors:

- It may be partly caused by the relatively low SL of the stimuli.
  Hearing-impaired people are usually tested at low SLs; higher SLs are
  not possible because of their loudness recruitment. ITD discrimination in normally hearing subjects worsens markedly when the sound
  level is below about 20 dB SL (Häusler, Colburn and Marr, 1983) and
  so poor performance would also be expected in hearing-impaired
  people when tested at low SLs.
- It may result from abnormalities in the propagation time of the travelling wave along the BM or in the phase of neural spike initiation, and
  from differences in travel time or phase of spike initiation between the
  two ears (Ruggero and Rich, 1987; Ruggero, Rich and Recio, 1993). As
  described above, discrimination of ITDs tends to be best for low-
  frequency sounds. The propagation time of the travelling wave to its
  point of maximum amplitude on the BM is probably in the range 5-9 ms
  for low-frequency sounds in a normal ear (Ruggero and Rich, 1987).
  Cochlear damage can result in marked changes in this propagation
  time, which may amount to as much as 1 ms (Ruggero, 1994). However,
  the direction of the change depends upon the exact nature of the underlying pathology (Ruggero, 1994). It seems likely that cochlear damage
  will often result in differences in propagation time along the BM,
  especially for asymmetric losses, and this will have an effect similar to
  introducing a time delay between the two ears. The difference in travel
  time may be large compared to the range of ITDs that occurs naturally
  (up to $650\,\mu s$) and this would adversely affect the discrimination of
  ITDs. It may also strongly affect the perceived location of sound sources.
- The people tested were often hearing-aid users. Hearing aids can
  introduce time delays that are a significant proportion of the ITDs
  that occur naturally. Extensive use of a monaurally fitted hearing aid
  could result in some form of adaptation to the abnormal ITD. This
  may impair discrimination of ITD when the aid is not worn.
- Poor discrimination of ITD may be the result of abnormalities in
  phase locking (see Chapter 1). If the precision of phase locking is
  reduced, then the timing of the sound at each ear will be coded less
  precisely, leading to impaired ITD discrimination.

Abnormalities in ILD discrimination may also have multiple causes:

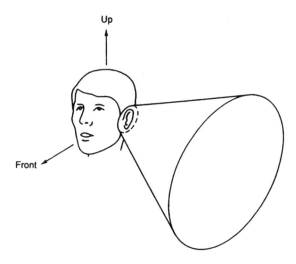

Figure 7.5: Illustration of the cone of confusion for a specific ITD. All points on the surface of the cone give rise to that same ITD.

- As for ITD discrimination, they may result from the relatively low SL of the stimuli.
- They may result from abnormal input-output functions on the BM, and from differences in input-output functions between the two ears. Put in another way, differences in loudness between the two ears, or in the rate of growth of loudness with increasing sound level, may impair the discrimination of ILDs. In this context it is noteworthy that ILD discrimination in normally hearing subjects can be markedly impaired by putting an earplug in one ear (Häusler, Colburn and Marr, 1983).

The cone of confusion, head movements and pinna cues

The cone of confusion

If the influence of the pinnae is ignored, then the head may be regarded as a pair of holes separated by a spherical obstacle. If the head is kept stationary, then a given ITD will not be sufficient to define uniquely the position of the sound source in space. For example, if the left ear leads the right ear by 50 μs, this indicates that the sound lies to the left, but the sound could be in front of or behind the head, and above or below the horizontal plane. In fact, there is a *cone of confusion* such that any sound source on the surface of this cone would give rise to the same ITD (see Mills, 1972, and Figure 7.5). A similar ambiguity arises for ILDs. One extreme case applies when both the ITD and ILD are zero, i.e. the sound is the same at the two ears. In this case, the sound could be located anywhere in the median plane; the cone 'expands' to become a plane.

The role of head movements

Ambiguities related to the cone of confusion may be resolved by head movements. Suppose, for example, that it is desired to resolve an ambiguity about the location of a sound source in the vertical direction, i.e. about its elevation. If the head is rotated about a vertical axis by, say, 20° and this results in a 20° shift in the apparent lateral position of the auditory image in relation to the head, then the sound source must be located in the horizontal plane. If the rotation of the head is accompanied by no change in the auditory image, then the sound must be located either directly above or directly below the head. Human listeners do seem to be able to use head movements to resolve ambiguities in this way (Wallach, 1940; Perrett and Noble, 1997). Intermediate shifts in the location of the auditory image lead to intermediate vertical height judgements (Wallach, 1940).

Information provided by the pinnae

Even when the head is fixed, or when the duration of a sound is too short to allow useful information to be gained from head movements, ambiguities associated with the cone of confusion do not seem to pose a problem in everyday situations. For example, a brief click can usually be localised accurately, without any confusion about whether it comes from in front or behind the head. The ambiguities are resolved by information provided by the pinnae. Some of the sound reaching the ear enters the meatus directly, but some enters the meatus after reflection from one or more of the folds in the pinna. There are also some reflections from the shoulders and the upper part of the torso. When the direct sound and the reflected sound are added together, this results in a change in the spectrum of the sound reaching the eardrum.

Say, for example, that the sound reflected from the pinna has a time delay of 75 μs (this is the time taken for a sound to travel a distance of about 2.5 cm), and that the sound source is a white noise, which contains a wide range of frequencies. For a frequency of 6667 Hz (period = 150 μs), the reflected sound is delayed by half of a period relative to the leading sound. The direct and reflected sounds therefore cancel, giving a dip in the spectrum at 6667 Hz. For a frequency of 13 333 Hz (period = 75 μs), the reflected sound is delayed by one whole period, so the direct and reflected sounds add, giving a peak in the spectrum. Because there are usually several reflections from the pinna, the spectrum of the sound reaching the eardrum is complex, containing multiple peaks and dips. The spectral pattern varies systematically with the direction of the sound source (Wightman and Kistler, 1989; Blauert, 1996).

The spectral changes produced by the pinna can be used to judge the location of a sound source. As it is the spectral *patterning* of the sound that is important, the information provided by the pinna is most effective when the sound has spectral energy over a wide frequency range. High frequencies, above 6 kHz, are especially important, since it is only at high frequencies that the wavelength of sound is sufficiently short for it to interact strongly with the pinna.

Localisation using pinna cues by normal and hearing-impaired people

Häusler, Colburn and Marr (1983) measured MAAs in the vertical direction for sounds coming from straight ahead, using broad-band noise as a stimulus; in other words, subjects had to detect shifts in elevation for sounds presented in the median plane. Stimuli were presented at levels ranging from 85 to 100 dB SPL. One ear was plugged, so presumably the only cue available was the spectral patterning provided by the pinna and head.

Subjects with normal hearing had MAAs in the range 1-10°. Subjects with bilateral cochlear hearing loss fell into two groups. One group had MAAs within the normal range and also had good speech discrimination. The other group had MAAs that were so large that they could not be measured and had poor speech discrimination. For subjects with unilateral losses due to Ménière's syndrome, some of the impaired ears also showed MAAs within the normal range, while others showed slightly larger than normal MAAs. MAAs were within the normal range for the normally hearing ear.

Noble, Byrne and Lepage (1994) required subjects to identify which loudspeaker from an array was emitting a broadband pink noise. They tested six normally hearing subjects and 87 subjects with sensorineural hearing loss. Of these, 66 subjects had a symmetrical loss that was assumed to be cochlear in origin. Generally, the hearing-impaired subjects performed more poorly than the normally hearing subjects. Differences in localisation accuracy in different regions of auditory space were related to different configurations of hearing loss. The ability to judge the elevation of sounds (i.e. to judge location in the up-down dimension) depended on high-frequency sensitivity; high absolute thresholds at high frequencies were correlated with poor localisation. Front-rear discrimination was correlated with absolute thresholds in the range 4 to 6 kHz, high thresholds being associated with poor discrimination.

In summary, hearing-impaired subjects can differ markedly in their ability to make use of the high-frequency spectral cues provided by the pinna. Some subjects appear to be completely unable to use these cues, whereas others use them almost normally. The poor performance, when it occurs, is probably due to two factors:

- The high frequencies that carry pinna cues may be inaudible, or at very low SLs.
- The peaks and dips in spectrum introduced by the pinna may be not be resolved because of reduced frequency selectivity.

General conclusions on sound localisation

The auditory system is capable of using several physical cues to determine the location of a sound source. Time and intensity differences at the two ears, changes in the spectral composition of sounds due to head shadow and pinna effects, and changes in all of these cues produced by head or sound source movements, can all influence the perceived direction of a sound source. In laboratory studies usually just one or two of these cues are isolated. In this way it has been shown that sometimes a single cue may be sufficient for accurate localisation of a sound source. For real sound sources, such as speech or music, all of the cues described above may be available simultaneously. In this situation, the multiplicity of cues makes the location of the sound sources more definite and more accurate.

Hearing-impaired people show considerable individual differences in their ability to localise sounds. Often, in studies measuring the horizontal MAA for broadband sounds at high levels, performance is nearly normal, especially in cases of symmetrical losses. In this situation several cues are available - ITDs, ILDs and pinna cues - and an ability to use any one of these, or any combination, is sufficient to give good performance. In studies using earphones, where usually only one cue is present at a time, the performance of hearing-impaired subjects is often poorer than normal, especially when narrowband stimuli are used.

Binaural masking level differences (MLDs)

MLDs for normally hearing people

The masked threshold of a signal can sometimes be markedly lower when listening with two ears than when listening with one (Hirsh, 1948). Consider the situation shown in Figure 7.6a. White noise from the same noise generator is fed to both ears via stereo headphones. Sinusoidal signals, also from the same signal generator, are fed separately to each ear and mixed with the noise. Thus the stimuli at the two ears are identical. Assume that the level of the tone is adjusted until it is just masked by the noise, i.e. it is at its masked threshold, and let its level at this point be L_0 dB. Assume now that the signal is inverted in phase (equivalent to a phase shift of 180° or π radians) in one ear only (see Figure 7.6b). The result is that the signal becomes audible again. The tone can be adjusted to a new level, L_π, so that it is once again at its masked threshold. The difference between the two levels, $L_0 - L_\pi$ (dB) is known as a masking level difference (MLD), and its value may be as large as 15 dB at low frequencies (around 500 Hz), decreasing to 2-3 dB for frequencies above 1500 Hz. Thus, simply by inverting the signal waveform at one ear the signal becomes considerably more detectable.

An example which is surprising at first sight is given in Figure 7.6c. The noise and signal are fed to one ear only, and the signal is adjusted to be at its masked threshold. Now the noise alone is added at the other ear; the tone becomes audible once again (Figure 7.6d). Further, the tone disappears when it, too, is added to the second ear, making the

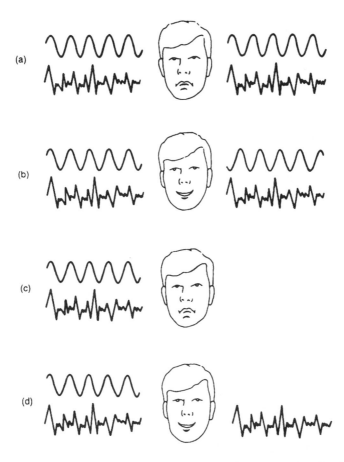

Figure 7.6: Illustration of two situations in which binaural masking level differences (MLDs) occur. In conditions (a) and (c) detectability is poor, while in conditions (b) and (d), where the interaural relations of the signal and masker are different, detectability is good (hence the smiling faces).

sounds at the two ears the same. Notice that it is important that the same noise is added to the non-signal ear; the noises at the two ears must be correlated or derived from the same noise generator. Release from masking is not obtained when an independent noise (derived from a second noise generator) is added to the non-signal ear.

The phenomenon of the MLD is not limited to pure tones. Similar effects have been observed for complex tones, clicks and speech sounds. Whenever the phase or level differences of the signal at the two ears are not the same as those of the masker, the ability to detect and identify the signal is improved relative to the case where the signal and masker have the same phase and level relationships at the two ears. Such differences only occur in real situations when the signal and masker are located in different positions in space. Thus, the detection and discrimination of signals, including speech, is better when the signal and masker are not coincident in space than when they are coincident (for example, when they come from the same loudspeaker).

To describe the conditions in experiments measuring MLDs, it is customary to use the symbols N (for noise) and S (for signal), each being followed by a suffix denoting relative phase at the two ears. A phase inversion is equivalent to a phase shift of 180° or π radians. Thus N_0S_π refers to the condition where the noise is in phase at the two ears and the signal is inverted in phase. N_u means that the noise is uncorrelated at the two ears. The suffix '$_m$' indicates monaural presentation, i.e. presentation to one ear only. Table 7.1 gives the magnitude of the MLD for a variety of combinations of signal and noise. Four conditions for which there is no binaural advantage, N_0S_0, N_mS_m, N_uS_m and $N_\pi S_\pi$, all give about the same 'reference' threshold. The MLDs for the conditions shown in the table are obtained by expressing thresholds relative to this reference threshold.

In addition to improving the detectability of tones, conditions that produce MLDs also favour other aspects of the ability to discriminate signals. For example, when speech signals are presented against noisy backgrounds, speech intelligibility is better under conditions when the speech and noise do not have the same interaural phase (Licklider, 1948). However, the advantage for intelligibility is not as large as the advantage for detection. For single words in broadband white noise, the speech-to-noise ratio required for 50% intelligibility is typically about 6 dB lower for N_0S_π than for N_0S_0, whereas the threshold for detecting the words is about 13 dB lower (Levitt and Rabiner, 1967).

Mechanisms underlying MLDs

Models of the mechanisms underlying MLDs are complex, and it is beyond the scope of this book to describe them fully. Briefly, most recent models assume that firing patterns are compared for neurones with

Table 7.1: Values of the MLD for various interaural phase relationships of the signal and masker. These results are typical of broadband maskers and low-frequency signals.

Interaural condition	MLD in dB
$N_u S_\pi$	3
$N_u S_0$	4
$N_\pi S_m$	6
$N_0 S_m$	9
$N_\pi S_0$	13
$N_0 S_\pi$	15

corresponding CFs in the two ears. It is assumed that, at each CF, there is an array of delay lines which can delay the neural spikes from one ear relative to those from the other; each delay line has a characteristic time delay. These are followed by coincidence detectors, which count the numbers of spikes arriving synchronously from the two ears. If a sound is delayed by a time τ at the left ear relative to the right, then a delay of τ in the neural spikes from the right ear will cause the spikes from the left and right ears to be synchronous at the point of binaural interaction. Thus the interaural delay of the signal is coded in terms of which delay line gives the highest response in the coincidence detectors.

This type of model was originally proposed to account for the ability to use interaural time delays in localising sounds (Jeffress, 1948), but it has since been extended to account for MLDs and other aspects of binaural processing. It is useful to think of the outputs of the coincidence detectors as providing a kind of two-dimensional display; one of the dimensions is CF and the other is the interaural delay. The response to any stimulus is a pattern of activity in this display. When a signal and a masker have the same interaural delay time, τ, then they produce activity at overlapping points in the pattern; most activity lies around a line of equal delay (τ) versus CF. When a signal and masker have different interaural delay times, the pattern is more complex. The addition of the signal to the masker may cause activity to appear at points in the pattern where there was little activity for the masker alone. This could enhance the detection of the signal, giving an MLD. For further details, the reader is referred to Colburn (1996) and Stern and Trahiotis (1995).

MLDs for people with cochlear hearing loss

A survey of studies of the MLD using hearing-impaired subjects was presented by Durlach, Thompson and Colburn (1981). While there was considerable variability in the results across studies, generally it was found that cochlear hearing loss leads to reduced MLDs, even when the hearing loss is reasonably symmetrical. For example, Quaranta and

Cervellera (1974) reported abnormally small MLDs in 86% of cases. However, the relative sizes of the MLDs in different conditions (see Table 7.1) were often similar to normal. In some cases with asymmetric hearing losses, the pattern of results can be very different from normal. For example, in the study of Schoeny and Carhart (1971), thresholds for the condition N_0S_m were lower (better) when the signal was delivered to the better-hearing ear than when it was delivered to the ear with poorer hearing, even though the N_mS_m thresholds were similar for the two ears.

Several more recent studies have confirmed that MLDs are typically smaller than normal in subjects with cochlear hearing loss (Hall, Tyler and Fernandes, 1984; Jerger, Brown and Smith, 1984; Staffel, Hall, Grose et al., 1990; Kinkel, Kollmeier and Holube, 1991). These studies have shown a trend for smaller MLDs in subjects with higher absolute thresholds, although the association is not generally strong, and subjects with similar absolute thresholds can have very different MLDs. MLDs also tend to be smaller the more asymmetrical is the loss (Jerger, Brown and Smith, 1984).

Possible reasons for smaller MLDs in people with cochlear damage

In normally hearing subjects, MLDs increase with increasing sound level, so the reduced MLDs in hearing-impaired subjects could be partly a consequence of the low SL of the stimuli; the loudness recruitment associated with cochlear damage prevents the use of high SLs. However, this cannot be a complete explanation, since reduced MLDs for subjects with cochlear hearing loss occur when the stimuli are at SLs where normally hearing subjects show large MLDs (Quaranta and Cervellera, 1974). Also reduced MLDs occur when the relative levels of the stimuli at the two ears are adjusted so that an in-phase stimulus produces an image centred in the head (Quaranta and Cervellera, 1974).

Hall, Tyler and Fernandes (1984) suggested that the small MLDs found for hearing-impaired subjects might be partly a consequence of poor coding of temporal fine structure. They tested six normally hearing subjects and ten subjects with mild-to-moderate cochlear hearing losses. They found a significant correlation between the MLD at 500 Hz and ITD thresholds for 500 Hz sinusoids, supporting their suggestion. Kinkel, Kollmeier and Holube (1991) also found a correlation between the MLD at 500 Hz and the ITD threshold at 500 Hz. However, the correlation might have been due to the fact that both the MLD and the ITD threshold were correlated with age and with the absolute threshold at 500 Hz (Kinkel and Kollmeier, 1992).

Staffel, Hall, Grose and Pillsbury (1990) suggested that the small MLDs found for hearing-impaired subjects might be partly a consequence of asymmetry of the auditory filters at the two ears at a given centre frequency. If the filters have different amplitude and phase responses at the two ears, because of differences in the underlying pathology (e.g. different patterns of OHC loss), this would lead to differences in the filter outputs in response to noise. Thus, the correlation of the noise would be reduced, which would in turn reduce the MLD; recall that MLDs do not occur when the noise is uncorrelated at the two ears. To test this hypothesis, they measured N_0S_0 and N_0S_π thresholds as a function of masker bandwidth, using a 500 Hz signal and noise centred at 500 Hz. Six normally hearing subjects and 18 subjects with cochlear hearing loss were tested; 10 of the latter had distinctly asymmetric hearing losses. Staffel et al. reasoned that interaural asymmetry of the auditory filters would have little effect for very small masker bandwidths, but would have an increasing effect as bandwidth increased. However, the results did not support this hypothesis. The MLDs of the hearing-impaired subjects were smaller than normal both for a masker with a very small bandwidth (25 Hz) and for maskers with much wider bandwidths (400 and 800 Hz). Thus, while auditory-filter asymmetry may play a small role in reducing MLDs in hearing-impaired subjects, it does not seem to be a major factor.

In summary, the causes of the reduced MLDs found for people with cochlear damage are not fully understood. The reduced SL of the stimuli, and reduced abilities to discriminate changes in interaural time and intensity may all play a role.

Head shadow effects

Benefits of head shadow for normally hearing people

Most studies of the MLD have used conditions where performance cannot be improved simply by attending to one ear only. Usually, this means that the sounds were presented over earphones. Hence, these studies have been specifically concerned with the benefit of binaural processing, where information from the two ears is combined and compared. However, when listening for a signal in background noise in everyday listening situations (i.e. not using earphones) it is often the case that the signal-to-noise ratio is much better at one ear than at the other. The differences in signal-to-noise ratio occur as a result of the head-shadow effects illustrated in Figure 7.2. For example, if a speech signal comes from the left and an interfering noise comes from the right, the speech-to-noise ratio will be higher at the left ear than at the right. The improved signal-to-noise ratio occurs mainly at high frequencies (above about 2 kHz). An advantage of having two ears is that the listener can effectively 'select' the ear giving the higher signal-to-masker ratio.

Bronkhorst and Plomp (1988) studied the effects of ITDs and head shadow on the intelligibility of speech in noise, under binaural listening conditions. The sounds were recorded using a realistic model of a human head and torso (KEMAR) (see Burkhard, 1975). The speech was presented from directly in front of KEMAR (0° azimuth), while the noise was presented at seven azimuths ranging from 0° (frontal) to 180°. The noise had the same long-term average spectrum as the speech. The recorded sounds were digitally processed to derive two signals, one containing only ITDs (identical intensity at the two ears at all frequencies) and the other containing only ILDs due to head shadow. The processed stimuli were presented via earphones. The speech-to-noise ratio required for 50% of sentences to be understood (the speech reception threshold, SRT) was determined for each noise azimuth. The decrease in SRT, relative to the case where both speech and noise came from 0° azimuth, is called the *binaural intelligibility level difference* (BILD). The BILD due to ITDs was between 3.9 and 5.1 dB (for noise azimuths between 30° and 150°). This BILD may be considered as a form of MLD resulting from comparison of the signals at the two ears, i.e. it reflects binaural processing. The BILD due to ILDs was 3.5 to 7.8 dB. This BILD probably has two components. One, like the BILD resulting from the ITDs alone, depends on binaural processing. The other depends on the fact that the signal-to-noise ratio at one ear is improved when the noise and speech are spatially separated. For example, for speech at 0° azimuth, when the noise is moved to the left, say to 45° azimuth, the signal-to-noise ratio improves at the right ear and worsens at the left ear. Performance can be improved by giving greater weight to the ear with the higher speech-to-noise ratio. In additional experiments, Bronkhorst and Plomp used the stimuli with ILDs alone, but they turned off the stimulus to one ear. Turning off the stimulus to the ear receiving the poorer signal-to-noise ratio produced little degradation in performance. They concluded that the advantage gained from ILDs mainly depends on the ear receiving the higher speech-to-noise ratio. However, this advantage decreases when the noise in the other ear is fairly loud.

When the unprocessed stimuli were used (i.e. when both ITDs and ILDs were present), the improvements were larger than for ITDs or ILDs alone, ranging from 5.8 to 10.1 dB. However, the overall effect was not as great as would be obtained if the BILDs gained from ITDs and ILDs simply added.

In summary, spatial separation of speech and background noise can lead to a BILD of up to 10 dB. A large part of this effect is due to the fact that the speech-to-noise ratio is improved at one ear by head shadow effects. A smaller part is due to binaural processing of ITDs.

Benefits of head shadow for hearing-impaired people

Bronkhorst and Plomp (1989) carried out similar experiments to those described above using 17 subjects with symmetrical hearing losses and 17 subjects with asymmetrical losses (differences in threshold between the two ears, averaged over 500, 1000 and 2000 Hz, ranging from 5 to 31 dB). Most subjects were diagnosed as having mild to moderate cochlear hearing losses. The noise level was adjusted for each subject so as to be as far as possible above absolute threshold without being uncomfortably loud. When the speech and noise both came from 0° azimuth, the SRTs were, on average, 2.5 dB higher than found for normally hearing subjects. Both groups of hearing-impaired subjects showed 2.6-5.1 dB less binaural gain than normal when the noise azimuth was changed to 90°. In other words, in this condition SRTs were 5.1-7.6 dB higher than normal, a considerable difference.

The BILDs due to ILDs alone ranged from 0 dB to normal values of 7 dB or more. The size of the BILDs depended on the high-frequency loss in the ear receiving the higher speech-to-noise ratio; greater high-frequency losses were associated with a reduced advantage. This makes sense, since head-shadow effects are greatest at high frequencies, and if those high frequencies are inaudible, little advantage can be gained. The average BILD due to ITDs alone was nearly normal (4.2 dB as compared to 4.7 dB for normally hearing subjects) for subjects with symmetrical hearing losses. However, subjects with asymmetrical losses showed smaller BILDs, averaging 2.5 dB. When ITDs were introduced in stimuli already containing ILDs, the gain was 2-2.5 dB for both groups, comparable to what was obtained for normally hearing subjects.

In summary, subjects with cochlear hearing loss are generally less able than normal to take advantage of spatial separation of speech and interfering noise. When tested under conditions where speech and noise are spatially separated, they perform more poorly, relative to normal, than when the speech and noise come from the same position in space. The disadvantage appears to arise mainly from the inaudiblity of high frequencies in the ear at which the speech-to-noise ratio is highest.

Diotic advantages

In many tasks, detection and discrimination performance is better when listening with two ears than with one, even when the same stimulus is delivered to the two ears. This is given the general name 'diotic summation'. For example, the absolute threshold is about 2 dB lower for diotic than for monaural stimulation (Shaw, Newman and Hirsh, 1947), and thresholds for the detection of changes in frequency or intensity are also lower for diotic stimulation (Jesteadt, Wier and Green, 1977a).

Of perhaps more interest is the fact that the intelligibility of speech in noise is usually greater for diotic than for monaural stimulation. For normally hearing subjects, the diotic advantage in intelligibility for key words in simple sentences is about 9% when baseline performance in the monaural condition is 70% (Davis, Haggard and Bell, 1990), and about 20% when monaural performance is 50% (Davis and Haggard,

1982). Plomp and Mimpen (1979) reported that the SRT for sentences presented in noise with the same long-term average spectrum as the speech was 1.4 dB lower for diotic presentation than for monaural presentation. This corresponds to an improvement in intelligibility in difficult listening situations (when about 50% of sentences are reported correctly) of about 20%.

People with cochlear hearing impairment also show better speech intelligibility for diotic stimulation than for monaural stimulation. Laurence, Moore and Glasberg (1983) measured SRTs in noise of eight subjects with moderate to severe cochlear losses under three conditions: unaided, with linear hearing aids, and with two-channel compression hearing aids (see Chapter 9 for more details of hearing aids with compression). For each condition they compared three cases: listening with both ears (either unaided or binaurally aided), listening with the left ear only, and listening with the right ear only. In the latter two cases, the unused ear was either plugged and muffed or fitted with a hearing aid that was turned off. For all three conditions, there was a significant advantage of binaural versus monaural listening, even when the speech and noise came from the same loudspeaker directly in front of the subject (this gives essentially diotic stimulation, at least for unaided listening). The advantage of using two ears was similar for unaided and aided conditions. On average, for the case where the speech and noise came from directly in front, the SRT was about 2 dB lower when listening binaurally than when listening with the better ear. For the speech material they used, this is equivalent to an improvement in intelligibility of about 22%. A similar average diotic advantage for subjects with cochlear hearing loss was reported by Moore, Johnson, Clark and Pluvinage (1992).

In summary, performance on many tasks, including the understanding of speech in noise, is better using two ears than with one, even when the stimuli at the two ears are essentially the same. This diotic advantage occurs for both normally hearing people and people with cochlear damage. If anything, it may be larger for hearing-impaired people.

Perceptual consequences of abnormal binaural and spatial hearing in people with cochlear damage

The most obvious consequence of abnormal binaural and spatial hearing is difficulty in localising sound sources. Some people with cochlear hearing loss have essentially no ability to use spectral cues provided by the pinna. This may happen either because the cues are inaudible, or because the patterns of spectral peaks and dips cannot be resolved. When pinna cues are lacking, this creates difficulty in deciding whether a sound comes from in front or behind, and from above or below. It should be noted that pinna cues are drastically altered or removed altogether by hearing aids; hearing aids alter the spectral patterns at the eardrum and usually do not amplify sounds in the frequency range above 6 kHz where pinna cues are most effective. Hence, hearing aid users are likely to suffer from difficulty in resolving the cone of confusion.

Some people with cochlear damage have higher than normal thresholds for detecting changes in ITD and ILD. This applies especially to people with asymmetrical losses, and to sounds with narrow bandwidths. This means that the precision with which the azimuth of a sound source can be determined is reduced, making it more difficult to orient to a sound and to decide what physical object gave rise to that sound.

Many studies comparing the intelligibility of speech in noise for normally hearing and hearing-impaired subjects have used speech and noise coming from the same loudspeaker. Such studies underestimate the difficulty experienced by hearing-impaired people in everyday life, as they fail to take into account the reduced ability of people with cochlear damage to take advantage of spatial separation of a desired sound and one or more interfering sounds. This reduced ability shows up both in studies of the MLD using earphones and in studies using stimuli presented in a free field. The disadvantage in free field depends partly on reduced binaural processing abilities, and partly on reduced audibility of high-frequency sounds at the ear receiving the higher signal-to-background ratio. For normally hearing subjects, spatial separation of speech and background noise can reduce the SRT by up to 10 dB. For people with moderate cochlear damage the advantage is 3-5 dB less. This is equivalent to a substantial loss in intelligibility.

Chapter 8
Speech Perception

Introduction

People with cochlear hearing loss frequently complain of difficulty with speech communication. The extent and nature of the difficulty depends partly on the severity of the hearing loss. People with mild or moderate losses can usually understand speech reasonably well when they are in a quiet room with only one person talking. However, they have difficulty when more than one person is talking at once, or when background noise or reverberation are present. People with severe or profound losses usually have difficulty even when listening to a single talker in a quiet room and they generally have severe problems when background noise is present. Hence their ability to understand speech relies heavily on lip reading and on the use of context.

There has been considerable controversy in the literature about the reasons for these difficulties in understanding speech. Some researchers have suggested that the difficulties arise primarily from reduced audibility; absolute thresholds are higher than normal, so the amount by which speech is above threshold, and the proportion of the speech spectrum that is above threshold, are both less than for normal listeners (Humes, Dirks and Kincaid, 1987; Zurek and Delhorne, 1987; Lee and Humes, 1993). In other words, it is argued that the difficulties occur mainly because part of the speech cannot be heard at all. Other researchers (Plomp, 1978; 1986; Dreschler and Plomp, 1980; 1985; Glasberg and Moore, 1989) have argued that the difficulty in understanding speech arises at least partly from reduced ability to discriminate sounds that are well above the absolute threshold. Many of the problems of discrimination have been reviewed in earlier chapters. According to this point of view, even if speech is amplified so that it is audible, the hearing-impaired person will still have problems in understanding speech.

The evidence reviewed below indicates that, for mild losses, audibility is the single most important factor. However, for severe to profound losses, poor discrimination of suprathreshold (audible) stimuli is also of major importance.

The magnitude of the noise problem

The issue considered next is: how much worse than normal are hearing-impaired people in their ability to understand speech in noise? This is often quantified by estimating the speech-to-noise ratio required to achieve a certain degree of intelligibility, such as 50% correct. This ratio is called the *speech reception threshold* (SRT) and it is usually expressed in dB. The higher the SRT, the poorer is performance. For many of the common speech materials used, and especially for sentence lists (Bench and Bamford, 1979; Plomp and Mimpen, 1979; Nilsson, Soli and Sullivan, 1994), the percent correct varies quite rapidly with changes in speech-to-noise ratio. For example, if the speech-to-noise ratio is set to a value giving about 50% correct, increasing the ratio by 1 dB typically gives an increase in percent correct of 7 to 19%. Correspondingly, even small differences in SRT between normally hearing and hearing-impaired listeners indicate substantial differences in the ability to understand speech in noise.

Plomp (1994) reviewed several studies which measured the SRT for sentences presented in a continuous background noise. The SRT was defined as the speech-to-noise ratio in dB required for 50% of sentences to be identified completely correctly. The noise had the same long-term average spectrum as the speech; such noise is referred to as *speech-shaped noise*. For high noise levels, people with cochlear hearing loss had higher SRTs than normally hearing people. The increase in SRT varied from about 2.5 dB for people with mild hearing losses caused by noise exposure or associated with ageing, to about 7 dB for people with moderate to severe losses caused by Ménière's syndrome or by unknown pathologies. An elevation in SRT of 2.5 dB is sufficient to create a substantial loss of intelligibility in difficult listening situations.

The elevation in SRT can be much greater when a fluctuating background noise or a single competing talker is used instead of a steady noise. Normally hearing subjects are able to take advantage of temporal and spectral 'dips' in the interfering sound to achieve a much lower SRT than when steady background noise is used (Duquesnoy, 1983; Festen and Plomp, 1990; Hygge, Rönnberg, Larsby et al., 1992; Baer and Moore, 1994; Moore, Glasberg and Vickers, 1995; Peters, Moore and Baer, 1998). For them, the SRT when the background is a single talker is 7 to 18 dB lower than when the background is speech-shaped noise. People with cochlear hearing loss are less able than normally hearing people to take advantage of the temporal and spectral dips. For the former, SRTs are not greatly different for a steady noise background and a single talker background (Duquesnoy, 1983; Festen and Plomp, 1990; Hygge, Rönnberg, Larsby et al., 1992; Peters, Moore and Baer, 1998). Hence, when the background is a single talker, the SRT is 12 dB or more higher for people with cochlear damage than for normally hearing people. This represents a very large deficit.

Finally, as described in Chapter 7, people with cochlear hearing loss are less able than normally hearing people to take advantage of spatial separation of the target speech and the interfering sound(s). This can lead to a further elevation in SRT, relative to that found for normally hearing subjects, of 5-7 dB.

In summary, in some listening situations common in everyday life, such as trying to listen to one person when another person is talking, people with cochlear hearing loss may require speech-to-background ratios 16 dB or more higher than normal (Duquesnoy, 1983). This represents a very substantial problem. However, the majority of laboratory experiments show a less severe problem as they have used as a background sound steady speech-shaped noise coming from the same direction as the target speech (or presented to the same ear via earphones).

The role of audibility

The articulation index

There is no doubt that audibility is crucial for speech intelligibility; if part of the speech spectrum is below the absolute threshold or is masked by background sound, then information is lost, and intelligibility will suffer to some extent. The *articulation index* (AI) provides a way of quantifying the role of audibility (French and Steinberg, 1947; Fletcher, 1952, Kryter, 1962; Pavlovic, 1984). In recent work, the term *speech intelligibility index* (SII) has been used instead of AI, but the underlying concepts are similar. The AI is based on the assumption that speech intelligibility is uniquely related to a quantity that, for a normally hearing person, can be calculated from the long-term average spectra of the speech and background sound reaching the ear of the listener. The frequency range from about 200 to 9000 Hz, which is the range most important for intelligibility, is divided into a number of bands. It is assumed that each band makes a certain contribution to speech intelligibility. That contribution is determined by the audibility of the speech in that band and by the relative importance of that band for intelligibility. The overall intelligibility is assumed to be related to a simple sum of the contributions from each band.

For a method using n bands, the AI is defined by the equation:

$$AI = \sum_{i=1}^{n} I_i A_i$$

(8.1)

The values of A_i represent the *audibility* of the different bands. For example, A_9 indicates the proportion of the speech spectrum that is audible in the ninth band. The values of A_i can vary between 0 and 1. The values of A_i depend on the spectra of the speech and the background, and on the level in each band relative to the absolute threshold. The values of I_i represent the relative importance of each band. The values of I_i add up to one. The values of I_i vary depending on the nature of the speech material used, for example whether it is composed of single words or sentences (Pavlovic, 1987). For each band the value of A_i is multiplied by the value of I_i. This gives an estimate of the contribution of the ith band to intelligibility. The products are then summed across bands, as indicated by the Σ symbol.

It is usually assumed that the speech in each band covers a 30 dB range of levels when measured using 125 ms samples. The speech peaks, specified as the level exceeded 1% of the time, have levels 12 dB above the level corresponding to the root mean square (rms) value of the speech. The speech minima have levels 18 dB below this mean level. A_i is the proportion of the 30 dB dynamic range in the ith band that is above both the absolute threshold and the masked threshold imposed by the background sound. For example, if no noise is present and the rms level of the speech in the ninth band is N dB above the absolute threshold for that band, then the value of A_9 is $(N + 12)/30$. If $N = 10$, then $A_9 = 0.73$. If N is greater than 18 dB, then the speech in that band is fully audible, and the value of A_9 is set to 1.0. If N is less than -12 dB, then the speech is completely inaudible in that band and A_9 is set to 0.

The AI gives a measure of the proportion of the speech spectrum that is audible, but a measure where the relative weighting of different frequencies reflects the relative importance of those frequencies for speech intelligibility. An AI value of 1.0 indicates that *all* of the speech spectrum is audible. For a hearing-impaired person, a hearing aid that resulted in an AI of 1.0 would be completely effective in restoring the audibility of speech. This would not ensure that the speech was intelligible. Indeed, sometimes the application of sufficient amplification to maximise the AI results in lower intelligibility of speech than when less amplification is used (Rankovic, 1991). However, achieving an AI of 1.0 would at least mean that intelligibility was not limited by part of the speech spectrum being below the absolute threshold. If a hearing aid gave an AI value less than 1.0, then intelligibility *might* be improved by increasing the amplification over the frequency range where part of the speech spectrum was inaudible.

To predict actual intelligibility scores, the empirical relationship between the value of the AI and intelligibility must first be determined for the specific speech material used and with a representative group of normally hearing subjects. This gives the 'intelligibility-articulation transfer function' (Fletcher, 1952). Provided the subjects in a given experiment have a similar amount of training to the subjects used to determine the transfer function, the transfer function can then be used to predict intelligibility from the AI. For clearly articulated sentence materials, an AI of 0.7 gives near-perfect (98%) intelligibility and an AI of 0.5 still gives scores above 90% correct. For nonsense syllables, an AI of 0.7 gives about 90% correct, and an AI of 0.5 gives about 70% correct (ANSI, 1969).

Use of the AI to predict speech intelligibility for the hearing impaired

Several researchers have examined the question of whether the AI can be used to predict speech intelligibility for hearing-impaired listeners. Obviously, in this case, the absolute thresholds of the individual listeners must be used in calculating the values of A_i. If the AI is successful in this respect, without any modification, this would imply that audibility is the main factor limiting intelligibility. While a few researchers have reported accurate predictions using the unmodified AI (Aniansson, 1974; Lee and Humes, 1993), most studies have shown that speech intelligibility is worse than would be predicted by the AI (Fletcher, 1952; Dugal, Braida and Durlach, 1978; Pavlovic, 1984; Pavlovic, Studebaker and Sherbecoe, 1986; Smoorenburg, 1992), especially for listeners with moderate or severe losses. The predictions are often quite accurate for those with mild losses.

An example of the results of this type of experiment is given in Figure 8.1; the data are from Pavlovic (1984). The speech materials were word lists presented under various conditions of filtering (broadband, lowpass and highpass) either with or without background white noise at a speech-to-noise ratio of 10 dB. Sixteen subjects with noise-induced hearing loss were used. For the eight subjects with the mildest losses (thresholds better than 50 dB HL at 4000 Hz), the mean scores across subjects for the eight different conditions, indicated by the numbers in the left panel of the figure, are close to the predictions based on the AI (solid curve). For the eight subjects with more severe losses (thresholds 55 dB HL or worse at 4000 Hz), the mean scores, shown in the right panel, fall consistently below the predicted values.

Overall, the results from studies using the AI suggest that, although audibility is of major importance, it is not the only factor involved, at least for people with moderate to severe cochlear losses. Supra-threshold discrimination abilities also need to be taken into account.

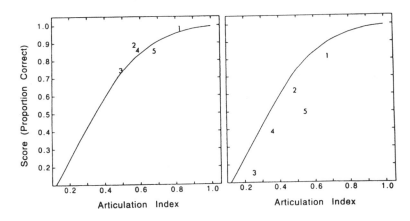

Figure 8.1: Results of Pavlovic (1984) comparing speech recognition scores of hearing-impaired subjects with predictions based on the AI. Each number represents the mean score across subjects for a specific condition of filtering/background noise. For subjects with mild losses, the predictions are accurate (left panel); for subjects with more severe losses, the obtained scores fall below the predicted values (right panel)

Additionally, it should be noted that the AI does not give accurate predictions of speech intelligibility under conditions where the background noise is fluctuating (e.g. when there is a single background talker) or when reverberation is present.

The intelligibility of speech in noise at high overall levels

Another way of evaluating the importance of audibility is to measure the SRT in noise as a function of overall noise level. If the performance of hearing-impaired subjects is limited by part of the speech spectrum being below absolute threshold, then the SRT, expressed as a speech-to-noise ratio, should decrease progressively with increasing noise level; as the noise level is increased, the speech level also has to be increased, and so more and more of the speech spectrum should lie above absolute threshold. Furthermore, the SRT for hearing-impaired subjects should approach that for normally hearing subjects at sufficiently high noise levels.

One study, using 20 elderly subjects with mild hearing losses (mean threshold about 20 dB HL at medium frequencies, increasing to 40 dB HL at 4000 Hz) reported results consistent with these predictions (Lee and Humes, 1993). However, the results of most other studies have not shown the predicted pattern: the SRT for hearing-impaired subjects remains approximately constant for noise levels above a certain value, and the SRT at high noise levels remains greater for hearing-impaired than for normally hearing subjects (Plomp, 1978, 1986, 1994; Smoorenburg, 1992).

There is, however, a difficulty in interpreting these results. For normally hearing people, the intelligibility of speech in noise decreases somewhat at high overall levels (Fletcher, 1953). This may happen partly because the auditory filters become broader with increasing level, as described in Chapter 3. The SRTs for hearing-impaired subjects tested at high noise levels have often been compared with SRTs measured at lower noise levels using normally hearing subjects. The discrepancy between the results for the hearing-impaired and the normally hearing subjects would be less if the normally hearing subjects were tested at higher levels. However, the effect of level is probably not sufficient to explain all of the difference in SRTs between normal and hearing-impaired listeners. Overall, these results lead to the same conclusions as those derived from studies using the AI. For people with moderate to severe losses, factors other than audibility contribute to their relatively poor ability to understand speech in noise.

Comparison of detection and recognition for speech in noise

Turner, Fabry, Barrett and Horwitz (1992) measured psychometric functions (percentage correct as a function of signal level) for the detection and recognition of stop consonants (p, t, k, b, d, g) followed by the vowel 'a' (as in 'Father') presented in white noise. They used two normally hearing subjects and three subjects with 'flat' moderate cochlear loss. They found that *detection* of the consonants occurred at the same speech-to-noise ratio for the normal and hearing-impaired subjects. However, for a given level of *recognition*, the hearing-impaired subjects required higher speech-to-noise ratios. They concluded that 'the poorer-than-normal speech recognition in noise exhibited by some hearing-impaired listeners is not due to a deficit in detecting the speech signal in noise. Instead, their poorer speech recognition performance in noise is due to their inability to efficiently utilise audible speech cues.' Some caution is needed, however, in drawing strong conclusions from these results. Detection can be based on audibility of a very limited part of the spectrum of the speech, but recognition of speech requires information to be audible over a wider frequency range.

The intelligibility of speech in quiet at high overall levels

As described earlier, hearing-impaired people with mild-to-moderate cochlear hearing losses do not generally have difficulty in understanding connected discourse in a quiet non-reverberant room. However, they may have some difficulty for isolated nonsense syllables. Subjects with severe losses can have considerable difficulty with speech in quiet. Turner and Robb (1987) tried to determine whether this difficulty could be explained in terms of audibility. They studied the identification of synthetic consonant-vowel syllables, composed of one of the six stop consonants (b, d, g, p, t, k) followed by the vowel 'a' (as in Father). A model of filtering in the peripheral auditory system was used to estimate the portion of the speech spectrum that was above the threshold of audibility for a given presentation level. Several presentation levels were used for each subject. They tested four normally hearing subjects and five subjects with moderate-to-severe hearing losses.

For the normally hearing subjects, recognition improved monotonically as the audible portion of the stimulus increased, and performance was perfect when most of the spectrum was above threshold. For four out of the five hearing-impaired subjects, recognition scores were consistently lower than for the normally hearing subjects at a given level of audibility. For these subjects, scores remained below 100%, even in cases where audibility was close to 100%. For the remaining subject, the hearing loss at low frequencies was too severe for even 50% audibility to be achieved. Overall, these results strongly suggest that reduced audibility is not sufficient to explain the relatively poor consonant recognition of the hearing-impaired subjects. It is noteworthy, however, that even presentation levels of 100 dB SPL were not sufficient to provide 100% audibility for subjects with severe losses (although appropriate frequency-dependent amplification could ensure 100% audibility at overall levels below 100 dB SPL).

Simulation of hearing loss by selective filtering (frequency-dependent attenuation)

Yet another approach for studying the effects of audibility is to subject the stimuli to frequency-dependent attenuation (filtering) so as to imitate the effect of a hearing loss on audibility. Say, for example, that a hearing-impaired subject has absolute thresholds of 30, 40, 45, 50, 70 and 70 dB HL at 250, 500, 1000, 2000, 4000 and 6000 Hz, respectively. The filter would be designed to attenuate by 30 dB at 250 Hz, 40 dB at 500 Hz, 45 dB at 1000 Hz, etc. The filtered stimuli are presented to normally hearing subjects. The filtering has the effect of matching the audiogram for the impaired ear (listening to unfiltered stimuli) and for the normal ears (listening to filtered stimuli). If audibility is the main cause of difficulty in speech understanding experienced by the hearing-impaired subject, then performance should be similar for the hearing-impaired subject listening to unfiltered speech and normally hearing subjects listening to filtered speech.

Only a few studies have used this approach. Sher and Owens (1974) compared consonant recognition in quiet for subjects with hearing loss above 2000 Hz and for normally hearing subjects listening to stimuli that were low-pass filtered at 2040 Hz. The filtering did not exactly simulate the reduced audibility for the hearing-impaired subjects. There were no significant differences between the two groups either in overall scores or in the patterns of consonant confusion.

Walden, Schwartz, Montgomery and Prosek (1981) used eight subjects with unilateral hearing losses. Consonant recognition in quiet was compared between the two ears. However, rather than using filtering to match audiograms in the two ears, they matched loudness in the two ears using tones at a suprathreshold level (60 dB HL in the normal ear). This meant that the filtering/attenuation of the stimuli presented to the normal ear was less than would be required to match the audiograms in the two ears. Large individual differences were observed but, on average, consonant recognition scores were 21% lower for the impaired than for the normal ears. This happened despite the fact that the proportion of the speech that was above threshold was greater for the impaired than for the normal ears (because the filtering/attenuation for the normal ears was less than would be required to match audibility). This strongly suggests that some factor other than audibility contributed to the relatively poor performance for the impaired ears.

Fabry and Van Tasell (1986) used six subjects with unilateral cochlear loss, filtering the stimuli to match the audiograms of the normal and impaired ears. Several of the subjects had absolute thresholds that were normal or near-normal at low frequencies, but increased markedly at high frequencies. They measured the identification of consonant-vowel nonsense syllables in quiet. For two subjects, scores were similar for unprocessed stimuli presented to the impaired ear and filtered stimuli presented to the normal ear. Patterns of errors were also similar for the two ears. For three subjects, performance was better for the impaired than for the normal ears by an average of about 8%. This may have happened because of the unfamiliarity of the filtered stimuli presented to the normal ears. Another possibility is that, for speech in quiet, loudness recruitment can actually have a small beneficial effect by increasing the loudness of sounds presented at low sensation levels (Gatehouse and Haggard, 1987); see the next section for further discussion of this point. For the remaining subject, the score was 11% worse for the impaired ear than for the normal ear.

Unfortunately, there do not seem to have been any studies of this type examining the intelligibility of speech in noise. Thus, it is not known whether selective filtering to match the audibility of the speech in noise for normal and hearing-impaired listeners would produce equal performance for the two groups.

Simulation of hearing loss by masking

Another approach uses masking noise with normal listeners to simulate the effects of the elevated thresholds associated with hearing impairment. The noise is spectrally shaped so that the masked audiograms of the normal listeners match the unmasked audiograms of the hearing-impaired listeners. This technique has been used by a number of different investigators (Fabry and Van Tasell, 1986; Humes, Dirks and Kincaid, 1987; Zurek and Delhorne, 1987; Humes and Roberts, 1990; Dubno and Schaefer, 1992). In some studies, speech intelligibility performance for the noise-masked normal ears has been reasonably close to that of the hearing-impaired subjects whose absolute thresholds were simulated. However, this was not the case for a study performed by Needleman and Crandell (1995). They measured SRTs for sentences in noise using ten subjects with mild-to-moderate sensorineural hearing loss. Two normally hearing subjects were matched with each hearing-impaired subject, using spectrally shaped noise. The noise-masked normal subjects obtained significantly lower (better) SRTs than the hearing-impaired subjects. This suggests that factors other than reduced audibility were responsible for the relatively high SRTs of the hearing-impaired subjects.

Two problems with the technique of noise masking should be noted. Firstly, the technique is limited to the simulation of mild-to-moderate hearing losses; the simulation of severe losses would require unacceptably loud noise. Secondly, the technique does not simulate the loss of audibility alone. The noise also produces an effect resembling loudness recruitment (see Chapter 4). Indeed, some researchers have suggested that noise may be regarded as simulating the combined effects of threshold elevation and loudness recruitment (Humes and Roberts, 1990). However, the nature of the recruitment produced by background noise is probably different from that produced by cochlear hearing loss (Phillips, 1987). More generally, the background noise may affect not only the detection thresholds, but also the perception of suprathreshold sounds. This idea is supported by the observation that using masking noise to match the audiograms of normal and impaired listeners has greater effects on speech intelligibility than using frequency-dependent attenuation (Fabry and Van Tasell, 1986).

Comparison of speech intelligibility for conductive and cochlear losses

Conductive hearing loss has the effect of attenuating sounds, reducing their effective levels, but it does not produce any substantial changes in the perception or discrimination of sounds that are presented at levels well above threshold. Therefore, comparisons of performance between people with conductive and cochlear losses of similar magnitude can provide some insight into the role of supra-threshold factors in cochlear hearing loss. Gatehouse and Haggard (1987) measured the intelligibility of isolated words in quiet as a function of presentation level, using subjects with 'pure' sensorineural losses of varying severity (presumably mainly cochlear losses) and subjects with varying degrees of conductive loss (sometimes in combination with sensorineural loss). They showed that, for a given degree of hearing loss, the results depended on overall level. At low stimulus levels, subjects with conductive loss showed poorer abilities to understand speech in quiet than subjects with cochlear loss; at high levels the reverse was true.

They interpreted their results as indicating a beneficial effect of loudness recruitment (in subjects with cochlear losses) for stimuli that are at low sensation levels; the recruitment has the effect of increasing the loudness of the speech, making the speech information more usable. However, at high levels, the benefit of recruitment is offset by the poor suprathreshold discrimination abilities of those with cochlear loss, so they perform more poorly than those with conductive loss. Gatehouse and Haggard emphasised that the beneficial effect of recruitment at low levels is only observed for speech in quiet. For speech in noise, people with cochlear loss perform more poorly than people with conductive loss, even at low presentation levels.

Conclusions on the role of audibility

Taken together, the results reviewed above strongly suggest that one or more factors other than audibility contribute to the difficulties of speech perception experienced by those with moderate or greater cochlear losses. This is especially true in situations where the stimuli are presented at high levels and/or in background noise. In other words, the difficulties arise partly from abnormalities in perception of sounds that are above the threshold of audibility. For those with mild losses, audibility is probably the dominant factor.

Correlation between psychoacoustic abilities and speech perception

Assuming that the speech perception difficulties of people with moderate or greater cochlear losses are partly caused by abnormalities in the perception of sounds that are above the threshold for detection, the question naturally follows: what psychoacoustical factors have the most influence on speech intelligibility. One method for studying this problem is to examine statistical relationships between measures of these abilities in hearing-impaired subjects. Typically, subjects have been given a battery of psychoacoustical and speech perceptual tests. Ideally, a large number of subjects should be tested (for statistical validity), the subjects should be given practice on each test until their performance is stable, and sufficient data should be gathered to give a reliable and accurate score on each test. Unfortunately, this would take an enormous amount of time and, in practice, compromises are inevitable. Either a large number of subjects can be tested, but with little time for practice on each test or for the execution of each test, or fewer subjects can be tested, with each given more training and more time per test.

Several researchers have conducted correlational studies (Dreschler and Plomp, 1980; 1985; Patterson, Nimmo-Smith, Weber et al., 1982; Tyler, Summerfield, Wood et al., 1982; Festen and Plomp, 1983; Horst, 1987; Glasberg and Moore, 1989; Van Rooij and Plomp, 1990; Lutman, 1991). Most studies have measured SRTs in noise and have assessed whether the SRTs can be 'accounted for' (in a statistical sense) by performance on various psychoacoustic tests. If the results of a given psychoacoustic test are highly correlated with the results of a measure of speech perception, then one might argue that the variations in performance on the speech perception test can be 'accounted for' by the variations on the psychoacoustic test. On the other hand, if performance on the two tests has a very low correlation, then some factor(s) other than that specific psychoacoustical measure must account for variability in the results of the speech perception test. Of course, causal relations cannot be inferred from correlations. A correlation between two measures does not necessarily imply that one causes the other.

The correlational studies indicate that a substantial part of the variability in SRTs is not explained by absolute thresholds. Most studies also agree that suprathreshold abilities such as frequency selectivity (Horst, 1987) or temporal resolution (Tyler, Summerfield, Wood et al., 1982) can account for a significant proportion of the variance in the SRTs. However, the effects of these variables are difficult to separate from the effects of absolute threshold.

Glasberg and Moore (1989) tested nine subjects with unilateral cochlear hearing loss; performance using the normal ear acted as a control for performance using the impaired ear, and the normal ear was compared with the impaired ear both at equal SL and at equal SPL. One possible drawback of using such subjects is that the impaired ear may become 'lazy' or 'neglected' in some sense, giving poorer discrimination abilities than might be expected from the pure-tone audiogram (Hood, 1984; Moore, Vickers, Glasberg et al., 1997). In addition, the pathologies producing unilateral loss may not be typical of hearing losses in general. Hence, Glasberg and Moore also tested six subjects with bilateral losses of cochlear origin. They measured SRTs in quiet and in two levels (60 and 75 dB SPL) of a noise with the same long-term average spectrum as the speech. They also measured performance on a variety of psychoacoustic tests, which were generally conducted at three centre frequencies: 0.5, 1.0 and 2.0 kHz. Most subjects had absolute thresholds for their impaired ears in the range 40 to 60 dB HL at these frequencies, but a few had thresholds as low as 30 dB HL or as high as 80 dB HL at one of the test frequencies.

The SRTs were higher for the impaired than for the normal ears, both in quiet and in noise. The elevation in quiet could be largely accounted for by the higher absolute thresholds for the impaired ears. Taking the results for all ears together, the SRT in quiet was highly correlated with the mean absolute threshold at 0.5, 1 and 2 kHz (r = 0.96, p < 0.001). For the impaired ears only, the corresponding correlation was r = 0.82 (p < 0.001).

The level of the 75 dB noise was sufficient to raise the SRTs well above those measured in quiet, and, at this noise level, the SRTs were higher for the impaired ears than for the normal ears. The mean SRT in the 75 dB noise, expressed as a speech-to-noise ratio, was –0.9 dB for the normal ears. For the impaired ears of the subjects with unilateral impairments the corresponding mean SRT was 7.1 dB. Thus the impaired ears required, on average, an 8 dB higher speech-to-noise ratio to achieve 50% intelligibility. For the subjects with bilateral impairments the mean SRT was 1.3 dB, which is 2.2 dB higher than normal. Taking the results for all ears together, the SRTs were correlated with the mean absolute threshold at 0.5, 1 and 2 kHz (r = 0.74, p < 0.001). For the impaired ears only the correlation reduced to r = 0.56 (p < 0.01). These correlations are lower than those found between the SRTs in quiet and the absolute thresholds. This indicates that, for noise levels sufficient to raise the SRT well above that measured in quiet, a significant proportion of the variance in the SRTs was not accounted for by variations in absolute threshold.

Although the SRTs in the 75 dB noise were correlated with the mean absolute thresholds at 0.5, 1 and 2 kHz, they were more highly correlated with three measures of supra-threshold discrimination. These measures were the frequency discrimination of pure tones, the frequency discrimination of complex tones, and the threshold for detecting temporal gaps in bands of noise. The higher correlations were found both for the results of all ears and for the impaired ears only. This is consistent with the hypothesis that, in high levels of background noise, the ability to understand speech is determined more by supra-threshold discrimination abilities than by absolute sensitivity.

Ching, Dillon and Byrne (1997) attempted to determine the importance of psychoacoustical factors for speech recognition after the effects of audibility had been taken into account. To do this, they presented speech in quiet over a wide range of levels and under various conditions of filtering. For each level and condition, the articulation index was calculated (they called it the speech intelligibility index, SII) and the number of key words in sentences that were correctly identified was measured. The results for eight normally hearing subjects were used to determine the transfer function relating the speech scores to the values of the SII. Twenty-two hearing-impaired subjects were tested. The speech scores for these subjects were expressed as *deviations* from the values predicted from the SII. These deviations represent the extent to which speech scores are better or worse than expected for a given amount of audibility of the speech. The deviations of the speech scores from the predicted values at high sensation levels were significantly correlated with a measure of frequency selectivity at 2 kHz (obtained using a notched-noise masker) and with a measure of temporal resolution (Zwicker, 1980).

Overall, the results of studies using the correlational approach have been somewhat inconclusive. They have provided evidence that the intelligibility of speech in noise for subjects with moderate or greater cochlear losses is influenced by suprathreshold discrimination abilities but they have not provided a clear indication of the relative importance of the various psychoacoustic factors that might be involved.

Assessing the effects of frequency selectivity on vowel and consonant perception

Some researchers have attempted to relate measures of frequency selectivity in specific frequency regions to the intelligibility of speech sounds for which important information is carried in those frequency regions. This more focused approach can yield useful insights into the importance of frequency selectivity for speech perception.

Consonant perception

Preminger and Wiley (1985) measured psychophysical tuning curves (see Chapter 3) for a 500 Hz signal and a 4000 Hz signal in subjects with cochlear hearing loss of various configurations. Losses were classified as high-frequency, flat, or low-frequency; there were two subjects in each group. The test stimuli were consonant-vowel syllables which were categorised into three groups on the basis of the predominant spectral energy in the consonant parts of the sounds; the three groups were low frequency (e.g. w, b, m, l), high frequency (e.g. t, d, k, z, s), and diffuse (e.g. v, f). The subjects with high-frequency loss had broadened PTCs at 4000 Hz, but normal PTCs at 500 Hz. These subjects achieved higher performance for low-frequency consonants than for high-frequency consonants. The subjects with flat hearing losses showed almost no frequency selectivity at 4000 Hz (the PTCs were 'flat') and they both performed poorly at identifying high-frequency consonants. One subject also had a very broad PTC at 500 Hz, and that subject performed poorly at identifying low-frequency consonants. The other subject showed some tuning at 500 Hz and achieved better identification of low-frequency consonants. For the subjects with low-frequency loss, the relation between PTC tuning and consonant identification was not so clear.

Thibodeau and Van Tasell (1987) estimated frequency selectivity at 2000 Hz by measuring the percentage correct detection of a 2000 Hz sinusoid as a function of the width of a spectral notch in a noise, the notch being centred at 2000 Hz. Two normally hearing subjects and seven subjects with moderate flat sensorineural (probably cochlear) losses were used. They also measured the ability to discriminate two synthetic stop-vowel syllables, 'di' and 'gi', which were identical except for spectral transitions (glides in the formant frequencies; see below for a description of formants) in the range 1800-2500 Hz. These spectral transitions provided the information necessary to distinguish the two consonants. Discrimination was measured both in broadband noise and in noise with a spectral notch around 2000 Hz. There was a significant correlation between scores on the two tasks; subjects with poorer frequency selectivity were also poorer at discriminating the syllables.

These results indicate that effects of reduced frequency selectivity on consonant discrimination can be observed when the information in the speech is restricted to a certain frequency range. Poor frequency selectivity is associated with poor consonant discrimination. However, natural speech contains information over a wide frequency range, making it much harder to show specific effects of reduced frequency selectivity.

Vowel perception

Vowel sounds are characterised by peaks in their spectra at certain frequencies. These peaks correspond to resonances in the vocal tract. They are called formants and are numbered, the lowest in frequency being called the first formant (F1), the next the second formant (F2), and so on. The pattern of frequencies at which the formants occur is thought to play an important role in determining the perceived vowel identity. The first three formants are the most important ones. The excitation pattern evoked by a vowel can be regarded as an internal representation of the spectral shape of the vowel. This is illustrated in Figure 8.2. The top panel shows the spectrum of a synthetic vowel 'I' (as in 'bid') on a linear frequency scale while the middle panel shows the same spectrum on an ERB scale (see Chapter 3). The bottom panel shows the excitation pattern for the vowel plotted on an ERB scale. This pattern was calculated as described in Chapter 3 for a normal auditory system.

Several aspects of the excitation pattern are noteworthy. Firstly, the lowest three peaks in the excitation pattern do not correspond to formant frequencies but rather to individual lower harmonics; these harmonics are resolved in the normal peripheral auditory system, and can be heard out as separate tones under certain conditions, as described in Chapter 3. Hence the centre frequency of the first formant is not directly represented in the excitation pattern; it must be inferred

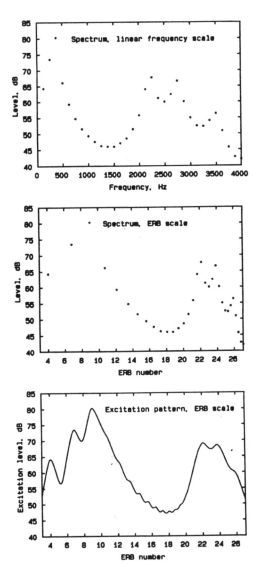

Figure 8.2: The top panel shows the spectrum of the synthetic vowel I, plotted on a linear frequency scale. The middle panel shows the spectrum plotted on an ERB scale. The bottom panel shows the excitation pattern for that vowel, calculated for a normal ear, and plotted on an ERB scale.

from the relative levels of the peaks corresponding to the individual lower harmonics.

A second noteworthy aspect of the excitation pattern is that the second, third and fourth formants, which are clearly separately visible in the original spectrum, are not well resolved. Rather, the second and third formants form a single prominence in the excitation pattern, with

only a small dip to indicate that two formants are present. The fourth
formant appears as a small 'shoulder' on the upper side of this prominence.

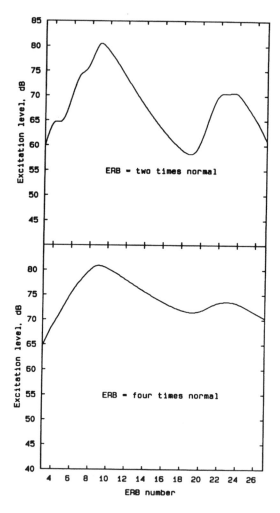

Figure 8.3: The excitation pattern for the same vowel as in Figure 8.2, but calculated
for an impaired ear with auditory filters two times broader than normal (top panel)
or four times broader than normal (bottom panel).

Figure 8.3 shows excitation patterns for the same vowel, but calculated for impaired auditory systems in which the auditory filters were
assumed to have ERBs twice as great as normal (top panel) or four times
as great as normal (bottom panel); these degrees of broadening are
typical of moderate and severe cochlear hearing losses, respectively. It is
obvious that spectral details are less well represented in these excitation

patterns; the peaks and dips corresponding to the lower harmonics are less clear, and the second, third and fourth formants are represented by only a single broad prominence. Indeed, in the lower panel, there is only a small, 2-3 dB, peak to indicate the presence of the second, third and fourth formants.

Given these considerations, one might expect that vowel identification would be less accurate in hearing-impaired subjects than in normally hearing subjects and that vowel identification would worsen progressively with decreasing frequency selectivity. There are at least some data to support this idea. Van Tasell, Fabry and Thibodeau (1987) measured confusions among seven synthetic steady state vowels for 10 normally hearing subjects and three subjects with cochlear hearing loss. Confusions were greater for the hearing-impaired than for the normal subjects. They also used some of the vowels as forward maskers; the threshold of a brief sinusoidal signal was measured at each harmonic frequency. These vowel masking patterns (VMPs) can be used to infer the internal representation of the vowels including the effects of suppression (see Chapter 3). The VMPs of the impaired subjects showed poorer preservation of the vowels' formant structure than did the VMPs of the normal subjects. Vowel identification accuracy appeared to be related mainly to the positions of peaks in the VMPs rather than to the levels of peaks or between-peak characteristics.

Turner and Henn (1989) also compared vowel identification with measures of frequency selectivity for two normally hearing subjects and three subjects with cochlear losses. For each of several frequencies of a sinusoidal signal, they measured the signal threshold in forward masking for a sinusoidal masker of variable frequency but fixed level of 95 dB SPL. The masking results were used to calculate the excitation patterns evoked by the vowels. They suggested that the more similar the excitation patterns of two vowels the more often they would be confused. This suggestion received some support when the measure of similarity was based on the entire shape of the calculated excitation patterns. However, it received stronger support when they used a measure that emphasised the similarities of spectral peak locations.

Although these experiments support the idea that reduced frequency selectivity can adversely affect vowel identification, everyday experience and studies using natural speech indicate that vowel identification by subjects with moderate cochlear hearing loss is often rather good. This may happen for at least two reasons. Firstly, the spectral differences between vowels are often very large, so that frequency selectivity has to be grossly impaired to prevent the differences being detected. Secondly, naturally produced vowels contain temporal cues (such as duration) as well as spectral cues and these cues may be used to compensate for the effects of reduced frequency selectivity.

The use of simulations to assess the importance of psychoacoustic factors in speech perception

Another approach to assessing the importance of suprathreshold discrimination abilities for speech perception is to simulate the effect of one specific aspect of hearing impairment by processing the stimuli in a way that mimics the effect of this aspect. The processed stimuli are then used in tests with normally hearing subjects. Provided the simulation is accurate, this makes it possible to study the effect of that aspect in isolation. This general strategy has been used to study the importance of three psychoacoustical factors: loudness recruitment combined with threshold elevation, frequency selectivity, and temporal resolution.

Simulations of loudness recruitment combined with threshold elevation

The effects of loudness recruitment combined with threshold elevation can be simulated by splitting the signal into a number of frequency bands and expanding the range of levels in each band before recombining the bands. Effectively, this simulation does the opposite of what happens in a normal cochlea, where stimuli are filtered along the BM, and fast-acting compression is applied at each CF (see Chapter 1). The goal of the simulation is to process the level of the stimulus in each band, on a moment-by-moment basis, so as to create loudness sensations in a normal ear that would resemble those produced in an impaired ear with recruitment. Say, for example, it is desired to simulate a hearing loss where the absolute threshold for a centre frequency of 1 kHz is 50 dB SPL, and 'normal' loudness is reached at 100 dB SPL. If the momentary level in the frequency band around 1 kHz is 50 dB SPL, then the signal in that band is attenuated by about 50 dB, so that its momentary level is close to the absolute threshold for normal hearing, i.e. roughly 0 dB SPL. If the momentary level is 100 dB or higher, no attenuation is applied; the signal level is unchanged. If the momentary level is at an intermediate value, say 75 dB SPL, then it is attenuated by an intermediate amount, 25 dB in this example.

Villchur (1974) used a three-band system to process speech so as to simulate the effects of recruitment associated with severe hearing loss. The stimulus in each band was processed using a fast-acting expander. Subjects with unilateral hearing impairments judged processed stimuli presented to their normal ear to sound 'similar' or 'very similar' to unprocessed stimuli presented to their impaired ear. The intelligibility of the processed speech was not measured in formal tests. However, Villchur concluded that recruitment is a sufficient cause for loss of intelligibility in cases of severe hearing loss.

In a later study (Villchur, 1977) he used a 16-band system, with computer-controlled attenuators to achieve expansion of the range of levels in each band. A severe sloping hearing loss was simulated. The intelligibility of speech in quiet at a level of 94 dB was adversely affected by the processing, both for isolated words and for sentences. The intelligibility of words and sentences in white noise was also adversely affected by the processing, the percentage correct decreasing from about 69% to 50%. An even greater effect was found for speech in speech-shaped noise.

Duchnowski (1989; Duchnowski and Zurek, 1995) used digital signal processing to implement a 14-band system. In one experiment, the processing was adjusted to simulate the hearing losses of the subjects tested by Zurek and Delhorne (1987); these subjects had mild-to-moderate hearing losses. The test stimuli were consonant-vowel (CV) syllables, presented in quiet and in various levels of speech-shaped noise. Generally, the pattern of results obtained using the simulation with normally hearing subjects matched the pattern obtained for the impaired subjects of Zurek and Delhorne. Thus, for these subjects, the threshold elevation and associated loudness recruitment appear sufficient to account for their difficulties in understanding speech.

In a second experiment, the hearing loss of subjects with more severe losses was simulated. The stimuli were amplified either by a constant amount across frequency (a 'flat' frequency-gain characteristic) or by an amount that increased with frequency (high-frequency emphasis). When the flat frequency-gain characteristic was used, the pattern of results from the impaired subjects closely matched the results from the normal subjects listening to the processed stimuli. However, when high-frequency emphasis was employed, the impaired subjects generally performed more poorly than their normal counterparts listening to processed stimuli. This suggests that some factor other than threshold elevation and loudness recruitment contributed to the speech perceptual problems of the hearing-impaired subjects.

Moore and Glasberg (1993) used digital signal processing to implement a 13-band system. They simulated a flat moderate hearing loss (condition R2), a flat severe hearing loss (condition R3) and a loss that increased with frequency, being mild at low frequencies and severe at high frequencies (condition RX). They also included a control condition (R1) in which stimuli were processed through the simulation, but no expansion of the range of levels was applied in any frequency band.

Moore and Glasberg also assessed whether there are deleterious effects of recruitment after the hearing loss has been corrected as far as possible by linear amplification, as would be used in a conventional hearing aid. To do this, they ran a set of conditions in which the stimuli in conditions (2) - (4) were subjected to the frequency-dependent gain recommended by the NAL revised procedure (Byrne and Dillon, 1986; see Chapter 9 for more details). This gain is appropriate for speech presented at a moderate conversational level of about 65 dB SPL. This gave three more conditions, R2+, R3+ and RX+.

For speech in quiet, the simulation produced, as expected, a reduction in the ability to understand low-level speech. The level of speech required for 50% intelligibility was 16 dB SPL in condition R1, 64 dB in condition R2, 79 dB in condition R3, and 53 dB in condition RX. However, speech at sufficiently high levels was highly intelligible in all conditions. Also, linear amplification according to the NAL prescription reduced the 50% intelligibility points to less than 50 dB SPL for all conditions, and gave high intelligibility for speech at normal conversational levels. Thus, linear amplification was rather effective in improving the intelligibility of speech in quiet, although it did not allow speech to be both intelligible and comfortable over a wide range of sound levels; speech with input levels above about 70 dB SPL was judged to be unpleasantly loud in the conditions involving linear amplification.

For speech presented at a fixed input level of 65 dB SPL, against a background of a single competing talker, simulation of hearing loss produced substantial decrements in performance. This is illustrated in Figure 8.4 for the case where the background speech had a level of 71 dB SPL. Performance was almost perfect for condition R1, but not for the conditions simulating threshold elevation and loudness recruitment. The speech-to-background ratios in conditions R2 and RX had to be 11-13 dB higher than in condition R1 to achieve similar levels of performance. Linear amplification according to the NAL prescription improved performance markedly for the conditions simulating flat losses, but was less effective for the condition simulating a sloping loss. Performance in this condition remained well below that in the control condition, even after linear amplification.

In a second study, Moore, Glasberg and Vickers (1995) used similar processing conditions (R1, R2, R3 and RX) but the speech was presented in a background of speech-shaped noise instead of a single competing talker. The input level of the speech was fixed at 65 dB SPL, whereas the level of the background noise varied from 65 to 74 dB SPL. The speech in condition R3 was inaudible. For conditions R2 and RX, the speech-to-noise ratios had to be up to 6 dB higher than in the control condition (R1, unprocessed stimuli) to achieve similar levels of performance. When linear amplification according to the NAL prescription was applied before the simulation, performance improved markedly for conditions R2 and RX, and did not differ significantly from that for R1. For condition R3, performance with simulated NAL amplification remained below that for condition R1; the decrement in performance was equivalent to about a 1 dB change in speech-to-noise ratio.

The results obtained using speech-shaped noise differ in two ways

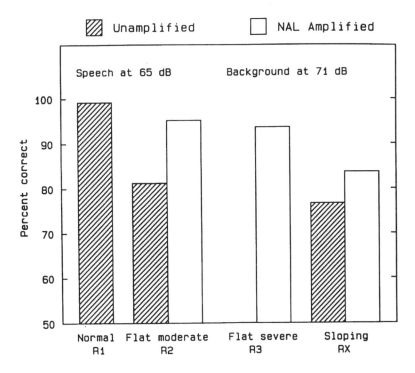

Figure 8.4: Comparison of percentage correct scores for the different conditions of Moore and Glasberg (1993), for a speech-to-background ratio of -6 dB. No score is shown for an unamplified condition R3, since the target speech was inaudible for that condition.

from the results obtained using a single talker as the interfering sound: firstly, the deleterious effects of the simulations were generally smaller with speech-shaped noise; secondly, linear amplification according to the NAL formula restored performance to normal for two of the three conditions tested (R2+ and RX+) using speech-shaped noise, whereas it did not when a single competing talker was used. In the remaining condition (R3+) the degradation in performance was significant, but was equivalent to a change of only 1 dB in speech-to-noise ratio.

The differences between the two sets of results can be understood in the following way. Normally hearing people can take advantage of spectral and temporal dips in a background of a single competing talker. Hence the speech-to-background ratio required to achieve a given level of performance is markedly lower than when the background is speech-shaped noise. However, 'dip listening' requires the ability to hear over a wide range of sound levels (a wide dynamic range). Consider as an example, a situation where the target speech has a level 10 dB lower than that of the interfering speech, and where the overall level is such that the interfering speech is loud but not uncomfortably so. The overall loudness is determined mainly by the levels of peaks in the interfering speech. In any given frequency band, the target speech may contain useful information at a level 40 dB below the peak level of the inter-fering speech (since for one voice the range of levels is about 30 dB - see the section on the AI). Such information may be audible during brief pauses in the interfering speech. Ideally, then, brief sounds should be audible and discriminable when their levels are 40 dB below the highest comfortable level.

Loudness recruitment, either real or simulated, reduces the range of levels over which sounds are both audible and comfortable. If the level of the speech is set so that the more intense parts of the speech are comfortably loud, the weaker parts may be inaudible. Hence, people with recruitment cannot exploit 'dip listening' as effectively as normally hearing people (Peters, Moore and Baer, 1998). When a background of speech-shaped noise is used, 'dip listening' is of much less importance, since the noise does not contain dips of sufficient magnitude or duration. Hence speech intelligibility depends more on the higher-level portions of the speech and these are less affected by reduced dynamic range. Furthermore, linear amplification, which ensures that the higher level portions of speech are clearly audible, is effective in compensating for the simulated recruitment, except when the hearing loss is severe (condition R3).

Moore, Glasberg, Vickers and Baer (1997) presented simulations of hearing impairment to the normal ears of subjects with moderate to severe unilateral cochlear hearing loss. The intelligibility of speech in quiet and in background sounds was compared with that obtained for the impaired ears using unprocessed stimuli. The results of loudness matches between the two ears were used to tailor a simulation of threshold elevation combined with loudness recruitment individually for each subject. The subjects reported that the simulation produced sounds with appropriate loudness and dynamics but the processed speech in the normal ear appeared markedly more clear than the unprocessed speech in the impaired ear. Performance for the impaired ears in identifying speech in quiet and in background sounds was markedly worse than for the normal ears using the simulation of threshold elevation and loudness recruitment. Moore et al. suggested that the relatively poor results for the impaired ears might be caused partly by a form of 'neglect' that is specific to subjects with unilateral or asymmetric loss (Hood, 1984). This idea was supported by results obtained using bilaterally hearing-impaired subjects, with similar amounts of hearing loss to the unilaterally hearing-impaired subjects. The speech identification scores of the bilaterally impaired subjects were markedly better than for the impaired ears of the unilaterally hearing-impaired subjects. However, the scores for identifying speech in background noise were still somewhat worse than those for the normal ears listening to the simulation of threshold elevation and loudness recruitment.

In one respect, the results of the simulations differ from those obtained using subjects who have 'real' cochlear hearing loss. When threshold elevation and loudness recruitment are simulated using normally hearing subjects, performance is markedly better when the interfering sound is a single talker than when it is speech-shaped noise. However, as described earlier, people with cochlear hearing loss often show little or no difference in intelligibility for these two backgrounds (Duquesnoy and Plomp, 1983; Festen and Plomp, 1990; Moore, Glasberg and Stone, 1991; Peters, Moore and Baer, 1998). This suggests that some factor other than recruitment contributes to the reduced ability of hearing-impaired people to 'listen in the dips'. A likely factor is reduced frequency selectivity, which may have especially strong effects on the ability to listen in spectral dips of the interfering sound (Baer and Moore, 1994).

In summary, the results of the simulations indicate that the reduced dynamic range associated with loudness recruitment can lead to difficulty in understanding speech in background sounds. When the background sound is a steady noise, the difficulty can be effectively compensated by linear amplification of the type commonly used in hearing aids, except when the loss is severe. When the background sound is fluctuating, as for a single talker, the deleterious effects of the reduced dynamic range are greater and are not fully compensated by linear amplification.

Simulations of reduced frequency selectivity

To simulate reduced frequency selectivity, the spectra of stimuli are 'smeared' or 'smoothed' on a moment-by-moment basis, so that the excitation pattern produced in a normal ear resembles (albeit crudely in many of the simulations) the pattern that would be produced in an impaired ear using unprocessed signals. Several different techniques have been used to perform the spectral smearing. Early studies used analogue signal processing (Villchur, 1977; Summers and Al-Dabbagh, 1982; Summers, 1991). In more recent studies, digital signal-processing techniques have been used. An illustration of this type of processing is shown in Figure 8.5. A short segment of the signal is taken, and its spectrum is calculated using a mathematical technique called the *Fast Fourier Transform* (FFT). The resulting spectrum is then smeared or blurred so as to decrease the contrast between peaks and valleys in the spectrum. The modified spectrum is transformed back into a temporal waveform using an *Inverse Fast Fourier Transform* (IFFT). This is repeated for a series of overlapping segments, and the resulting processed segments are added together. Hence this is referred to as the overlap-add method (Allen, 1977). The method has been used in several studies (Celmer and Bienvenue, 1987; Howard-Jones and Summers, 1992; ter Keurs, Festen and Plomp, 1992; 1993; Baer and Moore, 1993; 1994).

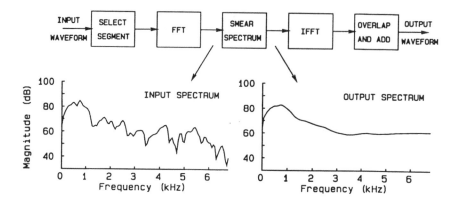

Figure 8.5: Schematic diagram of the sequence of operations used to perform spectral smearing. The upper part shows the overall sequence, while the lower part shows examples of short-term spectra at the input and output of the smearing process.

It should be noted that such spectral smearing does not simulate all of the effects of reduced frequency selectivity. Specifically, the time patterns at the outputs of the auditory filters are affected by reduced frequency selectivity in a way that is not reproduced by the simulations. Instead, the simulations alter the time patterns of the stimuli in a complex way that is a by-product of the specific processing used. Essentially, the simulations may be regarded as mimicking the consequences of reduced frequency selectivity in terms of place coding in the auditory system, but not in terms of temporal coding.

Ter Keurs, Festen and Plomp (1992) smeared the spectrum of each segment in such a way as to simulate the effect of broadened auditory filters whose bandwidth was a constant proportion of the centre frequency. They smeared the spectrum of speech and noise separately and then added the speech and noise together. The SRT for speech in noise increased once the filter bandwidth used in the simulation was increased beyond about 23% of the centre frequency (roughly double the normal bandwidth of the auditory filter). Vowel identification was affected more than consonant identification. In a second study (ter Keurs, Festen and Plomp, 1993) they compared the effects of the smearing using either speech-shaped noise or a single talker as the background sound. For both types of background, SRTs increased when the smearing bandwidth was increased. For unsmeared speech, SRTs were 5-7 dB lower when the background was a single talker than when it was speech-shaped noise. This difference decreased as the smearing bandwidth was increased. Hence, the effect of the spectral smearing on SRTs was greater for the speech masker than for the noise masker.

Baer and Moore (1993) measured the intelligibility of speech in quiet and in speech-shaped noise. Normally hearing subjects listened to sentence material that had been processed to simulate varying degrees of loss of frequency selectivity. When speech in noise was used, the speech was mixed with the noise prior to processing. The procedure for simulating impaired frequency selectivity used a realistic form of spectral smearing, based on measured characteristics of auditory filters in hearing-impaired people. It was based on a procedure that was previously validated using non-speech signals (Moore, Glasberg and Simpson, 1992). The stimuli were processed so that the excitation pattern produced in a normal ear, calculated over a short period of time, would resemble that found with unprocessed stimuli in an impaired ear.

Several different types of smearing were used, simulating specific degrees of broadening and asymmetry of the auditory filter. Sentences in quiet and in speech-shaped noise were smeared and presented to normally hearing listeners in intelligibility tests. Some of the results are illustrated in Figure 8.6. The intelligibility of speech in quiet (the three left-most bars in Figure 8.6) was hardly affected by spectral smearing, even for smearing that simulated auditory filters six times broader than normal. However, this probably reflects a ceiling effect, as scores were close to perfect in all conditions. The intelligibility of speech in noise was adversely affected by the smearing, especially for large degrees of smearing and at a low speech-to-noise ratio (–3 dB; see the three right-most bars in Figure 8.6). Simulation of asymmetrical broadening of the lower side of the auditory filter had a greater effect than simulation of asymmetrical broadening of the upper side, suggesting that upward spread of masking may be particularly important.

In a second study, Baer and Moore (1994) used a single competing talker as the background, instead of speech-shaped noise. The results were similar in form to those found using speech-shaped noise. Specifically, performance worsened with increasing smearing, and the worsening was greater at the more adverse speech-to-background ratio. The results agreed with those of ter Keurs, Festen and Plomp (1993) in showing that the deleterious effects of spectral smearing were greater for a speech masker than for a noise masker. Hence, the difference in masking produced by speech and noise maskers was less for spectrally smeared than for unprocessed stimuli. This is consistent with the finding noted earlier, that for normally hearing subjects SRTs are lower when the background is speech than when it is noise whereas, for hearing-impaired subjects, the difference is smaller or absent.

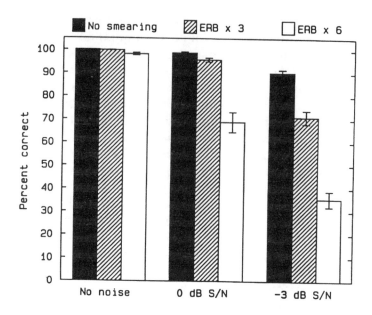

Figure 8.6: Results of Baer and Moore (1993) showing the percentage of key words correct for three amounts of spectral smearing and three different amounts of background noise. The three amounts of smearing were: no smearing (solid bars); simulation of auditory filters with bandwidths three times greater than normal (diagonally shaded bars); and simulation of auditory filters with bandwidths six times greater than normal (open bars). Error bars indicate +/– one standard error.

In summary, the results of experiments on spectral smearing suggest that reduced frequency selectivity does contribute significantly to the difficulties experienced by people with cochlear hearing loss in understanding speech in the presence of background sounds.

Simulation of the combined effects of threshold elevation, recruitment and reduced frequency selectivity

Nejime and Moore (1997) simulated the effect of loudness recruitment and threshold elevation together with reduced frequency selectivity. To implement the combined simulation they firstly applied the simulation of reduced frequency selectivity (as used by Baer and Moore, 1993) and then applied the simulation of threshold elevation combined with loudness recruitment (as used by Moore and Glasberg, 1993). In their first experiment, four conditions were simulated: a moderate flat loss with auditory filters broadened by a factor of three (B3R2); a moderate-to-severe sloping loss with auditory filters broadened by a constant factor of three (B3RX); and these conditions with linear amplification applied prior to the simulation processing (B3R2+, B3RX+). The amplification in these two latter conditions was similar to what might be used in a well-fitted linear hearing aid. For conditions B3R2 and B3RX, performance was markedly worse than for a control condition (normal hearing, condition R1) tested in a previous study. For conditions B3R2+ and B3RX+, linear amplification improved performance considerably. However, performance remained below that for condition R1 by between 5% and 19%. Thus, linear amplification did not fully compensate for the deleterious effects of the simulation.

In the second experiment of Nejime and Moore, the broadening of the auditory filters was made more realistic by making it a function of the absolute threshold at the centre frequency of the auditory filter; greater hearing loss was associated with a broader filter. Three different hearing losses were simulated: a moderate-to-severe sloping loss with variable broadening of the auditory filters (BXRX); the same moderate-to-severe sloping loss with linear amplification (BXRX+); and the same broadening of the auditory filters but without the simulation of loudness recruitment and threshold elevation (BX). For condition BXRX, performance was markedly worse than in condition R1, while performance in condition BX was somewhat worse than for condition R1. For condition BXRX+, linear amplification according to the NAL procedure improved performance to a large extent but it remained worse than for condition R1.

Comparison of the results with previous results using simulations only of recruitment and threshold elevation showed significantly poorer performance for the combined simulation. This was true both without and with linear amplification. The results suggest that the reduced frequency selectivity simulated by spectral smearing is a suprathreshold factor that is relatively unaffected by amplification and which combines roughly additively with the effects of loudness recruitment and threshold elevation.

Simulation of reduced temporal resolution

In Chapter 5, temporal resolution was described in terms of a four-stage model consisting of an array of bandpass filters (the auditory filters) each followed by a compressive non-linearity, a sliding temporal integrator and a decision device. It was argued that cochlear hearing loss can affect the first two stages, the filters and the non-linearity, but that it usually did not affect the last two. Cochlear hearing loss results in a broadening of the auditory filters and a reduction in the compressive non-linearity. The end result is that temporal resolution is reduced only for certain specific stimuli, namely those with slowly fluctuating envelopes. In some situations, temporal resolution may be poor simply because of the low sensation level of the stimuli for people with cochlear hearing loss.

The simulation of loudness recruitment described above effectively includes these effects; specifically, it models the effects of reduced sensation level and reduced compressive non-linearity. Indeed, as described in Chapter 5, simulation of loudness recruitment in this way results in poorer detection of temporal gaps in narrow bands of noise. One might question, therefore, whether it is appropriate to go any further in simulating the effects of abnormalities in temporal processing. However, some researchers have taken the approach of simulating the effects of reduced temporal resolution 'directly' by temporal smearing analogous to the spectral smearing used to simulate reduced frequency selectivity. Such work can be valuable because it provides a way of estimating the relative importance for speech intelligibility of temporal modulations at different rates.

Drullman, Festen and Plomp (1994) carried out a study of the effects of temporal envelope smearing on speech intelligibility. The study was not designed specifically as a simulation of reduced temporal resolution, but in effect the processing was equivalent to such a simulation. They split the input signal into a number of frequency bands covering the range 100-6400 Hz. The bands had widths of 0.25, 0.5 or 1 octave. The narrowest bandwidth corresponds roughly with the ERBs of normal auditory filters, while the wider bandwidths correspond roughly with the auditory filter bandwidths that might occur in people with moderate-to-severe cochlear losses. They extracted the envelope of the signal in each band and processed the envelope so as to smooth out rapid fluctuations. The envelope for each band was lowpass filtered with various cutoff frequencies. As the cut-off frequency was reduced, the envelope became more and more smeared in the time domain, simulating loss of temporal resolution. For all filtering bandwidths (0.25, 0.5 or 1 oct), the SRT of sentences in speech-shaped noise was almost unaffected by lowpass filtering the envelopes with cut-off frequencies of 64, 32 or 16 Hz; the SRT was elevated by only about one decibel relative to that for a control condition with no envelope filtering. However, lowpass filtering with cut-off frequencies of 8 or 4 Hz produced mean elevations in SRT of 2.4 and 5.6 dB relative to the control condition. Thus, removing very fast envelope fluctuations had little effect, but removing slow fluctuations led to impaired intelligibility. These results indicate that fluctuations of the envelopes of the filtered bands at rates of 16 Hz and above are relatively unimportant for speech intelligibility. Since most people with cochlear hearing loss can easily detect modulation at rates up to 16 Hz (see, for example, Figure 5.7), this suggests that reduced temporal resolution is not a factor limiting speech intelligibility for most people with cochlear hearing loss.

Hou and Pavlovic (1994) carried out a study that was aimed at directly simulating the effects of reduced temporal resolution in the auditory system. They first filtered the speech into 23 bands using simulated auditory filters with bandwidths corresponding to those found in normal ears. They then smeared the temporal envelope in each band using a sliding temporal integrator similar to that described in Chapter 5 for the model of temporal resolution (Moore, Glasberg, Plack et al., 1988; Plack and Moore, 1990). When the temporal integrator performed less smearing than the temporal integrator in the normal auditory system (see Chapter 5), the smearing had no effect on the intelligibility of nonsense syllables in quiet. When the temporal smearing was greater, small but significant decreases in intelligibility occurred. However, even when the smearing was about three times as large as that occurring in a normal auditory system, the decrease in intelligibility was only 5-10%.

The results of Hou and Pavlovic indicate that temporal smearing can produce reduced intelligibility of nonsense syllables in quiet. They argued that reduced temporal resolution in the impaired auditory system was probably as detrimental to speech recognition as reduced frequency selectivity. However, it remains unclear whether temporal smearing is an appropriate way to model reduced temporal resolution in hearing-impaired subjects. The temporal smearing of Hou and Pavlovic would lead to reduced temporal resolution for all types of stimuli whereas, as described in Chapter 5, reduced temporal resolution in people with cochlear hearing loss generally occurs only for stimuli at low SLs or with slowly fluctuating envelopes. In any case, the shape of the temporal integrator measured for hearing-impaired subjects is not usually markedly different from normal (Plack and Moore, 1991).

Conclusions

People with mild or moderate cochlear losses can usually understand speech reasonably well when they are in a quiet room with only one person talking. However, they have difficulty when more than one person is talking at once, or when background noise or reverberation are present. People with severe or profound losses usually have difficulty even when listening to a single talker in a quiet room and they generally have severe problems when background noise is present. The elevation of the SRT in noise, relative to the value for normally hearing subjects, is greater when the background sound is fluctuating (e.g. a single talker) than when it is a steady noise. This probably happens because people with cochlear hearing loss are less able than normally hearing people to take advantage of temporal and spectral dips in fluctuating background sounds. People with cochlear hearing loss are also less able than normally hearing people to exploit spatial separation between the target and interfering sounds.

The speech understanding difficulties of people with mild cochlear hearing losses can be accounted for primarily in terms of audibility. With suitable linear amplification, such people can usually understand speech almost as well as normally hearing people. However, for people with moderate-to-severe cochlear hearing losses, supra-threshold discrimination abilities also need to be taken into account. Although audibility is still of primary importance, it does not fully account for the difficulties experienced by such people.

It has proved difficult to determine the relative importance of different psychoacoustic factors that might affect speech intelligibility. However, evidence from a range of studies, including correlational studies, studies of the use of specific speech cues, and simulations, all indicates that reduced frequency selectivity plays a significant role. There is also evidence, mainly from simulations, that loudness recruitment is a significant factor. However, the most important aspect of loudness recruitment appears to be reduced dynamic range, rather than distorted loudness relationships.

Chapter 9
Hearing Aids

Introduction

Cochlear hearing loss can rarely be 'cured', although drugs can be of benefit in some cases; for a review of drug treatments, see Dobie (1997). Hearing aids are the primary method for alleviating problems associated with cochlear hearing loss. However, people with cochlear hearing loss frequently complain that their hearing aids are of limited benefit. They find that the aids are sometimes useful in helping them to hear weak sounds but that the aids do not help very much, if at all, when background noise is present. It seems clear that hearing aids are not like eyeglasses. A well-fitted pair of eyeglasses can give good vision if the problem is caused by poor focus of the image on the retina, as is usually the case. Hearing aids do not restore hearing to 'normal'. They can partially compensate for the loss of sensitivity produced by cochlear damage, but they do not compensate for the supra-threshold changes in perception caused, for example, by reduced frequency selectivity. This chapter reviews the capabilities and limitations of current hearing aids, and considers some ways in which hearing aids may be improved in the future. It also discusses methods of fitting hearing aids to suit the individual.

Restoration of audibility using linear amplification

The impossibility of fully restoring audibility using linear aids

The primary goal of most hearing aids is to restore audibility via frequency-selective amplification. Many hearing aids operate essentially as linear amplifiers; over most of their operating range they apply a gain that is independent of level. For example, an aid may amplify by 20 dB at 1 kHz, and that same gain is applied regardless of the input level. A 1 kHz sinusoid with an input level of 40 dB SPL would be amplified to a level of 60 dB SPL, whereas an input level of 80 dB SPL would be amplified to 100 dB SPL. In practice, most hearing aids incorporate some means for limiting the maximum output and if the limiter comes into operation the aid behaves in a non-linear manner; for example, significant harmonic and inter-modulation distortion may be produced (see Chapter 1). However, for convenience, aids that are normally used over the linear part of their operating range will be referred to as 'linear'.

It became apparent very soon after hearing aids first came into use that it was not practical to use linear amplification to compensate fully for the loss of audibility caused by cochlear hearing loss. The major factor preventing this was loudness recruitment and the associated reduced dynamic range. Say, for example, a person had a cochlear hearing loss of 60 dB at all frequencies. The highest comfortable level (HCL) for such a person would typically be around 90-100 dB HL. If the person had a hearing aid that fully compensated for the loss of audibility, the aid would apply a gain of 60 dB at all frequencies. However, that would mean that any sound with a level above about 40 dB HL would be amplified to a level exceeding the HCL. In practice, many sounds encountered in everyday life would become unpleasantly loud.

As mentioned above, most hearing aids incorporate a way of limiting their maximum output so as to avoid discomfort to the user. In early hearing aids, and in many current hearing aids, this is achieved by electronic peak clipping in the output stage of the aid. The voltage is prevented from exceeding a certain absolute value (either positive or negative), which results in the larger peaks in the electrical signal being clipped or flattened off; see Chapter 1, Figure 1.1, for an example of the effects of such clipping. Clipping introduces unpleasant-sounding distortion (Crain and Van Tasell, 1994) and, in practice, most users of hearing aids set the volume control to avoid clipping in everyday listening situations.

Prescriptive fitting rules for linear hearing aids

Even when hearing aids include output limiting, it has been found to be impractical to compensate fully for loss of audibility. Rather, various prescriptive rules have been developed that can be used to derive an appropriate frequency-gain characteristic from the pattern of hearing loss as a function of frequency (Lybarger, 1978; McCandless and Lyregard, 1983; Byrne and Dillon, 1986; Moore and Glasberg, 1998). These rules prescribe the amount of gain that is required as a function of frequency. Sometimes, suprathreshold measures such as the uncomfortable loudness level (ULL) or most comfortable level (MCL) are also taken into account. Such rules always prescribe less gain than the hearing loss at a given frequency. Typically, the rules prescribe a gain that is between one-third and one-half of the hearing loss. For example, if the hearing loss is 60 dB at 1 kHz, then the prescribed gain is between 20 and 30 dB.

The goal of most of these rules is to select a frequency-gain character-istic that will amplify speech so as to improve intelligibility while avoiding making speech uncomfortably loud. One rule that is quite widely used is the NAL(R) formula devised at the National Acoustics Laboratories of Australia (Byrne and Dillon, 1986). The rule works solely on the basis of the pure-tone audiogram. It was derived by dividing speech into a number of contiguous 1/3 octave bands or one-octave bands covering the range 250 to 6 kHz, and working out what gain would be required in each band to amplify the speech in that band to the MCL, assuming that the speech was at a normal conversational level (typically 65-70 dB SPL overall when the talker and listener are separated by about one metre). It should be noted that the user of a hearing aid is free to adjust the overall gain via the volume control on the aid. Hence, the main point of prescriptive rules, including NAL(R), is to select an appropriate *shape* for the frequency-gain characteristic. However, the NAL(R) formula prescribes a gain that is intended to corres-pond to the average gain actually used. The goal of the NAL(R) proced-ure seems very reasonable. Making each frequency band in speech equally loud can ensure that no single band contributes excessively to loudness. Thus the overall amplification can be increased, increasing the proportion of the speech spectrum that is audible while maintaining a comfortable loudness.

To check whether the NAL(R) procedure does actually meet its goal, Moore and Glasberg (1998) used the loudness model described in Chapter 4. They calculated specific loudness patterns evoked by a sound with a spectrum corresponding to the long-term average spectrum of speech (Byrne et al., 1994), assuming an overall speech level of 65 dB SPL. The specific loudness patterns were calculated for several hypothet-ical hearing losses, varying in severity and type (e.g. flat losses, losses increasing towards high frequencies, and so on). Specific loudness patterns were calculated both for the unamplified speech spectrum, and for speech spectra that had been subjected to frequency-selective ampli-fication according to various prescription rules, including NAL(R). In principle, the NAL(R) prescription should result in a specific loudness pattern that is flat (constant specific loudness) over the frequency range that is important for speech, namely 250 to 6000 Hz. However, Moore and Glasberg found that the specific loudness patterns were not flat; they usually showed a mid-frequency peak, with the specific loudness decreasing at higher frequencies. Moore and Glasberg proposed a new formula, the 'Cambridge' formula, which did lead to specific loudness patterns that were approximately flat, according to the loudness model. This formula calls for slightly less mid-frequency gain and slightly more high-frequency gain than the NAL(R) formula.

Although the various prescriptive rules do lead to different frequency-gain characteristics for a given hearing-impaired person, it has proved surprisingly difficult to demonstrate differences between the rules in terms of resulting speech recognition scores; for a review see Humes (1991). The intelligibility of speech in noise does not seem to be greatly affected by the shape of the frequency-gain characteristic, provided the amplification is sufficient to place most of the speech spectrum above absolute threshold. For example, Van Buuren, Festen and Plomp (1995) measured SRTs for speech in speech-shaped noise using a wide range of frequency-gain characteristics. These characteristics were chosen so that the average speech spectrum, after amplification, fell in the range from 5 dB above the absolute threshold to just below ULL. The SRTs were similar for most of the frequency-gain characteristics. However, performance was somewhat worse (SRTs were higher) when the amplified speech spectrum had high levels at low frequencies.

At first sight, these results appear to suggest that the frequency-gain characteristic is unimportant. However, in the study of Van Buuren et al., the speech was presented over a very restricted range of sound levels. A given frequency-gain characteristic might give satisfactory results over a small range of levels, but might be much less successful for speech covering a wide range of levels, such as occurs in everyday life. Say, for example, that a frequency-gain characteristic with low-frequency emphasis was used. The low-frequencies in the speech might be presented at a level just below the ULL, while the high frequencies might be only 5 dB above absolute threshold. If the overall level was increased, the low frequencies would become uncomfortably loud, whereas if the level was decreased by more than 5 dB, some of the high frequencies would become inaudible. In practice, it would be better to use a frequency-gain characteristic that placed speech with a moderate overall level more towards the middle of the listener's dynamic range at all frequencies. A formula such as the Cambridge formula does something close to that. If speech is at an equal comfortable level in all frequency bands, then increasing or decreasing the level of the speech by a *moderate* amount will not lead to the speech becoming uncomfortably loud or partly inaudible.

In any case, it should be realised that the goal of amplifying all bands of speech to the MCL could only be realised in practice for one specific speaker talking at one specific level. The long-term average spectrum of speech can vary markedly from one speaker to another. Also, the average shape of the speech spectrum for a given talker varies with vocal effort; a higher vocal effort leads to relatively more high-frequency emphasis (Pearsons, Bennett and Fidell, 1976). Thus, at best, a prescriptive rule can give a frequency-gain characteristic that will be appropriate for 'typical' listening situations encountered by a 'typical' user. In practice, it may be necessary to do some 'fine tuning' of a hearing aid around the frequency-gain characteristic recommended by a given rule (Moore and Glasberg, 1998).

Problems with linear hearing aids

A problem with linear amplification is connected with the gain selected by the user (i.e. the volume control setting) in everyday listening situations. There is evidence that the selected gain is often small, and certainly smaller than recommended by rules such as NAL(R) (Leijon, 1989). In many cases, the gain is probably insufficient to ensure audibility of speech at normal conversational levels over a wide frequency range. Low gains are probably selected because the user wishes to avoid unpleasantly loud sounds, or to avoid the distortion associated with peak clipping. Stone, Moore, Wojtczak and Gudgin (1997) found that, under conditions where subjects are sure that they will not be exposed to any unexpected loud or unpleasant sounds, they will elect to use rather high gains, sometimes about 10 dB higher those recommended by the NAL(R) formula. This can lead to better intelligibility than when lower gains are used. However, people do not use such high gains in everyday life. One may conclude that, in practice, the gain provided by linear hearing aids is usually less than would be required to provide optimum speech intelligibility.

A second problem with linear hearing aids is that users often find it necessary to adjust the volume control to deal with different listening situations. The overall level of speech and other sounds can vary considerably from one situation to another (Pearsons, Bennett and Fidell, 1976; Killion, 1997), and people with cochlear hearing loss do not have sufficient dynamic range to deal with this. However, adjustment of the volume control can be difficult, especially for elderly people who may have limited manual dexterity, and placing a hand near the aid changes the acoustical conditions and may induce feedback (see below for details). This situation has been somewhat improved by the introduction of hearing aids with remote control of volume, although such aids are not in widespread use. Even with remote control, the need to adjust the volume control frequently is irksome.

On the positive side, linear hearing aids can have beneficial effects other than restoring audibility. Consider, as an example, a person with a 'flat' hearing loss. Most prescriptive rules would recommend a gain that increased with frequency up to about 1 kHz, and flattened off above that. The reduced gain at low frequencies is partly introduced to allow for the fact that speech typically has more energy at low frequencies than at high frequencies; less amplification is necessary at frequencies where the speech has high energy. The reduced gain below 1 kHz has the beneficial effect of reducing upward spread of masking (the masking of medium and high frequencies by lower frequencies). This is important since many environmental sounds (e.g. car noise and air-conditioning noise) have most of their energy at low frequencies, and since many hearing-impaired people are particularly susceptible to masking by low-frequency sounds (see Chapter 3).

Some general problems with hearing aids

This section briefly discusses some problems that are inherent to most hearing aids, whether linear or not.

Inadequate gain at high frequencies

A common problem is inadequate gain at high frequencies relative to low or medium frequencies. This is a particularly the case when fitting aids to people with hearing losses that increase rapidly at high frequencies. Nowadays, it has become relatively common to check the real-ear gain of hearing aids using a probe-tube microphone whose tip is placed inside the ear canal, close to the eardrum. This can reveal 'errors' in fitting that can then sometimes be reduced by modifications to the aid. Preferably, this should be done electronically, using frequency-response shaping circuitry in the hearing aid. However, it is often necessary to resort to changes in the 'plumbing', for example by changing the tubing leading from a behind-the-ear aid to the earmould, or by the use of vents (small holes bored through the earmould. However, even after such modifications, the obtained frequency-gain characteristic may differ substantially from the one recommended by a prescriptive rule.

Sometimes it is impossible to achieve adequate gain at high frequencies because of problems with acoustic feedback, which is discussed in the next section. Indeed, the microphones and receivers (miniature loudspeakers) used in hearing aids often have a response that is deliberately reduced at high frequencies, to prevent acoustic feedback. Thus, many hearing aids produce little or no amplification above 5 to 6 kHz. This is not necessary or desirable from an auditory point of view. Skinner and Miller (1983) showed that speech intelligibility in quiet and in noise improved for people with sensorineural hearing loss when amplification was provided at frequencies above 6 kHz. Moreover, provided that the distortion of the hearing aid is kept low, a wide frequency range does not lead to a harsh or tinny sound quality (Killion, 1993).

An exception to this occurs in people with dead regions at high frequencies, as discussed in Chapters 2, 3, 4 and 6. For such people, high frequency tones are reported to sound highly distorted or noise-like (Villchur, 1973; Moore, Laurence and Wright, 1985; Murray and Byrne, 1986). In such cases, it appears that hearing aids work better if the frequencies corresponding to the dead region are attenuated, rather than amplified. This is especially true when background noise is present.

Acoustic feedback

Feedback occurs when the sound generated by a hearing aid leaks back to the microphone of the aid. The sound is then picked up by the microphone, and amplified further. This sets up a self-sustaining oscillation. It is usually heard as a 'whistling' sound. Feedback is usually unpleasant to listen to, and it may be accompanied by considerable distortion. In practice, feedback often limits the amount of gain that can be used in a hearing aid, especially at medium to high frequencies. Sometimes, the user of an aid does not hear feedback (for example, when it occurs at a high frequency where the audiometric loss may be severe) but becomes embarrassed about wearing the aid because he or she is aware that others can hear the feedback.

Feedback can be reduced in a number of ways. One way is to improve the seal of the aid or earmould to the ear canal, so that less sound leaks from the receiver (the miniature loudspeaker that generates the sound) to the microphone. This can be done by making a better-fitting aid or mould, or by smearing the ear canal or earmould with a substance like petroleum jelly before inserting the aid. For a behind-the-ear aid, increasing the thickness of the tubing leading from the aid to the earmould may reduce feedback. Another method is to increase the distance between the microphone and the receiver. Feedback can be reduced considerably if the microphone is some distance from the receiver, as is possible, for example, with chest-worn aids. However, if the microphone is not worn on the head, sound localisation may be markedly impaired (see Chapter 7). A third way of reducing feedback is by smoothing the frequency response of the aid. Feedback usually occurs at one specific frequency where there is a peak in the frequency-gain characteristic, or in the response of the transmission path from the ear canal to the microphone, or both. If the frequency-gain characteristic is smoothed, then the overall gain can often be increased before feedback starts again. The frequency response can be smoothed either by electronic filtering or by modifications to the earmould and tubing, for example by the use of acoustic resistors.

There is one commercial hearing aid, the 'Danavox DFS Genius', which achieves feedback reduction in a very different way, using digital signal processing. It adds a small amount of white noise to the amplified microphone signal, and uses this to estimate the characteristics of the feedback path from the receiver to the microphone. It then constructs a digital filter, which is used partially to cancel the feedback signal. This system typically allows an increase in high-frequency gain of about 10 dB before feedback occurs. The filter adapts slowly over time, so it can allow for changes in the feedback path caused, for example, by slight changes in the position of the earmould. However, it cannot handle rapid changes caused, for example, by chewing. A drawback of the system is that the added white noise may be audible and have disturbing effects. The noise is typically added at a level 12 to 18 dB below the level of the speech signal, and its level changes as the speech level changes. However, this aid is mainly intended for people with severe or profound losses who typically have a very small dynamic range. For these people, the added noise is usually barely audible but the 10 dB extra gain can be very beneficial in improving audibility.

Some other recent hearing aids also use digital signal processing to reduce feedback. The simplest way of doing this is by reducing the gain in a narrow frequency range around the frequency at which the feedback is occurring. Often, these aids have a method for detecting automatically when feedback is occurring. Assume, for example, that the signal is split into several frequency bands. When feedback occurs in a particular frequency band, the envelope of the signal in that band shows almost no modulation; the envelope remains constant as a function of time. In contrast, when feedback is absent, the envelope shows significant modulation whenever signals such as speech or music are present at the input to the aid. The amount of modulation of the envelope can thus be used to determine whether feedback is occurring or not. When feedback is detected in a band, the gain in that band can automatically be reduced.

Peakiness of frequency response

The frequency response of a hearing aid on a real ear often shows two or three distinct peaks caused by resonances in the acoustical delivery system. This is especially true for behind-the-ear aids. It is usually possible to reduce these peaks, smoothing the overall frequency response, by suitable modifications to the tubing and/or by the use of acoustic resistors (dampers) (Libby, 1981; Killion, 1982). It is now widely accepted that the frequency response should be smoothed in this way as far as possible. One study showed no significant differences in judged clarity and pleasantness between hearing aids with unsmoothed and smoothed responses (Cox and Gilmore, 1986), but most other studies have shown that hearing aids with smoothed frequency responses are preferred (Libby, 1981; Mertz, 1982; Dillon and Macrae, 1984; Van Buuren, Festen and Houtgast, 1996). For a review see Bornstein and Randolph (1983). For example, Van Buuren, Festen and Houtgast (1996) found that large peaks in the frequency response adversely affected intelligibility (more for impaired than for normal listeners) and subjective sound quality. Smooth responses gave the best results for intelligibility and pleasantness.

In any case, there are at least three benefits of smoothing the frequency response other than effects of sound quality:

- it can reduce acoustic feedback, as described above;
- it can reduce the distortion that often occurs at frequencies around peaks in the response;
- it can allow a greater proportion of the speech spectrum to be above threshold before the uncomfortable loudness level is reached.

In spite of these benefits, in clinical practice measures to smooth the frequency response are often not taken. This happens either because of ignorance or laziness on the part of the hearing-aid dispenser, or from the mistaken belief of the dispenser that there is no benefit in smoothing the response. It is to be hoped that this state of affairs will improve in the coming years, especially with the increasing use of real-ear probe tube measurement systems.

It should be noted that the acoustical delivery system can be important in other ways. The overall response of an aid at the eardrum can be markedly altered by changes in the tubing or by venting (introducing a small hole in the earmould). For example, the output of a behind-the-ear aid at high frequencies is reduced if tubing with a constant bore is used. The response can be maintained at high frequencies by using tubing whose bore increases progressively from the receiver to the inside end of the earmould (Libby, 1982). It is unfortunate that many dispensers of hearing aids do not make full use of the opportunities that this provides for extending the effective frequency range of a hearing aid and for tailoring the frequency response to match a target.

The occlusion effect

People who wear hearing aids often complain that that their own voice sounds unnatural, being excessively loud and 'hollow' sounding. This is sometimes called the *occlusion effect*. The effect occurs when an earmould is worn that blocks the entrance to the ear canal. The sound of the person's own voice is transmitted through the bones of the head into the ear canal (meatus). The transmission occurs mainly through the flexible (cartilaginous) outer part of the ear canal. When the ear canal is blocked, the sound cannot escape, and the resulting sound pressure at the eardrum is markedly higher than would occur for an unblocked ear. Using a probe tube microphone, Killion, Wilber and Gudmundsen (1988) showed that sound levels exceeding 90 dB SPL could occur for certain speech sounds such as /a/ as in 'Father'. An illustration of this effect is available on compact discs (Berlin, 1996; Moore, 1997a).

The traditional way of alleviating the occlusion effect is to vent the earmould, by drilling a small hole through it. However, this can lead to acoustic feedback. Indeed, feedback often limits the size of the vent that can be used, so that the occlusion effect remains a significant problem. This is especially so in cases of near-normal low-frequency hearing with moderate or severe hearing loss at high frequencies, as is common in elderly people. The large vent that would be required to alleviate the occlusion effect would prevent the aid from providing adequate gain at high frequencies.

Recently, a new solution to this problem has emerged, based on some observations by Zwislocki (1953). He showed that the transmission of bone-conducted sound into the ear canal was much less when an earplug was inserted deeply into the ear canal than when it was inserted only into the flexible outer part. The inner part of the ear canal is composed of rigid bone, which accounts for the reduced transmission. Zwislocki's observations have been confirmed by Schroeter and Poesselt (1986) and by Killion, Wilber and Gudmundsen (1988) who showed that the sound level in the ear canal produced by a person's own voice could be reduced by as much as 20 dB at low frequencies by using a deeply seated earplug or earmould, as compared to a shallow one. This effect is also illustrated on the CDs referred to above (Berlin, 1996; Moore, 1997a).

In the case of hearing aids, the occlusion effect can be markedly reduced either by using an aid that is fitted deeply inside the ear canal (all-in-the-ear devices), or by using an earmould that extends deeply into the ear canal. This means that a 'deep' ear impression has to be taken, which is difficult and may require special techniques. However, users of hearing aids that fit deeply inside the ear canal do report that their own voices sound much more natural.

Compression amplification

Linear amplification does not provide an effective way of dealing with the reduced dynamic range of people with cochlear hearing loss; with linear amplification it is not possible to restore audibility of weak sounds without intense sounds being over-amplified and becoming uncomfortably loud. It was suggested many years ago that this problem could be alleviated by the use of *automatic gain control* (AGC) (Steinberg and Gardner, 1937). With AGC, it is possible to amplify weak sounds more than stronger ones, with the result that the wide dynamic range of the input signal is compressed into a smaller dynamic range at the output. Hence AGC systems are also called *compressors*. Although this idea sounds simple, in practice there are many ways of implementing AGC and there is still no clear consensus as to the 'best' method, if there is such a thing. There is also considerable controversy about the efficacy of AGC systems. To understand why things are not so simple, it is helpful first to consider some of the basic characteristics of AGC systems.

Basic characteristics of AGC systems

An AGC amplifier is an amplifier whose gain is determined by a control signal. The gain is defined as output voltage divided by the input voltage or, if both are expressed in decibels, as the output level minus the input level. For example, if the output voltage is twice the input voltage, the gain is 2 (in linear terms) or 6 dB (since $20\log_{10}(2) = 6$). The control signal is derived either from the input to the amplifier or from its output. The gain is reduced as the input level is increased. For inputs below a certain level, most AGC amplifiers act as linear amplifiers. Over the range where the amplifier is linear, the output is directly proportional to the input. If the output level in decibels is plotted as a function of the input level in decibels, the result is a straight line with a slope of one; see Chapter 1. Once the input level exceeds a certain value, the gain is reduced, and the slope of the line becomes less than one. This is illustrated by the input-output function in Figure 9.1. The *compression threshold* is defined as the input level at which the gain is reduced by 2 dB, relative to the gain applied in the region of linear amplification. For example, if the gain was 25 dB for input levels well below the compression threshold, the compression threshold would be the input level at which the gain was reduced to 23 dB.

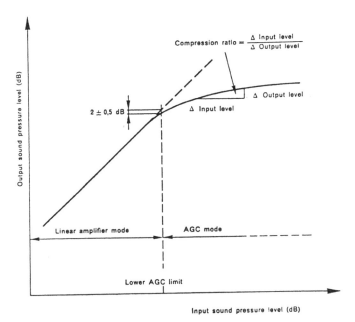

Figure 9.1: An input-output function for an automatic gain control (AGC) system. The output level in decibels is plotted as a function of the input level in decibels.

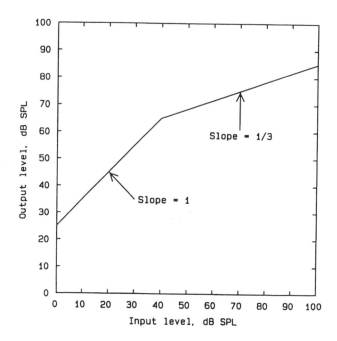

Figure 9.2: A schematic input-output function for an AGC system with a compression threshold of 43 dB SPL, and a compression ratio of 3. Notice that for input levels above about 78 dB SPL, the output level is lower than the input level, i.e. the system acts as an attenuator.

The 'amount' of compression is specified by the *compression ratio*, which is the change in input level (in decibels) required to achieve a 1 dB change in output level (for an input exceeding the compression threshold); the compression ratio is equal to the reciprocal of the slope of the input-output function in the range where the compression is applied. For example, a compression ratio of three means that the output grows by 1 dB for each 3 dB increase in input level. When the input level is high, the gain of an AGC amplifier, expressed in decibels, may actually become negative - i.e. the signal is attenuated rather than being amplified.

Consider the example shown in Figure 9.2. For input levels below 40 dB SPL, the AGC amplifier applies a gain of 25 dB. The gain starts to decrease for input levels above 40 dB SPL. For an input level of 43 dB SPL the gain is reduced to 23 dB. Therefore, the AGC amplifier has a compression threshold of 43 dB SPL. The compression ratio is assumed to be three. When the input level is increased from 40 to 100 dB (a 60 dB range) the output increases from 65 to 85 dB (a 20 dB range). Thus, for an input level of 100 dB, the signal is attenuated by 15 dB. This is not necessarily a bad thing. Many people, including both normally hearing and hearing-impaired people, find that sounds with levels of 100 dB and above are unpleasantly loud. Reducing the sound level can make the loudness more acceptable, without impairing the ability to detect or discriminate the sounds.

Automatic gain control amplifiers vary in how quickly they react to changes in input sound level. Typically, the speed of response is measured by using as an input a sound whose level changes abruptly between two values, normally 55 dB SPL and 80 dB SPL. When the sound level abruptly increases, the gain decreases, but this takes time to occur. Hence the output of the amplifier shows an initial 'spike' or 'overshoot', followed by a decline to a steady value. This is illustrated in Figure 9.3. The time taken for the output to get within 2 dB of its steady value is called the *attack time*, and is labelled t_a in Figure 9.3. When the sound level abruptly decreases, the gain increases, but again this takes time to occur. Hence the output of the amplifier shows an initial dip followed by an increase to a steady value. The time taken for the output to increase to within 2 dB of its steady value is called the *recovery time* or *release time*, and is labelled t_r in Figure 9.3.

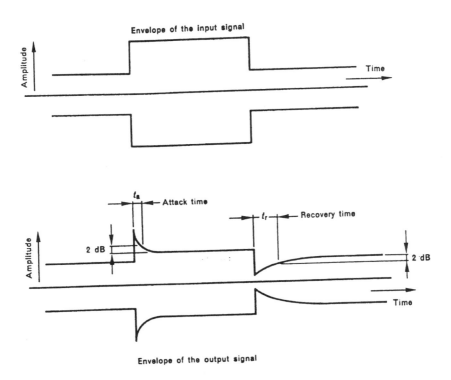

Figure 9.3: Illustration of the temporal response of an AGC system. The envelope of the input signal is shown at the top. The envelope of the response of the system is shown at the bottom.

Most hearing aids with AGC circuits still have a volume control, even though the AGC circuit can, in principle, adjust the volume 'automatically'. When the volume control is placed *after* the AGC circuit, the AGC is sometimes said to be input controlled; this configuration is sometimes called AGCi. In AGCi systems, adjustment of the volume control does not change the compression threshold. Decreasing the volume causes the whole input-output function to shift downwards vertically, without changing its shape. When the volume control is placed *before* the AGC circuit, the AGC is sometimes said to be output controlled; this configuration is sometimes called AGCo. In AGCo systems, adjustment of the volume control changes the compression threshold; decreasing the volume increases the compression threshold. When the volume is decreased, the whole input-output function is shifted to the right, without changing its shape.

In practice, the situation is often more complex than this. For example, the user-accessible volume control may be after the AGC circuit, but the gain before the AGC circuit may be adjustable by the dispenser, or may be adjustable via a remote control. For some hearing aids, adjustment of the volume affects the gain both before and after the AGC circuit. Some hearing aids incorporate more than one AGC circuit in series and the volume control may be between the two. In practice, the terms AGCi and AGCo can be more confusing than helpful. It is better to understand the specific form of processing used in a particular aid.

Varieties of AGC systems

Automatic gain control systems have been designed in many different forms, mostly on the basis of different rationales or design goals. For reviews see Moore (1990), Hickson (1994) and Dillon (1996). This section briefly describes some of the different types.

Some systems are intended to adjust the gain automatically for different listening situations. Essentially, they are intended to relieve the user of the need to adjust the volume control to deal with these situations. Usually, such systems change their gain slowly with changes in sound level; this is achieved by making t_r, or t_r and t_a, relatively long (usually t_r is a few hundred milliseconds). These systems are often referred to as 'automatic volume control' (AVC). Although it is generally accepted that AVC can be useful, relatively few commercial hearing aids incorporate AVC. Some reasons for this are discussed below.

Automatic gain control is often used primarily to limit the maximum output of hearing aids, to prevent discomfort and/or circuit overload at high input sound levels. The compression ratio is usually very large (10 or more) and the compression threshold is usually relatively high (typically around 85 dB SPL). Such systems are known as *compression limiters*. Compression limiters usually have a small value of the attack time, t_a, (1-10 ms) so as to respond rapidly to sudden increases in sound level. The recovery time, t_r, is also usually fairly small (20-100 ms). The function of compression limiters is similar to that of the peak clippers described earlier. However, peak clipping causes unpleasant-sounding distortion whereas the effects of compression limiting are not so noticeable. Hence compression limiters are quite widely used in hearing aids.

An alternative type of compressor, with lower compression ratios and lower compression thresholds, has been used in hearing aids in attempts to make the hearing-impaired person's perception of loudness more like that of a normal listener. These are sometimes called 'wide dynamic range' compressors, as the compression operates over a wide range of input sound levels. Typically, the compression threshold is about 45 dB SPL, and the compression ratio has values up to about 3. One aim of such systems is to ensure that the weaker consonant sounds of speech, such as 'p', 't' and 'k', are audible without the more intense sounds (e.g. vowels) being uncomfortably loud. To achieve this goal, the compressors usually have short time constants. The attack times are typically 2-10 ms and the recovery times are typically 20-150 ms. Systems with time constants in this range are often referred to as 'fast-acting compressors' or 'syllabic compressors', since the gain changes over times comparable to the durations of individual syllables in speech.

Rationales for the use of multi-band compression

Several authors (Villchur, 1973; Mangold and Leijon, 1979; Laurence, Moore and Glasberg, 1983) have proposed that syllabic compression should be applied separately in two or more frequency bands. The idea is that the signal picked up by the microphone is filtered to split it into several frequency bands, and each band has its own independent fast-acting AGC amplifier. There are at least two reasons why this might be beneficial. Firstly, the amount of hearing loss often varies markedly with frequency; typically, hearing loss is greater at high frequencies than at low frequencies and the dynamic range decreases with increasing frequency. Hence, the amount of compression should vary with frequency and this requires that compression be applied independently in more than one band. A second reason is that relatively weak high-frequency components in speech (e.g. those associated with 'k', 'p', 't'), which can be important for intelligibility, are often accompanied by, or follow rapidly after, relatively intense low-frequency components, often associated with vowels. This requires more gain at high frequencies than at low. However, other high frequency sounds (for example 's' sounds in speech, or the sound of cutlery on plates) can be relatively intense. To prevent these from becoming too loud, the gain at high frequencies must be adjusted rapidly from moment to moment. The use of fast-acting AGC in two or more separate bands can ensure that weak high-frequency components are always audible, even in the presence of intense low-frequencies, whereas the more intense high-frequency sounds do not become uncomfortably loud.

Another rationale for the use of multi-band compression, as opposed to single-band (broad-band) compression is to reduce the effects of interfering sounds (Ono, Kanzaki and Mizoi, 1983; Van Dijkhuizen, Festen and Plomp, 1991; Rankovic, Freyman and Zurek, 1992). Consider a hypothetical situation where a hearing-impaired person is trying to understand speech in the presence of an intense noise whose energy is concentrated in a narrow frequency range (a rather rare circumstance in everyday life). A broad-band AGC system would reduce its gain in response to the intense noise, thereby reducing the audibility of the speech. A multi-band AGC system would reduce the gain only for the frequency band(s) dominated by the noise, reducing the masking effect and loudness of the noise without affecting the audibility of the parts of the speech spectrum remote from the frequency of the noise. Van Dijkhuizen, Festen and Plomp (1991) have argued that the gain in such systems should change slowly with time (i.e. t_a and t_r should be large, at least several hundred milliseconds).

Several commercial hearing aids incorporate a form of multi-band AGC based on this rationale. Indeed, some digital hearing aids (such as the Widex Senso and the Siemens Prisma) have methods for detecting whether a particular frequency band is dominated by speech or by noise. If a band is dominated by noise then the gain in that band is reduced. At the time of writing, these aids have only a small number of bands (up to four). With such a small number of bands, reduction of gain to reduce the effects of interfering background sounds also results in reduced gain for a significant part of the speech spectrum. Probably, such systems do not improve intelligibility very much, although they can improve listening comfort considerably.

Research on the effectiveness of multi-band syllabic compression

This section is mainly concerned with research on the effectiveness of fast-acting (syllabic) multi-band compression. In principle, such compression could restore the loudness perception of a hearing-impaired person roughly to 'normal'; it could be thought of as replacing the fast-acting compression that occurs in a normal cochlea. The compression in the cochlea is lost or reduced when the OHCs are damaged, as described in earlier chapters. Research on the effectiveness of multi-band compression has given somewhat conflicting results. The conflict arises partly from differences in the way that the compression systems have been implemented and partly from differences in methods of evaluation. Individual differences between the subjects used may also have played a role.

Comprehensive reviews of results using multi-channel compression have been provided by Braida, Durlach, De Gennaro et al. (1982), Hickson (1994) and Dillon (1996). Some general trends can be discerned from the results:

- For speech in quiet, benefits of compression have often been found, in a variety of systems, when the speech materials used have covered a wide range of levels, as occurs in everyday life (Villchur, 1973; Lippmann, Braida and Durlach, 1981; Laurence, Moore and Glasberg, 1983; Moore, Laurence and Wright, 1985; Moore and Glasberg, 1986a; 1988a; Moore, 1987a; Moore, Glasberg and Stone, 1991; Moore, Johnson, Clark et al., 1992). When the speech material has been presented at one reasonably high level, and when the speech material has been carefully equalised in level during the recording process (as was the case in many studies), compression does not show benefits over linear amplification (Lippmann, Braida and Durlach, 1981).

- For speech in background noise, benefits of fast-acting compression have sometimes (but not always) been found for systems with a small number of bands (Villchur, 1973; Laurence, Moore and Glasberg, 1983; Moore, Laurence and Wright, 1985; Moore and Glasberg, 1986a; 1988a; Moore, 1987a; Ringdahl, Eriksson-Mangold, Israelsson et al., 1990; Moore, Glasberg and Stone, 1991; Moore, Johnson, Clark et al., 1992). Benefits have not usually been found for systems with a large number of bands (Lippmann, Braida and Durlach, 1981; Bustamante and Braida, 1987) although Yund and Buckles (1995a; 1995b) found some benefit of increasing the number of bands up to eight.

- The extent of the benefit of compression for the understanding of speech in noise depends upon how the frequency-gain characteristic was chosen for the control condition using linear amplification. Under laboratory conditions using speech in noise with carefully controlled levels and fixed spectra, it may be possible to use linear amplification to make the speech audible and comfortable over a wide frequency range. Under these conditions there may be little benefit from compression. However, if the linear condition is set up so that speech and/or environmental sounds with reasonably high input levels are not amplified to unpleasantly loud levels, then lower overall gains must be used. Under these conditions, benefits of compression may become apparent because the compression allows more amplification for weaker sounds while not amplifying intense sounds excessively.

- Most (but not all) of the studies showing benefits of compression for listening to speech in noise have used aids that the subjects could wear in their everyday lives. This is important, since if a person has had a hearing impairment for many years, it may take some time (weeks or months) for him or her to learn to use the new cues provided by a compression system (Gatehouse, 1992).

In summary, clear benefits have been demonstrated for multi-band compression under conditions that are representative of those occurring in everyday life. The benefits have also become clear from consumer acceptance; sales of hearing aids with multi-band compression have increased markedly over the last few years, and several major manufacturers now market such aids.

Fitting hearing aids with multi-band compression

Multi-band compression hearing aids can be rather complex to fit to the individual person. Many different parameters need to be adjusted and procedures for making these adjustments are not yet well established. Often, certain parameters are pre-set by the manufacturer, for example the attack and recovery times. However, gains and compression ratios in the individual frequency bands usually need to be adjusted by the dispenser. Several researchers and hearing aid companies have proposed the use of loudness scaling in the fitting of multi-band compression hearing aids (Pluvinage, 1989; Allen and Jeng, 1990; Cox, 1995; Cornelisse, Seewald and Jamieson, 1995; Cox, Alexander, Taylor et al., 1997; Kiessling, 1997). Loudness scaling methods were described in Chapter 4. Typically, the listener is required to judge the loudness of bands of noise or sinusoids. The stimuli are presented over a range of centre frequencies and sound levels. The loudness judgements are then used to calculate the level-dependent gains required in each band of a hearing aid, in order to restore loudness perception to 'normal' or 'near-normal'. The loudness scaling can be done prior to the fitting of the hearing aid. The level-dependent gains required in each band are then calculated based on the known electro-acoustic properties of the aid (Pluvinage, 1989). Alternatively, loudness scaling can be performed while the aid is being worn and the level-dependent gains in each band can be adjusted to achieve 'normal' or 'near-normal' loudness judgements (Kiessling, 1997). This has the advantage that any effects of the earmould and tubing, and of ear canal size, are automatically taken into account.

Although these procedures are now widely used, the rationale behind them can be questioned on several grounds. Firstly, even for normal listeners, the variability of loudness judgements for a given sound level can be considerable (Elberling and Nielsen, 1993; Cox, Alexander, Taylor et al., 1997; Kiessling, 1997). Similarly, the sound level required for a given category, such as 'comfortable' can vary markedly across normal listeners, both for a given procedure, and across procedures. For example, Cox, Alexander, Taylor and Gray (1997) reported that, for normally hearing listeners, the level of a 2 kHz 'warble' tone judged as 'comfortable' had a standard deviation of about 11 dB. Given this variability, it seems clear that 'normal' loudness is not well defined, at least using these procedures, so restoration of loudness to 'normal' is problematic. A second problem is that the results of loudness scaling procedures can be strongly influenced by the range of stimuli presented, as described in Chapter 4. However, there is no easy way of determining what is the 'correct' range to use for a particular person. A third problem is that judgements of loudness for artificial sounds such as tones or bands of noise may not be good predictors of the preferred loudness of everyday sounds, such as speech. For example, one person tested in my laboratory judged bands of noise as 'very loud' whenever their level exceeded 80 dB SPL. On the other hand, when speech was presented at 80 dB SPL, it was judged to be 'quiet'.

In addition to these problems, one might question whether restoration of loudness to 'normal' is an appropriate goal for multi-band compression systems. One can argue that the goal should be to give good audibility and intelligibility for speech over a wide range of input sound levels, while maintaining listening comfort. Of course, if this can be done by restoring loudness to 'normal', then there is no conflict between these two goals. However, it is not clear that restoration of 'normal' loudness should be a primary goal; loudness *per se* may not be of great importance.

An alternative approach to fitting multi-band compression hearing aids has been described by Moore, Alcántara and Glasberg (1998). The procedure has two parts: choice of initial values for the level-dependent gains in each band; and fine tuning to suit the individual person. The fine tuning is based on an adaptive procedure where the settings of the hearing aid are adjusted according to the responses of the listener to test signals. Broadband speech is used as the test signal, rather than tones or bands of noise. The fitting is done using the hearing aid(s) and earmoulds that the person will actually wear. This avoids problems associated with calibration, variability in microphones and receivers, and individual differences in ear-canal geometry.

Initial values for the level-dependent gains in each band are derived from the pure-tone audiogram. For example, gains for low-level inputs can be chosen, where possible, to give aided thresholds of about 20 dB HL at all frequencies; however, higher target aided thresholds are appropriate when the hearing loss is more than moderate. Gains for higher level inputs can be based on a prescriptive approach (Seewald, 1992; Killion and Fikret-Pasa, 1993) or on a loudness model, such as that described in Chapter 4 (Moore and Glasberg, 1997). For example, the gains for a 65 dB speech input can be chosen to give an equal comfortable loudness in all frequency bands; this approach was described earlier for the fitting of linear hearing aids. The initial parameter values are not critical as the adaptive procedure will perform the necessary fine tuning. However, the initial parameters should lead to frequency-response shapes for high and low input levels that are appropriate for the audiogram.

The goal of the adaptive fitting procedure is to 'fine tune' the level-dependent gain values to suit the preferences of the individual user, so that sounds are audible and comfortable in a wide range of everyday listening situations while giving a reasonable impression of loudness. The rationale for the procedure is based on the fact that hearing aid users will often want to listen to speech and therefore it is important that speech should have an acceptable loudness and tone quality over the range of sound levels that occurs in everyday life. Hence, the procedure involves both adjustment of the gains in all bands (affecting overall loudness) and adjustment of the relative gains at high frequencies and low frequencies (influencing perceived tone quality). The 'target' of the fitting procedure is that speech with an overall level of 60 dB SPL should be judged as 'quiet' and speech with a level of 85 dB SPL should be judged as 'loud'; in both cases the speech should have an appropriate tone quality (neither tinny nor boomy). The levels of 60 and 85 dB SPL do not reach the extremes encountered in everyday life, but they represent the boundaries of the range most commonly encountered.

The adaptive procedure works in the following way. Initially, sentences with a level of 85 dB are presented. If these are judged as loud, the gains are left unaltered. If the speech is judged as very loud or too loud, the gains in all bands are decreased. The gains are changed by the same amount for both high and low input levels; the effect is like adjusting a volume control after the AGC circuit. If the speech is judged as comfortable or quieter than comfortable, the gains in all bands are increased. Again, the gains are changed by the same amount for both high and low input levels. Then, the listeners are asked to make judgements about sound quality on a scale going from 'tinny' to 'boomy'. The relative gains at high and low frequencies are adjusted until the speech is judged as 'neither tinny nor boomy'. Then sentences with a level of 60 dB are presented. If these are judged as quiet, the gains are left unaltered. If the speech is judged as comfortable or louder, the *low-level* gains in all bands are decreased. Decreasing the low-level gains has the effect of decreasing the compression ratio. If the speech is judged as very quiet, the *low-level* gains in all bands are increased; this has the effect of increasing the compression ratio. Then, the listeners are asked to make judgements about sound quality on a scale going from 'shrill' to 'muffled'. The relative low-level gains at high and low frequencies are adjusted until the speech is judged as 'neither shrill nor muffled'. All of these steps are repeated until the listener consistently gives the target responses. Typically, this only takes between 5 and 10 minutes per ear, which is less than the time taken for most loudness scaling procedures. The result of this fitting procedure is that speech is audible, comfortable and has an acceptable tone quality for a wide range of input levels.

This procedure has not yet been evaluated extensively in clinical practice. However, the initial evaluation described by Moore, Alcántara and Glasberg (1998) showed very promising results. Subjects fitted with hearing aids using the procedure were very satisfied with the performance of their aids in everyday life, as evaluated using a questionnaire (Cox and Gilmore, 1990). Sounds were generally comfortable in loudness and acceptable in quality. Furthermore, laboratory measurements showed that settings that gave good comfort also gave good intelligibility for speech in quiet and in the presence of background sounds.

Bass increase at low levels (BILL) versus treble increase at low levels (TILL)

For people whose hearing loss increases at high frequencies, multi-band compression systems fitted using loudness scaling procedures, or using the procedure described immediately above, generally have a frequency-gain characteristic that gives relatively more high-frequency emphasis at low sound levels. For example, for speech with a low input level (say 50 dB SPL), the gain might be 20 dB at low frequencies and 40 dB at high frequencies; the high-frequency gain is 20 dB more than the low-frequency gain. On the other hand, for speech with a high input level (say, 85 dB SPL) the gain might be 5 dB at low frequencies and 10 dB at high frequencies; in this case the high-frequency gain is only 5 dB more than the low-frequency gain. This sort of sound processing is often described as 'treble increase at low levels' or *TILL*.

In contrast, some commercially available hearing aids do what appears to be the opposite; they have a frequency-gain characteristic that gives relatively more low-frequency emphasis at low sound levels. This type of sound processing is called 'bass increase at low levels' or *BILL*. It is also sometimes misleadingly called 'automatic signal processing' (ASP). The rationale behind BILL processing is that speech at high levels is often accompanied by background noise with most of its energy at low frequencies. The masking effect of the noise can be decreased by reducing the gain at low frequencies. Perhaps a better name for this type of processing would be 'bass decrease at high levels'.

One argument that is sometimes given to support the idea of BILL processing is based on the phenomenon of the 'upward spread of masking' that was described in Chapter 3. At high sound levels, low-frequency sounds produce considerable masking of medium and high-frequency sounds and the amount of masking grows in a non-linear way. For example, an increase in level of a low-frequency masker by 10 dB can increase the amount of masking of a high-frequency signal by more than 20 dB; see Figure 3.9. Reduction of low-frequency gain at high levels in a hearing aid could help to prevent the upward spread of masking. However, as described in Chapters 3 and 4, the non-linear growth of masking is reduced or absent in people with cochlear hearing loss; for them an increase in masker level of 10 dB gives an increase in signal threshold of about 10 dB. This weakens the rationale for reducing low-frequency gain at high levels; masking effects produced by low-frequency sounds do not become more pronounced at high overall levels for hearing-impaired subjects.

Experimental evaluations of hearing aids with BILL processing have given mixed results. Where benefits have been found, they can probably be attributed at least partly to the fact that the circuit reduces distortion that would otherwise be present at the output of the aids for high input sound levels (Van Tasell and Crain, 1992). In any case, it should be noted that multi-band compression systems that are set up as TILL sound processors will actually behave as BILL processors under conditions where intense low-frequency noise is present; such noise will automatically lead to a reduction of low-frequency gain. Thus, the distinction between BILL and TILL processors is not as clear cut as is often claimed. Multi-band compression systems can act either as TILL or as BILL processors, depending on how they are adjusted and on the nature of the input signal.

The dual front-end AGC system

Although benefits of fast-acting multi-band compression have been demonstrated, it is not clear that such compression is the best way to compensate for the effects of loudness recruitment. There is certainly some evidence that the use of high compression ratios (greater than 2 to 3) in such systems has deleterious effects on speech intelligibility in quiet and in noise (Plomp, 1994; Crain and Yund, 1995; Hohmann and Kollmeier, 1995; Verschuure and Dreschler, 1996). For people with severe to profound hearing loss, it may be necessary to use high compression ratios to make sure that speech is both audible and comfortable over the wide range of sound levels encountered in everyday life. However, such high compression ratios are not optimal for intelligibility at moderate input levels.

As described earlier, it has often been found that, for speech presented at a single level, an optimally adjusted linear amplifier gives speech intelligibility at least as good as, and sometimes better than, that provided by multi-band compression amplifiers. Therefore, an alternative approach to the problem of compensating for reduced dynamic range is to use slow-acting automatic volume control (AVC) to deliver speech at a single level, regardless of the input level. However, conventional AVC systems involve a compromise between conflicting requirements. For speech with a fixed average level, the level may fluctuate markedly from moment to moment and may drop to very low values during brief pauses in the speech. If the gain of an aid changes significantly during the speech itself, or during the pauses in the speech, then 'breathing' or 'pumping' noises may be heard that are objectionable to the user. These effects are particularly marked when moderate levels of background noise are present, as is often the case in everyday situations. The noise appears to come and go. It 'rushes up' during pauses in the speech, and becomes quieter when the speech starts again. In addition to these objectionable effects, the temporal envelope of the speech may be distorted by the changes in gain. To avoid these problems, the gain should change relatively slowly as a function of time, i.e. t_a and t_r should be long.

On the other hand, it is important to protect the user from sudden intense sounds, such as a door slamming or a cup being dropped. This requires the gain to change much more rapidly. This problem is usually dealt with by having an AVC system with a fast attack time (t_a in the range 1-10 ms), and a longer recovery time (t_r in the range 300-2000 ms). The fast attack time provides protection against sudden increases in sound level; the gain drops very quickly when the input sound level suddenly increases. However, such a system has the disadvantage that the gain of the aid drops to a low value immediately after an intense transient; the aid effectively goes 'dead' for a while. A further problem is that a recovery time of a few hundred ms is not sufficiently long to prevent 'breathing' and 'pumping' sounds from being heard.

An AVC system developed in my laboratory provides a better solution to these problems (Moore and Glasberg, 1988a; Moore, Glasberg and Stone, 1991; Moore, 1993; Stone, Moore, Wojtczak et al., 1997). This system, referred to as 'dual front-end AGC', is illustrated in Figure 9.4. The signal picked up by the microphone (1) is fed to an AGC amplifier (2) whose gain is determined by a control voltage. There are two control voltage generators (3 and 4). Both of these act in such a way that the amplifier (2) behaves as a 'compression limiter'; it amplifies without compression for input levels up to a certain compression threshold, and has effectively an infinite compression ratio for levels above that. One of the control voltage generators (4) has a lower compression threshold (about 63 dB SPL) than the other one, and it changes only slowly in response to changes in sound level; in our early work it had an attack time of roughly a few hundred ms and a recovery time of several seconds. Normally, the operation of the AGC amplifier is determined by this slow-acting control voltage. The effect is that the gain changes slowly as the listening situation changes, in a way that is almost unnoticed by the user and that avoids audible breathing noises. The overall output level of a speech signal is held almost constant for any input level above 63 dB SPL.

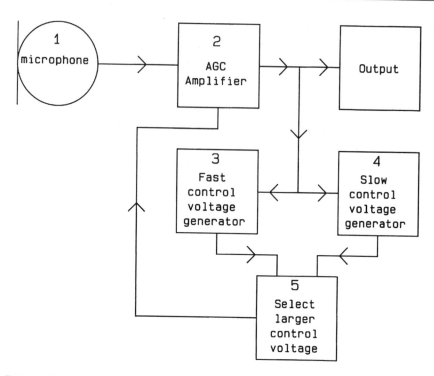

Figure 9.4: A block diagram of the dual front-end AGC system.

The fast-acting control voltage generator (3) has a compression threshold about 8 dB higher than that of the slower control voltage generator. It has an attack time of a few ms and a recovery time of about 100 ms. Normally it has little effect on the operation of the AGC amplifier. However, if an intense sound suddenly occurs, the fast-acting control voltage increases rapidly. When it exceeds the control voltage generated by (4), it is selected by circuit (5) to control the gain of the amplifier. The gain is rapidly reduced, thus protecting the user from over-amplification of the intense sound. However, the fast-acting control voltage decreases rapidly following the cessation of the intense sound, and control returns to the slow-acting control voltage. If the intense sound is brief, it does not significantly change the value of the slow-acting control voltage. Thus, following an intense transient, the gain returns to the original value determined by the overall level of the speech. In this way, intense transients are selectively attenuated, but the overall gain for the speech is held almost constant, except for a very brief period following the transient. Note that, although the transient is attenuated, it remains clearly audible, and can be identified, for example as a door slamming or cup being dropped.

We have conducted a series of experiments to optimise the time constants of the dual front-end AGC system (Moore, Glasberg and Stone,

1991; Moore, 1993). In the initial experiments, the dual front-end AGC was implemented as a laboratory prototype. Later experiments have employed chest-worn prototypes using both analogue and digital signal processing. The laboratory experiments showed that the optimum value of the recovery time of the fast component is about 80-150 ms and the optimum value of the attack time of the slow component is about 150-325 ms. Using these values, we were able to show significant benefits of the dual front-end AGC system. In situations where intense transient sounds (such as a door slamming or glass being tapped) were present, and there was either no background sound or continuous speech-shaped noise as a background, the dual front-end AGC gave significantly better speech intelligibility than linear amplification.

One significant problem with the dual front-end AGC was encountered in the laboratory experiments. The gain of the front-end AGC system was sometimes reduced as a result of the wearer of the aid talking. With the very long recovery time of the slow component, weak speech following soon after the wearer had been talking was sometimes inaudible. This problem was dealt with by making two changes in the design of the circuit. Firstly, the input signal was subjected to high-frequency emphasis prior to generation of the slow-acting control signal. The components of the wearer's voice reaching the ear-level hearing aid microphone have most of their energy at low frequencies. Thus, the introduction of high-frequency emphasis reduced the contribution of the wearer's own voice to the control signal. Secondly, the recovery of the slow component was itself given two components: a hold-off time of about 0.5 s during which the gain did not change at all, and a recovery time of about 0.8 s following the end of the hold-off time. During pauses in speech shorter than the hold-off time, the gain did not change. For longer pauses, the gain increased fairly rapidly following the hold off time. This system gave very satisfactory results in field trials.

Overall, the results indicate that the dual front-end AGC does achieve its design goals: it allows speech to be understood over a wide range of sound levels without any need to adjust the controls of the aid; it selectively reduces the gain for intense transients without affecting the long-term gain for speech and it changes the gain in such a way that breathing and pumping noises are not audible. The reactions of users in the field trial were highly favourable.

General conclusions about compression

It appears that compression can be beneficial in two ways. Firstly, it can allow speech in quiet to be understood over a wide range of sound levels without adjustment of the volume control and without the speech ever becoming uncomfortably loud. This can be achieved either by using a slow-acting AVC system, such as the dual front-end AGC (Moore,

Glasberg and Stone, 1991), or by using multi-channel syllabic compression (Moore, Johnson, Clark et al., 1992). Many people find it unnecessary to use the volume control with hearing aids incorporating compression. Indeed, some manufacturers produce compression aids without volume controls. Secondly, for speech at low to medium levels, compression can improve the intelligibility of speech in background noise, presumably by making speech cues more audible.

There is little evidence to support the idea that the benefits of compression accrue from restoring the perception of loudness to 'normal'. Indeed, if fast-acting compression is set up to do this, hearing aid users often complain that everything sounds too 'noisy'. In practice, the aids must be set up so as to 'under-compensate' for the loudness recruitment. Compression sufficient to restore loudness perception to 'normal' sometimes has deleterious effects on speech intelligibility and is not liked by users (Moore, Lynch and Stone, 1992; Plomp, 1994). It seems likely that the benefits of compression arise mainly from the fact that compression increases audibility while avoiding discomfort from loud sounds.

Methods for improving the speech-to-noise ratio

Directional microphones

It is widely acknowledged that the intelligibility of speech in background noise can be improved by increasing the signal-to-noise ratio. In fact, as mentioned in Chapter 8, under difficult listening conditions, each 1 dB improvement in speech-to-noise ratio typically gives an increase of intelligibility of 7 to 19%. One of the few ways of achieving a true improvement in speech-to-noise ratio is to use a directional microphone. Many hearing aids have *omni-directional* microphones that respond equally to sounds from all directions. In contrast, a directional microphone is more sensitive to sounds coming from certain directions than to sounds coming from other directions. In the case of a hearing aid microphone, it is assumed that the user will normally face towards the desired sound source, so the microphone is designed to be more sensitive to sounds coming from the front than to sounds coming from the sides or back. In practice the directional pattern is affected by placement of the microphone close to the head and body and the direction of maximum sensitivity is displaced somewhat away from straight ahead. For example, if the microphone is placed above the left ear, the direction of maximum sensitivity is usually at an azimuth of about 45° - i.e. 45° to the left of straight ahead.

The *directivity* of a microphone is a measure of the sensitivity to sounds coming from the desired direction relative to the sensitivity to sounds from other directions. In principle, a higher directivity gives a greater improvement in speech-to-noise ratio whenever the noise comes from one or more directions other than the desired direction. However, the beneficial effects of directional microphones are reduced in reverberant rooms, since, in such rooms, some of the interfering sound comes from the frontal direction.

Simple directional microphones have been used in hearing aids for many years. Their directivity has not generally been very high but they have been found to give worthwhile improvements in the ability to understand speech in noise. In a situation where the speech comes from in front (0° azimuth) and interfering sounds are used at various azimuths, the SRT in noise can be reduced by 2-3 dB compared to what is obtained with omni-directional microphones or unaided listening (Nielsen and Ludvigsen, 1978; Laurence, Moore and Glasberg, 1983; Hawkins and Yacullo, 1984; Leeuw and Dreschler, 1991). This is equivalent to improvements of intelligibility between 20 and 45% in difficult listening situations. Directional microphones can also improve the ability to localise sounds (Leeuw and Dreschler, 1991). In recent years, some manufacturers have developed directional microphone systems with somewhat improved directivity, and these have been found to give a high degree of user satisfaction (Kochkin, 1996).

Soede and his colleagues (Soede, Berkhout and Bilsen, 1993; Soede, Bilsen and Berkhout, 1993) have developed and evaluated two microphone arrays with improved directionality. The arrays consist of five microphones which can be mounted either along the front of a pair of spectacles (broadside array) or along the side (endfire array). The microphone signals are combined in such a way as to give high directivity. The arrays were evaluated using 30 normally hearing subjects and 45 hearing-impaired subjects listening to speech coming from the frontal direction. Independent speech-shaped noises were emitted from eight loudspeakers positioned on each side of the subject and below and above the subject. Initial tests were conducted using one ear only (the other ear being plugged). The results showed that SRTs in noise were substantially decreased (improved) relative to unaided listening or listening with an omni-directional microphone. Both the broadside array and the endfire array led to reductions in SRT averaging about 7 dB.

Subsequent tests using hearing-impaired subjects listening with two endfire arrays showed that SRTs were typically about 2 dB lower for binaural than for monaural listening. This is comparable to the diotic advantage usually found for listening to speech in noise, as described in Chapter 7. It can be concluded that this system is very effective in improving the ability to understand speech in background noise. Additional physical measurements indicated that the arrays were also effective in reverberant environments and would decrease the interfering effects of the reverberation. One drawback with the arrays is their physical size (14 cm for the broadside array and 10 cm for the endfire array), which is necessary to achieve high directivity. However, users may be willing to accept the large size given the substantial advantages in intelligibility that can be achieved.

Adaptive beamforming

When the outputs of two or more microphones are combined to give a specific directional characteristic, the resulting system is sometimes called a *beamformer* or *spatial filter*. The microphone arrays described above are called fixed beamformers or fixed spatial filters, because their directional characteristics are not time varying. A different type of system is called an adaptive beamformer or adaptive spatial filter (Griffiths and Jim, 1982; Hoffman, Trine, Buckley et al., 1994). Such systems adapt to the characteristics of the interfering sounds, so as to remove as much of the interference as possible. Generally, the goal is to preserve sounds coming from in front while removing sounds coming from other directions as much as possible. For example, if the interfering sound is coming predominantly from an azimuth of 90°, the directional characteristic is adapted so that there is a null in the response at that azimuth. In this way, the interfering sound is effectively suppressed. Adaptive beamformers can use any number of microphones, from two upwards. The microphones do not have to be widely spaced, so the microphone array can be quite compact.

The operation of a simple beamformer is illustrated in Figure 9.5. In this example, two microphones are used. One is the primary microphone, which picks up a mixture of the desired signal, usually speech (S), and the background interference (N1). The second microphone, the reference microphone, is intended to pick up mainly the interference. This can be achieved, for example, by using a microphone that responds to sounds from all directions *except* the frontal direction. Alternatively, a reference signal can be derived from two omni-directional microphones, equally distant from the desired signal, by subtracting their outputs; this cancels the desired signal while leaving most of the interfering sound. The reference signal, which contains a somewhat different version of the noise (N2), is passed through a digital filter whose amplitude and phase response can be adjusted. The output of this filter is subtracted from the primary signal. The basic idea is to adjust the characteristics of the digital filter so as to cancel as much as possible of the interference in the primary signal. This is done using an adaptive procedure that minimises the resultant output. In other words, the characteristics of the filter are adjusted to make the output as small as possible. The quantity that is minimised is usually the power at the output, although this is probably not the best criterion from a perceptual point of view.

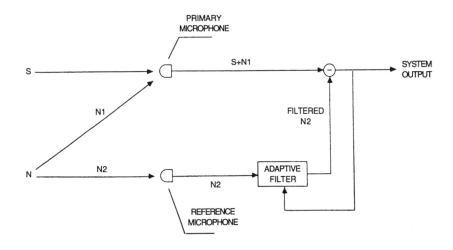

Figure 9.5: A block diagram of a simple adaptive beamformer. Redrawn from Weiss (1987).

Evaluations of such systems have shown that they can give substantial improvements (20 dB or more) in speech-to-background ratio provided that the listening room is not too reverberant (Peterson, Durlach, Rabinowitz et al., 1987; Schwander and Levitt, 1987; Weiss, 1987; Greenberg and Zurek, 1992; Hoffman, Trine, Buckley et al., 1994). However, under reverberant conditions, they do not work as well. Kompis and Dillier (1994) investigated the effect of combining directional microphones with an adaptive beamformer. They reported that the combination gave better intelligibility of speech in noise than either approach alone for sounds in an 'office' sized room with moderate reverberation (reverberation time = 0.4 s).

One significant problem with adaptive beamformers should be noted. The adaptation of the digital filter takes a certain time to occur. The more accurate the required cancellation of the interference, the longer is the response time. The changing response of the adaptive filter can have audible and disturbing effects, especially during head movements of the user.

Binaural processing algorithms

Kollmeier and his co-workers have described several methods of processing sounds that are based on the use of binaural cues to enhance speech-to-background ratios (Kollmeier, Peissig and Hohmann, 1993; Kollmeier and Koch, 1994; Wittkop, Hohmann and Kollmeier, 1996). These cues were described in Chapter 7; the main ones are interaural time differences (ITDs) and interaural level differences (ILDs). It is assumed that the user of the system would wear microphones mounted in or close to their ear canals. The simplest of their processing methods works in the following way. The sound is split into a large number of frequency bands. The ITD and ILD within each band are determined on a moment-by-moment basis. If the ITD and ILD are small within a given band, then the signal within that band probably came from directly in front of the head (although it could in fact come from any direction in the median plane - see Chapter 7). In that case, the signal in that band is passed unaltered. If the ITD and/or ILD are large within a given band, that indicates that the signal in that band is dominated by sound coming from a direction that is off to one side. In this case, the signal in that band is attenuated. In practice, the amount of attenuation is related to the magnitudes of the ITDs and ILDs, and the attenuation is made to vary smoothly over time and across frequency bands. The overall effect of the processing is that sounds from the frontal direction are preserved whereas sounds from other directions are attenuated.

Evaluations of this system (Kollmeier, Peissig and Hohmann, 1993) showed that it could give significant improvements in the intelligibility of speech in a 'cocktail party' situation (with several interfering speakers at various angles), provided that there was no reverberation; the improvements were roughly equivalent to those produced by a 5 dB change in speech-to-background ratio. However, the performance of the algorithm worsened when reverberation was present.

Several more complex schemes have been developed and evaluated, with promising results (Kollmeier, Peissig and Hohmann, 1993; Kollmeier and Koch, 1994; Wittkop, Hohmann and Kollmeier, 1996). However, the schemes are computationally intensive, and they introduce time delays in the signal that may be unacceptable. Further evaluations are necessary to assess how well such schemes may work in everyday situations.

Concluding remarks on schemes to improve the speech-to-noise ratio

Of the schemes described above, directional microphones are the most practical and straightforward. The microphone arrays described by Soede and co-workers (Soede, Berkhout and Bilsen, 1993; Soede, Bilsen and Berkhout, 1993) can be implemented without elaborate electronics. They produce a true improvement in speech-to-background ratio in both reverberant and non-reverberant environments and they do this without introducing processing artifacts. Furthermore, they do not introduce significant time delays. However, they are physically rather large, and this may limit their acceptability.

One other problem should be noted. High directionality is useful in noisy situations but it can be a problem in other situations, as the user

becomes effectively 'deaf' for certain directions. This makes it more difficult to detect voices coming from non-frontal directions and to detect
environmental sounds such as approaching cars. A highly directional
characteristic may also be undesirable when listening to music. This
problem can be alleviated by allowing the user to select either a directional characteristic or an omni-directional characteristic (as in some
aids made by Phonak, or incorporating the 'D-mic' system made by
Etymõtic Research).

Schemes based on digital signal processing are computationally
intensive, but may appear soon in digital hearing aids. The schemes
sometimes introduce processing artifacts, which may be audible and
disturbing. Furthermore, they can introduce significant time delays. This
may be a problem when the user is trying to combine visual information
(lip-reading) with auditory information. The delay may also affect
perception of the user's own voice, since their voice will often be heard
both via bone conduction and via the aid. The interference of delayed
and non-delayed sound can create disturbing echoes and coloration.
Processing algorithms will need to be designed so as to minimise time
delays, preferably keeping them below a few tens of milliseconds.

Signal-processing aids for severe and profound hearing loss

People with severe or profound hearing loss often derive little or no
benefit from conventional hearing aids. They usually have very small
dynamic ranges so extreme compression may be required to make
speech audible without it being uncomfortably loud. In people with
profound losses, residual hearing may be limited to a small frequency
range, say up to 1000 Hz. Even when speech is made audible, as far as
possible, the residual auditory capacities, such as frequency selectivity
and frequency discrimination, may be very poor (Faulkner, Fourcin and
Moore, 1990; Faulkner, Rosen and Moore, 1990), so the ability to understand speech, in quiet or in noise, is greatly diminished in comparison to
normally hearing people.

One approach to designing more effective hearing aids for such
people is based on the concept of extraction and presentation of speech
features. The basic idea is to extract simple features or patterns from
speech, such as the fundamental frequency of the speech, and to present
those features in a simplified form that is matched to the auditory abilities of the user. The extracted features may be designed specifically to
be used in conjunction with lip-reading. For example, the presence or
absence of voicing (vibration of the vocal folds) is difficult or impossible
to determine by looking at the face of the talker but it conveys important
linguistic information. By supplementing lip-reading with an auditory
signal that indicates the presence or absence of voicing, speech under-

standing may be improved. The improvement can be larger if information about the fundamental frequency (F0) of the voice is also conveyed (Rosen, Fourcin and Moore, 1981).

Faulkner, Ball, Rosen et al. (1992) described an evaluation of an aid based on this principle, called the SiVo (Sinusoidal Voice) aid. The aid detects when voicing occurs and extracts the F0 of the speaker's voice on a period-by-period basis. A sinusoid is synthesised whose period is equal to that of the extracted F0 and this synthesised signal is presented to the user. Optionally, the frequency of the synthesised sinusoid can be shifted downwards. This is useful in cases where the speaker has a voice with a high average F0 (for example a child); shifting F0 downwards can have the effect of making the sinusoid more audible and of increasing the discriminability of changes in F0, which convey intonation and linguistic structure (see Chapter 8). The synthesised sinusoid is generated with an output level that is independent of the input level of the speech; rather it is set to the user's most comfortable listening level for the specific frequency being generated. This ensures that the signal is always audible and comfortable. One rationale for synthesising a sinusoid rather than a complex periodic signal is that, for people with profound hearing loss, frequency discrimination is sometimes better for sinusoids than it is for complex tones.

Faulkner et al. evaluated the SiVo aid by comparing it with 'conventional' hearing aids with AGC and an extended low-frequency output (to make optimal use of the residual hearing of the subjects), using an audio-visual consonant recognition task. Out of eleven profoundly hearing-impaired subjects, four scored more highly with the SiVo aid, five performed better with the conventional aids and two achieved similar scores for the two types of aids.

In a second study, they evaluated a more complex laboratory prototype version of the SiVo aid, that presented more speech features. The amplitude envelope of the whole speech signal was used to modulate the output sinusoid, with appropriate compression so as to map the amplitude fluctuations into the user's available dynamic range. The presence of noise-like speech sounds (e.g. s, sh, p, t, k) was signalled by low-frequency noise. This compound speech-pattern aid was demonstrated to give better consonant identification than the simple SiVo aid. Of five subjects tested with this aid, three showed better speech recognition than with a 'conventional' aid and two showed similar performance for the speech-pattern aid and the conventional aid. The better performance for the speech-pattern aid was obtained both for consonant identification and for the tracking of connected discourse.

In a more recent study, Faulkner, van Son, Beijk et al. (1998) evaluated a wearable aid called the SiVo-3, similar to the laboratory prototype described above. The aid was implemented using a digital signal processor, and information about voicing and fundamental frequency were extracted using a 'neural network' (also called a multi-layer percep-tron), which worked well in the presence of background noise. The aid could also be programmed as a 'conventional' aid fitted according to the POGO prescription (McCandless and Lyregard, 1983). The SiVo-3 and 'conventional' aids were compared using 12 profoundly hearing-impaired subjects, after a training period of about three months, using measures of audio-visual consonant and sentence perception. For speech in quiet, performance did not differ significantly between the two aids. However, when speech-shaped noise was present at speech-to-noise ratios between 5 and 10 dB, performance was better for the SiVo-3 aid. Subjective ratings indicated a preference for the SiVo-3 aid over the 'conventional' aid when listening to speech in noise or in a group.

Overall, these results seem promising. Speech-pattern hearing aids may prove to be a useful alternative to conventional aids or to cochlear implants (see below) for those with profound hearing loss.

Cochlear implants

Cochlear implants represent a form of treatment for severe to total deafness arising from damage to the cochlea. Such deafness is usually associated with loss of function of the outer and inner hair cells, but the auditory nerve survives to some extent. The treatment involves the implantation of electrodes so as to stimulate the surviving neurones electrically. This results in sensations of sound.

It is beyond the scope of this book to give more than a brief overview of this topic. For reviews see Clark, Tong and Patrick (1990), Tyler (1993) and Parkins (1997). Briefly, the systems currently in use have two major parts. One part is external to the patient. It consists of a microphone to pick up the sound, and a processor (that may be analogue or digital) that analyses the sound and derives from it signals appropriate for delivery to the individual electrodes. These signals are transmitted through the skin to the implanted part of the system. This consists of a receiver of the transmitted signals, and a device which separates the signals intended for the individual electrodes and delivers each of these signals to its appropriate electrode. The electrodes are usually implanted within the cochlea, by insertion through the round window.

The majority of cochlear implants currently in use are multi-channel devices, using several electrodes, although some devices have only one channel. The multi-channel devices attempt to exploit the tonotopic or 'place' organisation of the cochlea - see Chapter 1. The electrodes are distributed as far as possible along the length of the cochlea and each is intended to stimulate neurones with a limited range of CFs (here, CF is used to refer to the frequency that would best excite a given neurone if the cochlea were not damaged). In practice, it is difficult to insert the electrode array very deeply into the cochlea, so the electrodes mainly lie close to neurones with medium and high CFs. The electrical current from a given electrode or electrode pair also spreads out within the cochlea, so the stimulation is not confined to neurones with a small range of CFs.

In a cochlear implant, information is transmitted in two basic ways: in terms of which electrode is active or of the distribution of current across electrodes ('place' coding) and in terms of the amplitude and time pattern of stimulation on individual electrodes ('temporal' coding). Changes in the place of stimulation generally give rise to changes in perceived timbre; stimulation at the basal end gives a 'sharp' timbre whereas stimulation towards the apical end gives a more mellow or bass-like timbre. Sometimes the percepts associated with stimulation of different places are described in terms of differences in pitch rather than differences in timbre (McDermott and McKay, 1997). Changes in the rate of stimulation on a single electrode can give rise to changes in perceived pitch, if the rate is below a few hundred Hertz (Pijl and Schwarz, 1995; Pijl, 1997). If an electrode is stimulated with brief electrical pulses at a high rate (say 1000 pulses per second), amplitude modulation of the pulses can lead to the percept of a pitch related to the modulation rate (McKay, McDermott and Clark, 1994; McDermott and McKay, 1997).

Many different coding 'strategies' have been used in cochlear implants. Some strategies are based on the extraction of certain speech features, an approach similar to that used with the SiVo aid described above. For example, one version of the 'Nucleus' device (Clark and al., 1987) extracts F0 and the frequencies of the first two formants. The value of F0 is signalled by the rate of electrical pulses, whereas the formant frequencies are signalled according to which electrodes are stimulated. The device also detects the presence of frication and signals this by an irregular pulse pattern on electrodes towards the base of the cochlea.

Other devices filter the signal into frequency bands; the output from each band is used to derive a signal that stimulates a specific electrode. In one coding strategy, called compressed analogue (CA), the input waveform is first compressed, then filtered, and the resulting analogue waveforms are applied directly to the electrodes (Eddington, 1983). In another strategy, the envelopes of the outputs of the filters are used to control the amplitudes of brief electrical pulses that are delivered at a constant high rate (typically about 800 pulses per second). The pulses are interleaved on the different electrodes, hence the name 'continuous interleaved sampling' (CIS) (Wilson, Finley, Lawson et al., 1991). The interleaving is done to reduce interactions of electrical fields between electrodes, so as to improve the specificity of place coding (Parkins, 1997). This type of processing has been found to be very effective, and it is incorporated in several commercial devices, for example the Clarion, Med-El, and Laura devices.

Nucleus has moved away from an approach based on feature extraction to an approach based on presenting information about momentary spectral peaks in the signal. One recent processor incorporates 20 bandpass filters with centre frequencies distributed over a range from roughly 150 to 10 800 Hz. About every 4 ms, between one and 10 (typically six) filters with the largest outputs are selected and corresponding electrodes are stimulated by current pulses whose amplitudes are determined by the respective filter outputs. This is referred to as the 'SPEAK' processing strategy.

Results obtained using cochlear implants vary widely across patients even for a single type of implant. However, it is remarkable that for each of the different types of implants described above, some patients have achieved good levels of speech understanding without lip-reading. Almost all patients find that the quality of their lives has been improved by the implants. It is difficult to determine which system is the 'best'. Current evidence suggests that CIS gives better speech intelligibility than CA (Wilson, Finley, Lawson et al., 1991) and the SPEAK processor gives better speech intelligibility than the earlier processor based on feature extraction (McKay and McDermott, 1993; Skinner, Fourakis, Holden et al., 1996).

When cochlear implants were first introduced they were restricted to people with total or near-total hearing loss. However, the results have been sufficiently good that their use has been extended to people with a small amount of residual hearing. An important area for future research is to devise criteria to decide on the most effective treatment for a specific person with a profound hearing loss; should they be given a 'conventional' aid (with AGC), a speech-pattern aid, or a cochlear implant? Cochlear implants are now being widely used with children (McCormick, Archbold and Sheppard, 1994). The results have been very promising, with especially good results for children who are implanted at an early age.

Some concluding remarks

Hearing aids have improved considerably in recent years. Aids are available with low distortion and with smooth wideband frequency responses. Many aids, and especially the newer programmable aids, have a high degree of flexibility in shaping their frequency-gain characteristic. In principle it is usually possible to tailor the frequency response of a linear aid to suit an individual patient. Hearing aids are also available that offer reasonably effective compensation for loudness recruitment. In practice, however, many hearing-impaired people are still being fitted with hearing aids that have significant distortion, that have an irregular frequency response with an inappropriate shape, and that do not offer effective compensation for loudness recruitment.

Even the best possible current hearing aids do not restore hearing to normal; especially when listening to speech in noise or competing speech, hearing-impaired people listening through hearing aids perform more poorly than normally hearing people. This situation may be improved in the future through the use of directional microphones and through the use of digital signal processing to improve speech-to-background ratios. Digital hearing aids also offer the possibility of very precise frequency response shaping and compensation for loudness recruitment. People with severe or profound hearing losses may benefit from future developments in speech-pattern hearing aids and cochlear implants.

References

Allen JB (1977) Short term spectral analysis, synthesis and modification by discrete Fourier transform. IEEE Trans Acoust Speech Sig Proc 25: 235–38.

Allen JB, Jeng PS (1990) Loudness growth in 1/2–octave bands (LGOB); a procedure for the assessment of loudness. J Acoust Soc Am 88: 745–753.

American Standards Association (1960) Acoustical Terminology. SI, 1–1960. New York: American Standards Association.

Aniansson G (1974) Methods for assessing high-frequency hearing loss in everyday situations. Acta Otolaryngol Suppl 320: 1–50.

ANSI (1969) S.3.5. American national standard methods for the calculation of the articulation index. New York: American National Standards Institute.

Arehart KH (1994) Effects of harmonic content on complex-tone fundamental-frequency discrimination in hearing-impaired listeners. J Acoust Soc Am 95: 3574–85.

Arthur RM, Pfeiffer RR, Suga N (1971) Properties of 'two-tone inhibition' in primary auditory neurones. J Physiol 212: 593–609.

Ashmore JF (1987) A fast motile response in guinea pig outer hair cells: the cellular basis of the cochlear amplifier. J Physiol 388: 323–47.

Attneave F, Olson RK (1971) Pitch as a medium: a new approach to psychophysical scaling. Am J Psychol 84: 147–166.

Bachem A (1950) Tone height and tone chroma as two different pitch qualities. Acta Psychol 7: 80–8.

Bacon SP, Gleitman RM (1992) Modulation detection in subjects with relatively flat hearing losses. J Speech Hear Res 35: 642–53.

Bacon SP, Viemeister NF (1985) Temporal modulation transfer functions in normal-hearing and hearing-impaired subjects. Audiology 24: 117–34.

Baer T, Moore BCJ (1993) Effects of spectral smearing on the intelligibility of sentences in the presence of noise. J Acoust Soc Am 94: 1229–41.

Baer T, Moore BCJ (1994) Effects of spectral smearing on the intelligibility of sentences in the presence of interfering speech. J Acoust Soc Am 95: 2277–80.

Bench J, Bamford J (1979) Speech-Hearing Tests and the Spoken Language of Hearing-Impaired Children. London: Academic Press.

Berlin CI (1996) Hair Cells and Hearing Aids. San Diego: Singular.

Beveridge HA, Carlyon RP (1996) Effects of aspirin on human psychophysical tuning curves in forward and simultaneous masking. Hear Res 99: 110–18.

Blauert J (1996) Spatial Hearing: The Psychophysics of Human Sound Localization. Cambridge MA: MIT Press.

Bonding P (1979a) Critical bandwidth in loudness summation in sensorineural hearing loss. Brit J Audiol 13: 23–30.

Bonding P (1979b) Frequency selectivity and speech discrimination in sensorineural hearing loss. Scand Audiol 8: 205–16.

Bonding P, Elberling C (1980) Loudness summation across frequency under masking and in sensorineural hearing loss. Audiology 19: 57–74.

Bornstein SP, Randolph KJ (1983) Research on smooth wideband frequency responses: current status and unresolved issues. Hear Inst 34: 12–16.

Braida LD, Durlach NI, De Gennaro SV, Peterson PM, Bustamante DK (1982) Review of recent research on multiband amplitude compression for the hearing impaired. In GA Studebaker and FH Bess (eds) The Vanderbilt Hearing-Aid Report. Upper Darby PA: Monographs in Contemporary Audiology.

Brokx JPL, Nooteboom SG (1982). Intonation and the perceptual separation of simultaneous voices. J Phonetics 10: 23–36.

Bronkhorst AW, Plomp R (1988) The effect of head-induced interaural time and level differences on speech intelligibility in noise. J Acoust Soc Am 83: 1508–16.

Bronkhorst AW, Plomp R (1989) Binaural speech intelligibility in noise for hearing-impaired listeners. J Acoust Soc Am 86: 1374–83.

Burkhard MD, Sachs RM (1975) Anthropometric manikin for acoustic research. J Acoust Soc Am 58: 214–22.

Burns EM, Keefe DH, Ling R (1998) Energy reflectance in the ear canal can exceed unity near spontaneous otoacoustic emission frequencies. J Acoust Soc Am 103: 462–74.

Burns EM, Turner C (1986) Pure-tone pitch anomalies. II. Pitch-intensity effects and diplacusis in impaired ears. J Acoust Soc Am 79: 1530–40.

Bustamante DK, Braida LD (1987) Multiband compression limiting for hearing-impaired listeners. J Rehab Res Devel 24: 149–60.

Buus S, Florentine M (1985) Gap detection in normal and impaired listeners: the effect of level and frequency. In A Michelsen (ed.) Time Resolution in Auditory Systems. New York: Springer-Verlag.

Buus S, Florentine M, Poulsen T (1997) Temporal integration of loudness, loudness discrimination, and the form of the loudness function. J Acoust Soc Am 101: 669–80.

Buus S, Florentine M, Redden RB (1982a) The SISI test: A review. Part I. Audiology 21: 273–93.

Buus S, Florentine M, Redden RB (1982b) The SISI test: A review. Part II. Audiology 21: 365–85.

Buus S, Schorer E, Florentine M, Zwicker E (1986) Decision rules in detection of simple and complex tones. J Acoust Soc Am 80: 1646–57.

Byrne D, Dillon H (1986) The National Acoustic Laboratories' (NAL) new procedure for selecting the gain and frequency response of a hearing aid. Ear Hear 7: 257–65.

Byrne D et al (1994) An international comparison of long-term average speech spectra. J Acoust Soc Am 96: 2108–20.

Cariani PA, Delgutte B (1996a) Neural correlates of the pitch of complex tones. I: Pitch and pitch salience. J Neurophysiol 76: 1698–716.

Cariani PA, Delgutte B (1996b) Neural correlates of the pitch of complex tones. II: Pitch shift, pitch ambiguity, phase invariance, pitch circularity, rate pitch and the dominance region for pitch. J Neurophysiol 76: 1717–34.

Carlyon RP (1997) The effects of two temporal cues on pitch judgements. J Acoust Soc Am 102: 1097–105.

Carlyon RP, Buus S, Florentine M (1990) Temporal integration of trains of tone pulses by normal and by cochlearly impaired listeners. J Acoust Soc Am 87: 260–8.

Carlyon RP, Shackleton TM (1994) Comparing the fundamental frequencies of resolved and unresolved harmonics: Evidence for two pitch mechanisms? J Acoust Soc Am 95: 3541–54.

Carney AE, Nelson DA (1983) An analysis of psychophysical tuning curves in normal and pathological ears. J Acoust Soc Am 73: 268–78.

Celmer RD, Bienvenue GR (1987) Critical bands in the perception of speech signals by normal and sensorineural hearing loss listeners. In MEH Schouten (ed.) The Psychophysics of Speech Perception. Dordrecht: Nijhoff.

Ching T, Dillon H, Byrne D (1997) Prediction of speech recognition from audibility and psychoacoustic abilities of hearing-impaired listeners. In W Jesteadt (ed.) Modeling Sensorineural Hearing Loss. Mawah NJ: Erlbaum.

Chistovich LA (1957) Frequency characteristics of masking effect. Biophys 2: 743–55.

Chung DY (1981) Masking, temporal integration, and sensorineural hearing loss. J Speech Hear Res 24: 514–20.

Clark GM et al. (1987) The University of Melbourne-Nucleus Multi-electrode Cochlear Implant. Basel: Karger.

Clark GM, Tong YC, Patrick JF (1990). Cochlear Prostheses. Edinburgh: Churchill Livingstone.

Cokely CG, Humes LE (1993) Two experiments on the temporal boundaries for the non-linear additivity of masking. J Acoust Soc Am 94: 2553–9.

Colburn HS (1996) Computational models of binaural processing. In H Hawkins, T McMullin (eds) Auditory Computation. New York: Springer-Verlag.

Colburn HS, Trahiotis C (1992) Effects of noise on binaural hearing. In A Dancer, D Henderson, R Salvi, R Hamernik (eds) Noise-Induced Hearing Loss. St Louis: Mosby.

Cooper NP, Rhode WS (1992) Basilar membrane mechanics in the hook region of cat and guinea-pig cochleae: sharp tuning and non-linearity in the absence of baseline position shifts. Hear Res 63: 163–190.

Cornelisse LE, Seewald RC, Jamieson DG (1995) The input/output formula: a theoretical approach to the fitting of personal amplification devices. J Acoust Soc Am 97: 1854–64.

Cox RM (1995) Using loudness data for hearing aid selection. The IHAFF approach. Hear J 48: 1039–44.

Cox RM, Alexander GC, Taylor IM, Gray GA (1997) The contour test of loudness perception. Ear Hear 18: 388–400.

Cox RM, Gilmore C (1986) Damping and the hearing aid frequency response: effects on speech clarity and preferred listening level. J Speech Hear Res 29: 357–65.

Cox RM, Gilmore C (1990) Development of the profile of hearing aid performance. J Speech Hear Res 33: 343–57.

Crain TR, Van Tasell D J (1994) Effect of peak clipping on speech recognition threshold. Ear Hear 15: 443–53.

Crain TR, Yund EW (1995) The effect of multichannel compression on vowel and stop-consonant discrimination in normal-hearing and hearing-impaired subjects. Ear Hear 16: 529–43.

Culling JF, Darwin CJ (1993) Perceptual separation of simultaneous vowels: Within and across-formant grouping by F0. J Acoust Soc Am 93: 3454–67.

Dallos P (1973) The Auditory Periphery: Biophysics and Physiology. New York: Academic Press.

Davis A, Haggard M, Bell I (1990) Magnitude of diotic summation in speech-in-noise tasks: Performance region and appropriate baseline. Brit J Audiol 24: 11–16.

Davis AC, Haggard MP (1982) Some implications of audiological measures in the population for binaural aiding strategies. Scand Audiol Suppl 15.

Davis H (1962) Advances in the neurophysiology and neuroanatomy of the cochlea. J Acoust Soc Am 34: 1377–85.

De Filippo CL, Snell KB (1986) Detection of a temporal gap in low-frequency narrowband signals by normal hearing and hearing-impaired listeners. J Acoust Soc Am 80: 1354–8.

De Mare G (1948). Investigations into the functions of the auditory apparatus in perception deafness. Acta Otolaryngol Suppl 74: 107–16.

Delgutte B (1988) Physiological mechanisms of masking. In H Duifhuis, J W Horst, HP Wit (eds) Basic Issues in Hearing. London: Academic Press.

Delgutte B (1990) Physiological mechanisms of psychophysical masking: Observations from auditory-nerve fibers. J Acoust Soc Am 87: 791–809.

Delgutte B (1996) Physiological models for basic auditory percepts. In HL Hawkins, TA McMullen, AN Popper, RR Fay (eds) Auditory Computation. New York: Springer.

Dillon H (1996) Compression? Yes, but for low or high frequencies for low or high intensities and with what response times? Ear Hear 17: 287–307.

Dillon H, Macrae J (1984) Derivation of design specifications for hearing aids (NAL report number 102). Canberra: Australian Government Publishing Service.

Dix M, Hallpike C, Hood J (1948) Observations upon the loudness recruitment phonemenon with especial reference to the differential diagnosis of disorders of the internal ear and VIIIth nerve. J Laryngol Otol 62: 671–86.

Dobie RA (1997) Drug treatments for sensorineural hearing loss and tinnitus. In CI Berlin (ed.) Neurotransmission and Hearing Loss. San Diego: Singular.

Dreschler WA, Plomp R (1980) Relations between psychophysical data and speech perception for hearing-impaired subjects. I. J Acoust Soc Am 68: 1608–15.

Dreschler WA, Plomp R (1985) Relations between psychophysical data and speech perception for hearing-impaired subjects. II. J Acoust Soc Am 78: 1261–70.

Drullman R, Festen JM, Plomp R (1994) Effect of temporal envelope smearing on speech reception. J Acoust Soc Am 95: 1053–64.

Dubno JR, Dirks DD (1989) Auditory filter characteristics and consonant recognition for hearing-impaired listeners. J Acoust Soc Am 85: 1666–75.

Dubno JR, Schaefer AB (1992) Comparison of frequency selectivity and consonant recognition among hearing-impaired and masked normal-hearing listeners. J Acoust Soc Am 91: 2110–21.

Duchnowski P (1989) Simulation of sensorineural hearing impairment. MS Thesis, MIT, Cambridge MA.

Duchnowski P, Zurek PM (1995) Villchur revisited: Another look at automatic gain control simulation of hearing loss. J Acoust Soc Am 98: 3170–81.

Dugal R, Braida LD, Durlach NI (1978) Implications of previous research for the selection of frequency-gain characteristics. In GA Studebaker, I Hochberg (eds) Acoustical Factors Affecting Hearing Aid Performance. Baltimore: University Park Press.

Duifhuis H (1973) Consequences of peripheral frequency selectivity for nonsimultaneous masking. J Acoust Soc Am 54: 1471–88.

Duquesnoy AJ (1983) Effect of a single interfering noise or speech source on the binaural sentence intelligibility of aged persons. J Acoust Soc Am 74: 739–43.

Duquesnoy AJ, Plomp R (1983) The effect of a hearing aid on the speech-reception threshold of hearing-impaired listeners in quiet and in noise. J Acoust Soc Am 73: 2166–73.

Durlach NI, Thompson CL, Colburn HS (1981) Binaural interaction in impaired listeners. Audiology 20: 181–211.

Dye RH, Hafter ER (1984) The effects of intensity on the detection of interaural differences of time in high-frequency trains of clicks. J Acoust Soc Am 75: 1593–8.

Eddington DK (1983) Speech recognition in deaf subjects with multichannel intracochlear electrodes. Ann New York Acad Sci 405: 241–58.

Eddins DA, Green DM (1995) Temporal integration and temporal resolution. In BCJ Moore (ed.) Hearing. San Diego: Academic Press.

Eddins DA, Hall JW, Grose JH (1992) Detection of temporal gaps as a function of frequency region and absolute noise bandwidth. J Acoust Soc Am 91: 1069–77.

Egan JP, Hake HW (1950) On the masking pattern of a simple auditory stimulus. J Acoust Soc Am 22: 622–30.

Elberling C, Nielsen C (1993) The dynamics of speech and the auditory dynamic range in sensorineural hearing impairment. In J Beilin, GR Jensen (eds) Recent Developments in Hearing, Instrument Technology. Copenhagen: Stougaard Jensen.

Elliott LL (1975) Temporal and masking phenomena in persons with sensorineural hearing loss. Audiology 14: 336–53.

Evans EF (1975) The sharpening of frequency selectivity in the normal and abnormal cochlea. Audiology 14: 419–42.

Evans EF (1978) Place and time coding of frequency in the peripheral auditory system: some physiological pros and cons. Audiology 17: 369–420.

Evans EF, Harrison RV (1976) Correlation between outer hair cell damage and deterioration of cochlear nerve tuning properties in the guinea pig. J Physiol 252: 43–44.

Exner S (1876) Zur Lehre von den Gehörsempfindungen. Pflügers Archiv 13: 228–53.

Fabry DA, Van Tasell DJ (1986) Masked and filtered simulation of hearing loss: Effects on consonant recognition. J Speech Hear Res 29: 170–8.

Fastl H (1976) Temporal masking effects: I. Broad band noise masker. Acustica 35: 287–302.

Faulkner A, Ball V, Rosen S, Moore BCJ, Fourcin AJ (1992) Speech pattern hearing aids for the profoundly hearing impaired: Speech perception and auditory abilities. J Acoust Soc Am 91: 2136–55.

Faulkner A, Fourcin AJ, Moore BCJ (1990) Psychoacoustic aspects of speech pattern coding for the deaf. Acta Otolaryngol Suppl 469: 172–80.

Faulkner A, Rosen S, Moore BCJ (1990) Residual frequency selectivity in the profoundly hearing-impaired listener. Brit J Audiol 24: 381–92.

Faulkner A, Van Son N, Beijk C, Smith K, Wei J, Walliker JR (1998) Speech perception in quiet and noise: Speech-analytic processing for the profoundly impaired listener. Brit J Audiol 32: 40–1.

Feddersen WE, Sandel TT, Teas DC, Jeffress LA (1957) Localization of high-frequency tones. J Acoust Soc Am 29: 988–91.

Festen JM, Plomp R (1983) Relations between auditory functions in impaired hearing J Acoust Soc Am 73: 652–62.

Festen JM, Plomp R (1990) Effects of fluctuating noise and interfering speech on the speech-reception threshold for impaired and normal hearing. J Acoust Soc Am 88: 1725–36.

Fitzgibbons PJ (1983) Temporal gap detection in noise as a function of frequency, bandwidth and level. J Acoust Soc Am 74: 67–72.

Fitzgibbons PJ, Gordon-Salant S (1987) Minimum stimulus levels for temporal gap resolution in listeners with sensorineural hearing loss. J Acoust Soc Am 81: 1542–5.

Fitzgibbons PJ, Wightman FL (1982) Gap detection in normal and hearing-impaired listeners. J Acoust Soc Am 72: 761–5.

Flanagan JL, Saslow MG (1958) Pitch discrimination for synthetic vowels. J Acoust Soc Am 30: 435–42.

Fletcher H (1940) Auditory patterns. Rev Mod Phys 12: 47–65.

Fletcher H (1952) The perception of sounds by deafened persons. J Acoust Soc Am 24: 490–7.

Fletcher H (1953) Speech and Hearing in Communication. New York: Van Nostrand.

Fletcher H, Munson WA (1933) Loudness: Its definition, measurement and calculation. J Acoust Soc Am 5: 82–108.

Fletcher H, Munson WA (1937) Relation between loudness and masking. J Acoust Soc Am 9: 1–10.

Florentine M, Buus S (1984) Temporal gap detection in sensorineural and simulated hearing impairment. J Speech Hear Res 27: 449–55.

Florentine M, Buus S, Hellman RP (1997) A model of loudness summation applied to high-frequency hearing loss. In W Jesteadt (ed.) Modeling Sensorineural Hearing Loss. Mahwah NJ: Erlbaum.

Florentine M, Buus S, Scharf B, Zwicker E (1980) Frequency selectivity in normally-hearing and hearing-impaired observers. J Speech Hear Res 23: 643–69.

Florentine M, Fastl H, Buus S (1988) Temporal integration in normal hearing, cochlear impairment and impairment simulated by masking. J Acoust Soc Am 84: 195–203.

Florentine M, Houtsma A J M (1983) Tuning curves and pitch matches in a listener with a unilateral low-frequency hearing loss. J Acoust Soc Am 73: 961–5.

Florentine M, Zwicker E (1979) A model of loudness summation applied to noise-induced hearing loss. Hear Res 1: 121–32.

Formby C (1982) Differential sensitivity to tonal frequency and to the rate of amplitude modulation of broad-band noise by hearing-impaired listeners. PhD Thesis. Washington University, St Louis.

Fowler E P (1936) A method for the early detection of otosclerosis. Arch Otolaryngol 24: 731–41.

French NR, Steinberg JC (1947) Factors governing the intelligibility of speech sounds. J Acoust Soc Am 19: 90–119.

Freyman RL, Nelson DA (1986) Frequency discrimination as a function of tonal duration and excitation-pattern slopes in normal and hearing-impaired listeners. J Acoust Soc Am 79: 1034–44.

Freyman RL, Nelson DA (1987) Frequency discrimination of short- versus long-duration tones by normal and hearing-impaired listeners. J Speech Hear Res 30: 28–36.

Freyman RL, Nelson DA (1991) Frequency discrimination as a function of signal frequency and level in normal-hearing and hearing-impaired listeners. J Speech Hear Res 34: 1371–86.

Gabriel B, Kollmeier B, Mellert V (1997). Influence of individual listener, measurement room and choice of test-tone levels on the shape of equal-loudness level contours. Acustica – Acta Acustica 83: 670–83.

Gabriel KJ, Koehnke J, Colburn HS (1992) Frequency dependence of binaural performance in listeners with impaired binaural hearing. J Acoust Soc Am 91: 336–47.

Gaeth J, Norris T (1965) Diplacusis in unilateral high frequency hearing losses. J Speech Hear Res 8: 63–75.

Garner WR (1954) Context effects and the validity of loudness scales. J Exp Psychol 48: 218–24.

Garner WR, Miller GA (1947) The masked threshold of pure tones as a function of duration. J Exp Psychol 37: 293–303.

Gatehouse S (1992) The time course and magnitude of perceptual acclimatization to frequency responses: Evidence from monaural fitting of hearing aids. J Acoust Soc Am 92: 1258–68.

Gatehouse S, Haggard MP (1987) The effects of air-bone gap and presentation level on word identification. Ear Hear 8: 140–6.

Gengel RW (1973) Temporal effects on frequency discrimination by hearing-impaired listeners. J Acoust Soc Am 54: 11–15.

Gengel RW, Watson CS (1971) Temporal integration: I. Clinical implications of a laboratory study. II. Additional data from hearing-impaired subjects. J Speech Hear Disord 36: 213–24.

Giguère C, Woodland PC (1994) A computational model of the auditory periphery for speech and hearing research: Ascending path. J Acoust Soc Am 95: 331–42.

Glasberg BR, Moore BCJ (1986) Auditory filter shapes in subjects with unilateral and bilateral cochlear impairments. J Acoust Soc Am 79: 1020–33.

Glasberg BR, Moore BCJ (1989) Psychoacoustic abilities of subjects with unilateral and bilateral cochlear impairments and their relationship to the ability to understand speech. Scand Audiol Suppl 32: 1–25.

Glasberg BR, Moore BCJ (1990) Derivation of auditory filter shapes from notched-noise data. Hear Res 47: 103–38.

Glasberg BR, Moore BCJ (1992) Effects of envelope fluctuations on gap detection. Hear Res 64: 81–92.

Glasberg BR, Moore BCJ, Bacon SP (1987) Gap detection and masking in hearing-impaired and normal-hearing subjects. J Acoust Soc Am 81: 1546–56.

Glasberg BR, Moore BCJ, Nimmo-Smith I (1984) Comparison of auditory filter shapes derived with three different maskers. J Acoust Soc Am 75: 536–44.

Goldstein JL (1973) An optimum processor theory for the central formation of the pitch of complex tones. J Acoust Soc Am 54: 1496–516.

Goldstein JL, Srulovicz P (1977) Auditory-nerve spike intervals as an adequate basis for aural frequency measurement. In EF Evans, JP Wilson (eds) Psychophysics and Physiology of Hearing. London: Academic Press.

Goodman A (1965) Reference zero levels for pure-tone audiometer. ASHA 7: 262–63.

Gorga MP, Neely ST, Ohlrich B, Hoover B, Redner J, Peters J (1997) From laboratory to clinic: a large scale study of distortion product otoacoustic emissions in ears with normal hearing and ears with hearing loss. Ear Hear 18: 440–55.

Grant KW (1987) Frequency modulation detection by normally hearing and profoundly hearing-impaired listeners. J Speech Hear Res 30: 558–63.

Grant KW, Ardell LH, Kuhl PK, Sparks D W (1985) The contributions of fundamental frequency, amplitude envelope and voicing duration cues to speechreading in normal-hearing subjects. J Acoust Soc Am 77: 671–7.

Grantham DW (1995) Spatial hearing and related phenomena. In BCJ Moore (ed.) Hearing. New York: Academic Press.

Green DM (1985) Temporal factors in psychoacoustics. In A Michelsen (ed.) Time Resolution in Auditory Systems. New York: Springer-Verlag.

Green DM, Swets JA (1974) Signal Detection Theory and Psychophysics. New York: Krieger.

Greenberg JE, Zurek PM (1992) Evaluation of an adaptive beamforming method for hearing aids. J Acoust Soc Am 91: 1662–76.

Greenwood DD (1961) Critical bandwidth and the frequency coordinates of the basilar membrane. J Acoust Soc Am 33: 1344–56.

Greenwood DD (1971) Aural combination tones and auditory masking. J Acoust Soc Am 50: 502–43.

Griffiths LJ, Jim CW (1982) An alternative approach to linearly constrained adaptive beamforming. IEEE Trans Antennas Propag AP-30: 27–34.

Hall JW, Fernandes MA (1983) Temporal integration, frequency resolution and off-frequency listening in normal-hearing and cochlear-impaired listeners. J Acoust Soc Am 74: 1172–7.

Hall JW, Haggard MP, Fernandes MA (1984) Detection in noise by spectro-temporal pattern analysis. J Acoust Soc Am 76: 50–6.

Hall JW, Tyler RS, Fernandes MA (1984) Factors influencing the masking level difference in cochlear hearing-impaired and normal-hearing listeners. J Speech Hear Res, 27, 145–154.

Hall JW, Wood EJ (1984) Stimulus duration and frequency discrimination for normal-hearing and hearing-impaired subjects. J Speech Hear Res 27: 252–6.

Handel S. (1995). Timbre perception and auditory object identification. In BCJ Moore (ed.) Hearing. San Diego: Academic Press.

Harris JD (1963) Loudness discrimination. J Speech Hear Disord Monographs Supplement 11: 1–63.

Harrison RV, Evans EF (1979) Some aspects of temporal coding by single cochlear fibres from regions of cochlear hair cell degeneration in the guinea pig. Arch Otolaryngol 224: 71–8.

Häusler R, Colburn HS, Marr E (1983) Sound localization in subjects with impaired hearing. Acta Otolaryngol Suppl 400: 1–62.

Hawkins DB, Wightman FL (1980). Interaural time discrimination ability of listeners with sensori-neural hearing loss. Audiol 19: 495–507.

Hawkins DB, Yacullo WS (1984) Signal-to-noise ratio advantage of binaural hearing aids and directional microphones under different levels of reverberation. J Speech Hear Disord 49: 278–86.

Hawkins JE Jr, Stevens SS (1950) The masking of pure tones and of speech by white noise. J Acoust Soc Am 22: 6–13.

Hellbrück J (1993) Hören. Göttingen: Hogrefe Verlag.

Hellbrück J, Moser LM (1985) Hörgeräte Audiometrie: Ein Computer-unterstütztes psychologisches Verfahren zur Hörgeräteanpassung. Psychologische Beiträge 27: 494–509.

Heller O (1991) Oriented category scaling of loudness and speech audiometric validation. In A Schick (ed.) Contributions to Psychological Acoustics. Oldenburg: BIS.

Hellman RP (1978) Dependence of loudness growth on skirts of excitation patterns. J Acoust Soc Am 63: 1114–19.

Hellman RP (1994) Relation between the growth of loudness and high-frequency excitation. J Acoust Soc Am 96: 2655–63.

Hellman RP, Meiselman CH (1986) Is high-frequency hearing necessary for normal loudness growth at low frequencies? 12th ICA Paper B11-5.

Hellman RP, Meiselman CH (1990) Loudness relations for individuals and groups in normal and impaired hearing. J Acoust Soc Am 88: 2596–2606.

Hellman RP, Meiselman CH (1993) Rate of loudness growth for pure tones in normal and impaired hearing. J Acoust Soc Am 93: 966–75.

Hellman RP, Zwislocki JJ (1961) Some factors affecting the estimation of loudness. J Acoust Soc Am 35: 687–94.

Henning GB (1967) A model for auditory discrimination and detection. J Acoust Soc Am 42: 1325–34.

Henning GB (1974) Detectability of interaural delay in high-frequency complex waveforms. J Acoust Soc Am 55: 84–90.

Hickson LMH (1994) Compression amplification in hearing aids. Am J Audiol 3: 51–65.

Hind JE, Rose JE, Brugge JF, Anderson DJ (1967) Coding of information pertaining to paired low-frequency tones in single auditory nerve fibres of the squirrel monkey. J Neurophysiol 30: 794–816.

Hirsh IJ (1948). Influence of interaural phase on interaural summation and inhibition. J Acoust Soc Am 20: 536–44.

Hoekstra A, Ritsma RJ (1977) Perceptive hearing loss and frequency selectivity. In EF Evans, JP Wilson (eds) Psychophysics and Physiology of Hearing. London: Academic.

Hoffman MW, Trine TD, Buckley KM, Van Tasell DJ (1994) Robust adaptive microphone array processing for hearing aids: Realistic speech enhancement. J Acoust Soc Am 96: 759–70.

Hohmann V (1993) Dynamikkompression für Hörgeräte – Psychoakustische Grundlagen und Algorithmen. Düsseldorf: VDI-Verlag.

Hohmann V, Kollmeier B (1995) The effect of multichannel dynamic compression on speech intelligibility. J Acoust Soc Am 97: 1191–5.

Hood JD (1984) Speech discrimination in bilateral and unilateral loss due to Ménière's disease. Brit J Audiol 18: 173–8.

Horst JW (1987) Frequency discrimination of complex signals, frequency selectivity and speech perception in hearing-impaired subjects. J Acoust Soc Am 82: 874–85.

Hou Z, Pavlovic CV (1994) Effects of temporal smearing on temporal resolution, frequency selectivity and speech intelligibility. J Acoust Soc Am 96: 1325–40.

Houtgast T (1972) Psychophysical evidence for lateral inhibition in hearing. J Acoust Soc Am 51: 1885–94.

Houtgast T (1973) Psychophysical experiments on 'tuning curves' and 'two-tone inhibition'. Acustica 29: 168–79.

Houtgast T (1974) Lateral Suppression in Hearing. PhD thesis. Free University of Amsterdam.

Houtsma AJM, Smurzynski J (1990) Pitch identification and discrimination for complex tones with many harmonics. J Acoust Soc Am 87: 304–10.

Howard-Jones PA, Summers IR (1992) Temporal features in spectrally degraded speech. Acoust Lett 15: 159–63.

Hughes JW (1946) The threshold of audition for short periods of stimulation. Phil Trans R Soc Lond B 133: 486–90.

Humes LE (1991) Prescribing gain characteristics of linear hearing aids. In GA Studebaker, FH Bess, LB Beck (eds) The Vanderbilt Hearing Aid Report. II. Parkton MD: York Press.

Humes LE, Dirks DD, Kincaid GE (1987) Recognition of nonsense syllables by hearing-impaired listeners and by noise masked normal listeners. J Acoust Soc Am 81: 765–73.

Humes LE, Jesteadt W, Lee LW (1992) Modeling the effects of sensorineural hearing loss on auditory perception. In Y Cazals, L Demany, K Horner (eds) Auditory Physiology and Perception. Oxford: Pergamon.

Humes LE, Roberts L (1990) Speech-recognition difficulties of the hearing-impaired elderly: the contributions of audibility. J Speech Hear Res 33: 726–35.

Hygge S, Rönnberg J, Larsby B, Arlinger S (1992) Normal-hearing and hearing-impaired subjects' ability to just follow conversation in competing speech, reversed speech and noise backgrounds. J Speech Hear Res 35: 208–15.

ISO 389–7 (1996) Acoustics – Reference zero for the calibration of audiometric equipment. Part 7: Reference threshold of hearing under free-field and diffuse-field listening conditions. Geneva: International Organization for Standardization.

Javel E (1980) Coding of AM tones in the chinchilla auditory nerve: Implications for the pitch of complex tones. J Acoust Soc Am 68: 133–46.

Jeffress LA (1948) A place theory of sound localization. J Comp Physiol Psychol 41: 35–9.

Jerger J (1962) The SISI test. Int Audiol 1: 246–7.

Jerger J, Brown D, Smith S (1984) Effect of peripheral hearing loss on the MLD. Arch Otolaryngol 110: 290–6.

Jerger J, Shedd J, Harford E (1959) On the detection of extremely small changes in sound intensity. Arch Otolaryngol 69: 200–11.

Jesteadt W, Bilger RC, Green DM, Patterson JH (1976) Temporal acuity in listeners with sensorineural hearing loss. J Speech Hear Res 19: 357–70.

Jesteadt W, Wier CC, Green DM (1977a) Comparison of monaural and binaural discrimination of intensity and frequency. J Acoust Soc Am 61: 1599–603.

Jesteadt W, Wier CC, Green DM (1977b). Intensity discrimination as a function of frequency and sensation level. J Acoust Soc Am 61: 169–77.

Johnson-Davies D, Patterson RD (1979) Psychophysical tuning curves: Restricting the listening band to the signal region. J Acoust Soc Am 65: 675–770.

Kemp DT (1978) Stimulated acoustic emissions from within the human auditory system. J Acoust Soc Am 64: 1386–91.

Khanna SM, Leonard DGB (1982) Basilar membrane tuning in the cat cochlea. Science 215: 305–6.

Kiang NY-S, Moxon EC, Levine RA (1970) Auditory nerve activity in cats with normal and abnormal cochleas. In GEW Wolstenholme, JJ Knight (eds) Sensorineural Hearing Loss. London: Churchill.

Kiang NY-S, Watanabe T, Thomas EC, Clark LF (1965) Discharge Patterns of Single Fibers in the Cat's Auditory Nerve. Cambridge MA: MIT Press.

Kidd G, Feth LL (1982) Effects of masker duration in pure-tone forward masking. J Acoust Soc Am 72: 1384–6.

Kiessling J (1997) Scaling methods for the selection, fitting and evaluation of hearing aids. In B Kollmeier (ed.) Psychoacoustics, Speech and Hearing Aids. Singapore: World Scientific.

Kiessling J, Steffens T, Wagner I (1993) Untersuchungen zur praktischen Anwendbarkeit der Lautheitsskalierung. Audiologische Akustik 4/93: 100–15.

Killion MC (1978) Revised estimate of minimal audible pressure: Where is the 'missing 6 dB'? J Acoust Soc Am 63: 1501–10.

Killion MC (1982) Transducers, earmolds and sound quality considerations. In GA Studebaker, FH Bess (eds) The Vanderbilt Hearing-Aid Report. Upper Darby PA: Monographs in Contemporary Audiology. .

Killion MC (1993) An attempt to present high fidelity for the hearing impaired. In J Beilin, GR Jensen (eds) Recent Developments in Hearing Instrument Technology. Copenhagen: Stougaard Jensen.

Killion MC (1997) Hearing aids: Past, present and future: Moving toward normal conversations in noise. Brit J Audiol 31: 141–8.

Killion MC, Fikret-Pasa S (1993) Three types of sensorineural hearing loss: loudness and intelligibility considerations. Hear J 46: 31–6.

Killion MC, Wilber LA, Gudmundsen GI (1988) Zwislocki was right: A potential solution to the 'hollow voice' problem (the amplified occlusion effect) with deeply sealed earmolds. Hear Inst 39: 14–18.

Kinkel M, Kollmeier B (1992) Binaurales Hören bei Normalhörenden und Schwerhörigen. II. Analyse der Ergebnisse. Audiologishe Akustik, 1/92: 22–33.

Kinkel M, Kollmeier B, Holube I (1991) Binaurales Hören bei Normalhörenden und Schwerhörigen. I. Meßmethoden und Meßergebnisse. Audiologishe Akustik 6/91: 192–201.

Klump RG, Eady HR (1956) Some measurements of interaural time difference thresholds. J Acoust Soc Am 28: 859–60.

Kochkin S (1996) Customer satisfaction and subjective benefit with high performance hearing aids. Hear Rev 3: 16–26.

Kohlrausch A (1988) Masking patterns of harmonic complex tone maskers and the role of the inner ear transfer function. In H Duifhuis, J W Horst, H P Wit (eds) Basic Issues in Hearing. London: Academic Press.

Kollmeier B, Hohmann V (1995) Loudness estimation and compensation employing a categorical scale. In GA Manley, GM Klump, C Köppl, H Fastl, H Oeckinghaus (eds) Advances in Hearing Research. Singapore: World Scientific Publishers.

Kollmeier B, Koch R (1994) Speech enhancement based on physiological and psychoacoustical models of modulation perception and binaural interaction. J Acoust Soc Am 95: 1593–602.

Kollmeier B, Peissig J, Hohmann V (1993) Binaural noise-reduction hearing aid scheme with real-time processing in the frequency domain. Scand Audiol Suppl 38: 28–38.

Kompis M, Dillier N (1994) Noise reduction for hearing aids: combining directional microphones with an adaptive beamformer. J Acoust Soc Am 96: 1910–13.

Kryter KD (1962). Methods for the calculation and use of the Articulation Index. J Acoust Soc Am 34, 467–77.

Lacher-Fougère, Demany L (1998) Modulation detection by normal and hearing-impaired listeners. Audiology 37, 109–21.

Laming D (1997) The Measurement of Sensation. Oxford: Oxford University Press.

Lamore PJJ, Verweij C, Brocaar MP (1984) Reliability of auditory function tests in severely hearing-impaired and deaf subjects. Audiology 23: 453–66.

Laroche C, Hétu R, Quoc HT, Josserand B, Glasberg B (1992) Frequency selectivity in workers with noise-induced hearing loss. Hear Res 64: 61–72.

Launer S (1995) Loudness perception in listeners with sensorineural hearing impairment. PhD Thesis. Oldenburg, Germany.

Launer S, Hohmann V, Kollmeier B (1997) Modeling loudness growth and loudness summation in hearing-impaired listeners. In W Jesteadt (ed.) Modeling Sensorineural Hearing Loss. Mahwah NJ: Erlbaum.

Laurence RF, Moore BCJ, Glasberg BR (1983) A comparison of behind-the-ear high-fidelity linear aids and two-channel compression hearing aids in the laboratory and in everyday life. Brit J Audiol 17: 31–48.

Lee LW, Humes LE (1993) Evaluating a speech-reception threshold model for hearing-impaired listeners. J Acoust Soc Am 93: 2879–85.

Leek MR, Summers V (1993) Auditory filter shapes of normal-hearing and hearing-impaired listeners in continuous broadband noise. J Acoust Soc Am 94: 3127–37.

Leeuw AR, Dreschler WA (1991) Advantages of directional hearing aid microphones related to room acoustics. Audiology 30: 330–44.

Leeuw AR, Dreschler WA (1994) Frequency-resolution measurements with notched noise for clinical purposes. Ear Hear 15: 240–55.

Leijon A (1989) Optimization of Hearing-Aid Gain and Frequency Response for Cochlear Hearing Losses. PhD Thesis, Chalmers University of Technology, Sweden.

Leijon A (1990) Hearing aid gain for loudness-density normalization in cochlear hearing losses with impaired frequency resolution. Ear Hear 12: 242–50.

Leonard DGB, Khanna SM (1984) Histological evaluation of damage in cat cochleas used for measurement of basilar membrane mechanics. J Acoust Soc Am 75: 515–27.

Leshowitz B, Linstrom R, Zurek P (1975) Psychophysical tuning curves in normal and impaired ears. J Acoust Soc Am 58: 71.

Levitt H, Rabiner LR (1967) Binaural release from masking for speech and gain in intelligibility. J Acoust Soc Am 42: 601–8.

Libby ER (1981) Achieving a transparent, smooth, wideband hearing aid response. Hear. Inst 32: 9–12.

Libby ER (1982). In search of transparent hearing aid responses. In GA Studebaker, FH Bess (eds) The Vanderbilt Hearing Aid Report. Upper Darby PA: Monographs in Contemporary Audiology.

Liberman MC (1978) Auditory-nerve response from cats raised in a low-noise chamber. J Acoust Soc Am 63: 442–55.

Liberman MC, Dodds LW (1984) Single neuron labeling and chronic cochlea pathology. III. Stereocilia damage and alterations in threshold tuning curves. Hear Res 16: 54–74.

Liberman MC, Dodds LW, Learson DA (1986) Structure-function correlation in noise-damaged ears: a light and electron-microscopic study. In RJ Salvi, D Henderson, RP Hamernik, V Colletti (eds) Basic and Applied Aspects of Noise-Induced Hearing Loss. New York: Plenum Press.

Licklider JCR (1948) The influence of interaural phase relations upon the masking of speech by white noise. J Acoust Soc Am 20: 150–9.

Licklider JCR (1956) Auditory frequency analysis. In C Cherry (ed.) Information Theory. New York: Academic Press.

Lindsay PH, Norman DA (1972) Human Information Processing. New York and London: Academic Press.

Lippmann RP, Braida LD, Durlach NI (1981) Study of multi-channel amplitude compression and linear amplification for persons with sensorineural hearing loss. J Acoust Soc Am 69: 524–34.

Loeb GE, White MW, Merzenich MM (1983) Spatial cross correlation: a proposed mechanism for acoustic pitch perception. Biol Cybern 47: 149–63.

Lundeen C, Small AM (1984) The influence of temporal cues on the strength of periodicity pitches. J Acoust Soc Am 75: 1578–87.

Lüscher E, Zwislocki JJ (1949) A simple method for indirect determination of the recruitment phenomenon (difference limen in intensity in different types of deafness). Acta Otolaryngol Suppl 78: 156–68.

Lutman ME (1991) Degradations in frequency and temporal resolution with age and their impact on speech identification. Acta Otolaryngol (Stockh) Suppl 4: 120–26.

Lybarger SF (1978) Selective amplification – a review and evaluation. J Am Aud Soc 3: 258–66.

Mangold S, Leijon A (1979) Programmable hearing aid with multi-channel compression. Scand Audiol 8: 121–6.

McCandless GA, Lyregard PE (1983) Prescription of gain/output (POGO) for hearing aids. Hear Inst 34: 16–21.

McCormick B, Archbold S, Sheppard S (1994) Cochlear Implants for Young Children. London: Whurr.

McDermott HJ, McKay CM (1997) Musical pitch perception with electrical stimulation of the cochlea. J Acoust Soc Am 101: 1622–31.

McKay CM, McDermott HJ (1993) Perceptual performance of subjects with cochlear implants using the spectral maxima sound processor (SMSP) and the mini speech processor (MSP). Ear Hear 15: 350–67.

McKay CM, McDermott HJ, Clark GM (1994) Pitch percepts associated with amplitude-modulated current pulse trains in cochlear implantees. J Acoust Soc Am 96: 2664–73.

Meddis R, Hewitt M (1991) Virtual pitch and phase sensitivity studied using a computer model of the auditory periphery: Pitch identification. J Acoust Soc Am 89: 2866–82.

Meddis R, O'Mard L (1997) A unitary model of pitch perception. J Acoust Soc Am 102: 1811–20.

Mertz P (1982) Clinical applications of innovative earmold coupling systems. Audecibel 31: 24–6.

Miller GA (1947) Sensitivity to changes in the intensity of white noise and its relation to masking and loudness. J Acoust Soc Am 191, 609–19.

Miller RL, Schilling JR, Franck KR, Young ED (1997) Effects of acoustic trauma on the representation of the vowel /ɛ/ in cat auditory nerve fibers. J Acoust Soc Am 101: 3602–16.

Mills AW (1958) On the minimum audible angle. J Acoust Soc Am 30: 237–46.

Mills AW (1960) Lateralization of high-frequency tones. J Acoust Soc Am 32: 132–34.

Mills AW (1972) Auditory localization. In JV Tobias (ed.) Foundations of Modern Auditory Theory, Vol II. New York: Academic Press.

Mills JH, Schmeidt RA (1983) Frequency selectivity: physiological and psychophysical tuning curves and suppression. In JV Tobias, ED Schubert (eds) Hearing Research and Theory, Vol 2. New York: Academic Press.

Miskolczy-Fodor F (1960) Relation between loudness and duration of tonal pulses. Response in cases of abnormal loudness function. J Acoust Soc Am 32: 486–92.

Moore BCJ (1973) Some experiments relating to the perception of complex tones. QJ Exp Psych 25: 451–75.

Moore BCJ (1974) Relation between the critical bandwidth and the frequency-difference limen. J Acoust Soc Am 55: 359.

Moore BCJ (1977) Effects of relative phase of the components on the pitch of three-component complex tones. In EF Evans, JP Wilson (eds) Psychophysics and Physiology of Hearing. London: Academic Press.

Moore BCJ (1978) Psychophysical tuning curves measured in simultaneous and forward masking. J Acoust Soc Am 63: 524–32.

Moore BCJ (1980) Detection cues in forward masking. In G van den Brink, FA Bilson (eds) Psychophysical, Physiological and Behavioural Studies in Hearing. Delft: Delft University Press.

Moore BCJ (1981). Interactions of masker bandwidth with signal duration and delay in forward masking. J Acoust Soc Am 70: 62–8.

Moore BCJ (1982) An Introduction to the Psychology of Hearing. 2 edn. London: Academic Press.

Moore BCJ (1987a) Design and evaluation of a two-channel compression hearing aid. J Rehab Res Devel 24: 181–92.

Moore BCJ (1987b) Distribution of auditory-filter bandwidths at 2 kHz in young normal listeners. J Acoust Soc Am 81: 1633–5.

Moore BCJ (1988) Dynamic aspects of auditory masking. In G Edelman, W Gall, W Cowan (eds) Auditory Function: Neurobiological Bases of Hearing. New York: Wiley.

Moore BCJ (1989) An Introduction to the Psychology of Hearing. 3 edn. London: Academic Press.

Moore BCJ (1990) How much do we gain by gain control in hearing aids? Acta Otolaryngol Suppl 469: 250–6.

Moore BCJ (1993) Signal processing to compensate for reduced dynamic range. In J Beilin, GR Jensen (eds) Recent Developments in Hearing Instrument Technology. Copenhagen: Stougaard Jensen.

Moore BCJ (1997a) A compact disc containing simulations of hearing impairment. Brit J Audiol 31: 353–7.

Moore BCJ (1997b) An Introduction to the Psychology of Hearing. 4 edn. San Diego: Academic Press.

Moore BCJ, Alcántara JI, Glasberg BR (1998) Development and evaluation of a procedure for fitting multi-channel compression hearing aids. Brit J Audiol 32: 177–95.

Moore BCJ, Glasberg BR (1982) Contralateral and ipsilateral cueing in forward masking. J Acoust Soc Am 71: 942–945.

Moore BCJ, Glasberg BR (1983a) Growth of forward masking for sinusoidal and noise maskers as a function of signal delay: Implications for suppression in noise. J Acoust Soc Am 73: 1249–59.

Moore BCJ, Glasberg BR (1983b) Masking patterns of synthetic vowels in simultaneous and forward masking. J Acoust Soc Am 73: 906–17.

Moore BCJ, Glasberg BR (1983c) Suggested formulae for calculating auditory-filter bandwidths and excitation patterns. J Acoust Soc Am 74: 750–3.

Moore BCJ, Glasberg BR (1985) The danger of using narrowband noise maskers to measure suppression. J Acoust Soc Am 77: 2137–41.

Moore BCJ, Glasberg BR (1986a) A comparison of two-channel and single-channel compression hearing aids. Audiology 25: 210–26.

Moore BCJ, Glasberg BR (1986b) Comparisons of frequency selectivity in simultaneous and forward masking for subjects with unilateral cochlear impairments. J Acoust Soc Am 80: 93–107.

Moore BCJ, Glasberg BR (1986c) The relationship between frequency selectivity and frequency discrimination for subjects with unilateral and bilateral cochlear impairments. In BCJ Moore, RD Patterson (eds) Auditory Frequency Selectivity. New York: Plenum Press.

Moore BCJ, Glasberg BR (1986d) The role of frequency selectivity in the perception of loudness, pitch and time. In BCJ Moore (ed.) Frequency Selectivity in Hearing. London: Academic Press.

Moore BCJ, Glasberg BR (1987) Formulae describing frequency selectivity as a function of frequency and level and their use in calculating excitation patterns. Hear Res 28: 209–25.

Moore BCJ, Glasberg BR (1988a) A comparison of four methods of implementing automatic gain control (AGC) in hearing aids. Brit J Audiol 22: 93–104.

Moore BCJ, Glasberg BR (1988b) Gap detection with sinusoids and noise in normal, impaired and electrically stimulated ears. J Acoust Soc Am 83: 1093–101.

Moore BCJ, Glasberg BR (1988c) Pitch perception and phase sensitivity for subjects with unilateral and bilateral cochlear hearing impairments. In A Quaranta (ed.) Clinical Audiology. Bari, Italy: Laterza.

Moore BCJ, Glasberg BR (1989) Mechanisms underlying the frequency discrimination of pulsed tones and the detection of frequency modulation. J Acoust Soc Am

86: 1722–32.

Moore BCJ, Glasberg BR (1990) Frequency selectivity in subjects with cochlear loss and its effects on pitch discrimination and phase sensitivity. In F Grandori, G Cianfrone, DT Kemp (eds) Advances in Audiology. Basel: Karger.

Moore BCJ, Glasberg BR (1993) Simulation of the effects of loudness recruitment and threshold elevation on the intelligibility of speech in quiet and in a background of speech. J Acoust Soc Am 94: 2050–62.

Moore BCJ, Glasberg BR (1996) A revision of Zwicker's loudness model. Acustica – Acta Acustica 82: 335–45.

Moore BCJ, Glasberg BR (1997) A model of loudness perception applied to cochlear hearing loss. Auditory Neurosci 3: 289–311.

Moore BCJ, Glasberg BR (1998) Use of a loudness model for hearing aid fitting. I. Linear hearing aids. Brit J Audiol (in press).

Moore BCJ Glasberg BR, Baer T (1997) A model for the prediction of thresholds, loudness and partial loudness. J Audio Eng Soc 45: 224–40.

Moore BCJ, Glasberg BR, Donaldson E, McPherson T, Plack C J (1989) Detection of temporal gaps in sinusoids by normally hearing and hearing-impaired subjects. J Acoust Soc Am 85: 1266–75.

Moore BCJ, Glasberg BR, Hess RF, Birchall JP (1985) Effects of flanking noise bands on the rate of growth of loudness of tones in normal and recruiting ears. J Acoust Soc Am 77: 1505–15.

Moore BCJ, Glasberg BR, Peters RW (1985) Relative dominance of individual partials in determining the pitch of complex tones. J Acoust Soc Am 77: 1853–60.

Moore BCJ, Glasberg BR, Plack CJ, Biswas AK (1988) The shape of the ear's temporal window. J Acoust Soc Am 83: 1102–16.

Moore BCJ, Glasberg BR, Roberts B (1984) Refining the measurement of psychophysical tuning curves. J Acoust Soc Am 76: 1057–66.

Moore BCJ, Glasberg BR, Shailer MJ (1984) Frequency and intensity difference limens for harmonics within complex tones. J Acoust Soc Am 75: 550–61.

Moore BCJ, Glasberg BR, Simpson A (1992) Evaluation of a method of simulating reduced frequency selectivity. J Acoust Soc Am 91: 3402–23.

Moore BCJ, Glasberg BR, Stone MA (1991) Optimization of a slow-acting automatic gain control system for use in hearing aids. Brit J Audiol 25: 171–82.

Moore BCJ, Glasberg BR, Vickers DA (1995) Simulation of the effects of loudness recruitment on the intelligibility of speech in noise. Brit J Audiol 29: 131–43.

Moore BCJ, Johnson JS, Clark TM, Pluvinage V (1992) Evaluation of a dual-channel full dynamic range compression system for people with sensorineural hearing loss. Ear Hear 13: 349–70.

Moore BCJ, Laurence RF, Wright D (1985) Improvements in speech intelligibility in quiet and in noise produced by two-channel compression hearing aids. Brit J Audiol 19: 175–87.

Moore BCJ, Lynch C, Stone MA (1992) Effects of the fitting parameters of a two-channel compression system on the intelligibility of speech in quiet and in noise. Brit J Audiol 26: 369–79.

Moore BCJ, Ohgushi K (1993) Audibility of partials in inharmonic complex tones. J Acoust Soc Am 93: 452–61.

Moore BCJ, O'Loughlin B J (1986) The use of nonsimultaneous masking to measure frequency selectivity and suppression. In BCJ Moore (ed.) Frequency Selectivity in Hearing. London: Academic Press.

Moore BCJ, Oxenham AJ (1998) Psychoacoustic consequences of compression in the peripheral auditory system. Psych Rev 105: 108–24.

Moore BCJ, Peters R W (1992) Pitch discrimination and phase sensitivity in young and elderly subjects and its relationship to frequency selectivity. J Acoust Soc Am 91: 2881–93.

Moore BCJ, Peters RW, Glasberg BR (1990) Auditory filter shapes at low center frequencies. J Acoust Soc Am 88: 132–40.

Moore BCJ, Peters RW, Glasberg BR (1993) Detection of temporal gaps in sinusoids: effects of frequency and level. J Acoust Soc Am 93: 1563–70.

Moore BCJ, Peters RW, Glasberg BR (1996) Detection of decrements and increments in sinusoids at high overall levels. J Acoust Soc Am 99: 3669–77.

Moore BCJ, Rosen SM (1979) Tune recognition with reduced pitch and interval information. Q J Exp Psychol 31: 229–40.

Moore BCJ, Sek A (1995) Effects of carrier frequency modulation rate and modulation waveform on the detection of modulation and the discrimination of modulation type (AM vs FM). J Acoust Soc Am 97: 2468–78.

Moore BCJ, Sek A (1996) Detection of frequency, modulation at low modulation rates: evidence for a mechanism based on phase locking. J Acoust Soc Am 100: 2320–31.

Moore BCJ, Shailer MJ, Schooneveldt GP (1992) Temporal modulation transfer functions for band-limited noise in subjects with cochlear hearing loss. Brit J Audiol 26: 229–37.

Moore BCJ, Vickers DA (1997) The role of spread of excitation and suppression in simultaneous masking. J Acoust Soc Am 102: 2284–90.

Moore BCJ, Vickers DA, Glasberg BR, Baer T (1997) Comparison of real and simulated hearing impairment in subjects with unilateral and bilateral cochlear hearing loss. Brit J Audiol 31: 227–45.

Moore BCJ, Wojtczak M, Vickers DA (1996) Effect of loudness recruitment on the perception of amplitude modulation. J Acoust Soc Am 100: 481–9.

Murray N, Byrne D (1986) Performance of hearing-impaired and normal hearing listeners with various high-frequency cut-offs in hearing aids. Aust J Audiol 8: 21–8.

Needleman A R, Crandell C C (1995) Speech recognition in noise by hearing-impaired and noise-masked normal-hearing listeners. J Am Acad Audiol 6: 414–24.

Neff DL (1985) Stimulus parameters governing confusion effects in forward masking. J Acoust Soc Am 78: 1966–76.

Nejime Y, Moore BCJ (1997) Simulation of the effect of threshold elevation and loudness recruitment combined with reduced frequency selectivity on the intelligibility of speech in noise. J Acoust Soc Am 102: 603–15.

Nelson DA (1991) High-level psychophysical tuning curves: Forward masking in normal-hearing and hearing-impaired listeners. J Speech Hear Res 34: 1233–49.

Nelson DA, Schroder AC (1997) Linearized response growth inferred from growth-of-masking slopes in ears with cochlear hearing loss. J Acoust Soc Am 101: 2186–201.

Nelson DA, Stanton ME, Freyman RL (1983) A general equation describing frequency discrimination as a function of frequency and sensation level. J Acoust Soc Am 73: 2117–23.

Nelson PB, Thomas SD (1997) Gap detection as a function of stimulus loudness for listeners with and without hearing loss. J Speech Lang Hear Res 40: 1387–94.

Nielsen HB, Ludvigsen C (1978) Effect of hearing aids with directional microphones in different acoustic environments. Scand Audiol 7: 217–24.

Nilsson M, Soli SD, Sullivan JA (1994) Development of the Hearing in Noise Test for the measurement of speech reception thresholds in quiet and in noise. J Acoust Soc Am 95: 1085–99.

Noble W, Byrne D, Lepage B (1994) Effects on sound localization of configuration and type of hearing impairment. J Acoust Soc Am 95: 992–1005.

Nordlund B (1964) Directional Audiometry. Acta Otolaryngol 57: 1–18.

Ohgushi K, Hatoh T (1991) Perception of the musical pitch of high frequency tones. In Y Cazals, L Demany, K Horner (eds) Ninth International Symposium on Hearing: Auditory Physiology and Perception. Oxford: Pergamon.

Ohm GS (1843) Über die Definition des Tones nebst daran geknüpfter Theorie der Sirene und ähnlicher tonbildender Vorrichtungen. Annalen der Physik und Chemie 59: 513–65.

O'Loughlin BJ, Moore BCJ (1981a) Improving psychoacoustical tuning curves. Hear Res 5: 343–6.

O'Loughlin BJ, Moore BCJ (1981b) Off-frequency listening: Effects on psychoacoustical tuning curves obtained in simultaneous and forward masking. J Acoust Soc Am 69: 1119–25.

Ono H, Kanzaki J, Mizoi K (1983) Clinical results of hearing aid with noise-level-controlled selective amplification. Audiology 22: 494–515.

Oxenham AJ, Moore BCJ (1994) Modeling the additivity of nonsimultaneous masking. Hear Res 80: 105–18.

Oxenham AJ, Moore BCJ (1995) Additivity of masking in normally hearing and hearing-impaired subjects. J Acoust Soc Am 98: 1921–35.

Oxenham AJ, Moore BCJ (1997) Modeling the effects of peripheral non-linearity in listeners with normal and impaired hearing. In W Jesteadt (ed.) Modeling Sensorineural Hearing Loss. Mawah NJ: Erlbaum.

Oxenham AJ, Plack CJ (1997) A behavioral measure of basilar-membrane non-linearity in listeners with normal and impaired hearing. J Acoust Soc Am 101: 3666–75.

Palmer AR (1987) Physiology of the cochlear nerve and cochlear nucleus. In MP Haggard, EF Evans (eds) Hearing. Edinburgh: Churchill Livingstone.

Palmer AR, Russell IJ (1986) Phase-locking in the cochlear nerve of the guinea-pig and its relation to the receptor potential of inner hair-cells. Hear Res 24: 1–15.

Parkins CW (1997) Compensating for hair cell loss with cochlear implants. In CI Berlin (ed.) Neurotransmission and Hearing Loss. San Diego: Singular.

Pascoe DP (1978) An approach to hearing aid selection. Hear Inst 29: 12–16.

Patterson RD (1973) The effects of relative phase and the number of components on residue pitch. J Acoust Soc Am 53: 1565–72.

Patterson RD (1974) Auditory filter shape. J Acoust Soc Am 55: 802–9.

Patterson RD (1976) Auditory filter shapes derived with noise stimuli. J Acoust Soc Am 59: 640–54.

Patterson RD (1987a) A pulse ribbon model of monaural phase perception. J Acoust Soc Am 82: 1560–86.

Patterson RD (1987b) A pulse ribbon model of peripheral auditory processing. In WA Yost, CS Watson (eds) Auditory Processing of Complex Sounds. Mawah NJ: Erlbaum.

Patterson RD, Henning GB (1977) Stimulus variability and auditory filter shape. J Acoust Soc Am 62: 649–64.

Patterson RD, Moore BCJ (1986) Auditory filters and excitation patterns as representations of frequency resolution. In BCJ Moore (ed.) Frequency Selectivity in Hearing. London: Academic Press.

Patterson RD, Nimmo-Smith I (1980) Off-frequency listening and auditory filter asymmetry. J Acoust Soc Am 67: 229–45.

Patterson RD, Nimmo-Smith I, Weber DL, Milroy R (1982) The deterioration of hearing with age: Frequency selectivity, the critical ratio, the audiogram, and speech threshold. J Acoust Soc Am 72: 1788–803.

Patuzzi R, Sellick PM, Johnstone BM (1984) The modulation of the sensitivity of the mammalian cochlea by low-frequency tones. III. Basilar membrane motion. Hear Res 13: 19–27.

Patuzzi RB (1992) Effects of noise on auditory nerve fiber response. In A Dancer, D Henderson, R Salvi, R Hamernik (eds) Noise Induced Hearing Loss. St Louis: Mosby Year Book.

Pavlovic C (1987) Derivation of primary parameters and procedures for use in speech intelligibility predictions. J Acoust Soc Am 82: 413–22.

Pavlovic C, Studebaker G, Sherbecoe R (1986) An articulation index based procedure for predicting the speech recognition performance of hearing-impaired individuals. J Acoust Soc Am 80: 50–57.

Pavlovic CV (1984) Use of the articulation index for assessing residual auditory function in listeners with sensorineural hearing impairment. J Acoust Soc Am 75: 1253–8.

Pearsons KS, Bennett RL, Fidell S (1976) Speech Levels in Various Environments. Report No 3281. Cambridge Massachusetts: Bolt Beranek & Newman.

Pedersen CB, Elberling C (1973) Temporal integration of acoustic energy in patients with presbyacusis. Acta Otolaryngol 75: 32–7.

Pedersen CB, Poulsen T (1973) Loudness of brief tones in hearing-impaired ears. Acta Otolaryngol 76: 402–9.

Penner MJ (1972) Neural or energy summation in a Poisson counting model. J Math Psychol 9: 286–93.

Penner M J (1980a) The coding of intensity and the interaction of forward and backward masking. J Acoust Soc Am 67: 608–16.

Penner MJ (1980b) Two-tone forward masking patterns and tinnitus. J Speech Hear Res 23: 779–86.

Penner MJ, Shiffrin RM (1980) Non-linearities in the coding of intensity within the context of a temporal summation model. J Acoust Soc Am 67: 617–27.

Perrett S, Noble W (1997) The effect of head rotations on vertical plane localization. J Acoust Soc Am 102: 2325–32.

Peters RW, Moore BCJ (1992) Auditory filter shapes at low center frequencies in young and elderly hearing-impaired subjects. J Acoust Soc Am 91: 256–66.

Peters RW, Moore BCJ, Baer T (1998) Speech reception thresholds in noise with and without spectral and temporal dips for hearing-impaired and normally hearing people. J Acoust Soc Am 103: 577–87.

Peters RW, Moore BCJ, Glasberg BR (1995) Effects of level and frequency on the detection of decrements and increments in sinusoids. J Acoust Soc Am 97: 3791–9.

Peterson PM, Durlach NI, Rabinowitz WM, Zurek PM (1987) Multimicrophone adaptive beamforming for interference reduction in hearing aids. J Rehab Res Devel 24: 103–10.

Phillips DP (1987) Stimulus intensity and loudness recruitment: Neural correlates. J Acoust Soc Am 82: 1–12.

Pickles JO (1984) Frequency threshold curves and simultaneous masking functions in single fibers of the guinea pig auditory nerve. Hear Res 14: 245–56.

Pijl S (1997) Pulse rate matching by cochlear implant patients: effects of loudness randomization and electrode position, Ear Hear 18: 316–25.

Pijl S, Schwarz DWF (1995) Melody recognition and musical interval perception by deaf subjects stimulated with electrical pulse trains through single cochlear implant electrodes. J Acoust Soc Am 98: 886–95.

Plack CJ, Carlyon RP (1995) Differences in frequency modulation detection and fundamental frequency discrimination between complex tones consisting of resolved and unresolved harmonics. J Acoust Soc Am 98: 1355–64.

Plack CJ, Moore BCJ (1990) Temporal window shape as a function of frequency and level. J Acoust Soc Am 87: 2178–87.

Plack CJ, Moore BCJ (1991) Decrement detection in normal and impaired ears. J Acoust Soc Am 90: 3069–76.

Plomp R (1964a) The ear as a frequency analyzer. J Acoust Soc Am 36: 1628–36.

Plomp R (1964b) The rate of decay of auditory sensation. J Acoust Soc Am 36: 277–82.

Plomp R (1967) Pitch of complex tones. J Acoust Soc Am 41: 1526–33.

Plomp R (1976) Aspects of Tone Sensation. London: Academic Press.

Plomp R (1978) Auditory handicap of hearing impairment and the limited benefit of hearing aids. J Acoust Soc Am 63: 533–49.

Plomp R (1986) A signal-to-noise ratio model for the speech-reception threshold of the hearing impaired. J Speech Hear Res 29: 146–54.

Plomp R (1994) Noise, amplification and compression: considerations of three main issues in hearing aid design. Ear Hear 15: 2–12.

Plomp R, Mimpen AM (1968) The ear as a frequency analyzer. II. J Acoust Soc Am 43: 764–7.

Plomp R, Mimpen AM (1979) Improving the reliability of testing the speech reception threshold for sentences. Audiol 18: 43–53.

Plomp R, Steeneken HJM (1973) Place dependence of timbre in reverberant sound fields. Acustica 28: 50–9.

Pluvinage V (1989) Clinical measurement of loudness growth. Hear Inst 39: 28–29, 32.

Preminger J, Wiley T L (1985) Frequency selectivity and consonant intelligibility in sensorineural hearing loss. J Speech Hear Res 28: 197–206.

Puria S, Rosowski JJ, Peake WT (1997) Sound-pressure measurements in the cochlear vestibule of human-cadaver ears. J Acoust Soc Am 101: 2754–70.

Quaranta A, Cervellera G (1974) Masking level differences in normal and pathological ears. Audiology 13: 428–31.

Rankovic CM (1991) An application of the articulation index to hearing aid fitting. J Speech Hear Res 34: 391–402.

Rankovic CM, Freyman RL, Zurek PM (1992) Potential benefits of adaptive frequency-gain characteristics for speech reception in noise. J Acoust Soc Am 91: 354–62.

Rayleigh Lord (1907) On our perception of sound direction. Phil Mag 13: 214–32.

Rhode WS (1971) Observations of the vibration of the basilar membrane in squirrel monkeys using the Mössbauer technique. J Acoust Soc Am 49: 1218–31.

Rhode WS (1977) Some observations on two-tone interaction measured with the Mössbauer effect. In EF Evans, JP Wilson (eds) Psychophysics and Physiology of Hearing. London: Academic Press.

Rhode WS, Robles L (1974) Evidence from Mössbauer experiments for non-linear vibration in the cochlea. J Acoust Soc Am 55: 588–96.

Riesz RR (1928) Differential intensity sensitivity of the ear for pure tones. Physical Reviews 31: 867–75.

Ringdahl A, Eriksson-Mangold M, Israelsson B, Lindkvist A, Mangold S (1990) Clinical trials with a programmable hearing aid set for various listening environments. Brit J Audiol 24: 235–42.

Risberg A (1974) The importance of prosodic elements for the lipreader. In HB Nielson, E Klamp (eds) Visual and Audio-visual Perception of Speech. Stockholm: Almquist & Wiksell.

Ritsma RJ (1962) Existence region of the tonal residue. I. J Acoust Soc Am 34: 1224–9.

Ritsma RJ (1963) Existence region of the tonal residue. II. J Acoust Soc Am 35: 1241–5.

Ritsma RJ (1967) Frequencies dominant in the perception of the pitch of complex sounds. J Acoust Soc Am 42: 191–8.

Robertson D, Manley GA (1974) Manipulation of frequency analysis in the cochlear ganglion of the guinea pig. J Comp Physiol 91: 363–75.

Robles L, Ruggero MA, Rich NC (1986) Basilar membrane mechanics at the base of the chinchilla cochlea. I. Input–output functions tuning curves and response phases. J Acoust Soc Am 80: 1364–74.

Robles L, Ruggero MA, Rich NC (1991) Two-tone distortion in the basilar membrane of the cochlea. Nature 349: 413–14.

Rose JE, Brugge JF, Anderson DJ, Hind JE (1968) Patterns of activity in single auditory nerve fibres of the squirrel monkey. In AVS de Reuck, J Knight (eds) Hearing Mechanisms in Vertebrates. London: Churchill.

Rosen S (1986) Monaural phase sensitivity: frequency selectivity and temporal processes. In BCJ Moore, RD Patterson (eds) Auditory Frequency Selectivity. New York: Plenum.

Rosen S (1987) Phase and the hearing impaired. In MEH Schouten (ed.) The Psychophysics of Speech Perception. Dordrecht: Martinus Nijhoff.

Rosen S, Baker RJ, Darling AM (1998) Auditory filter non-linearity at 2 kHz in normal hearing listeners. J Acoust Soc Am 103: 2539–50.

Rosen S, Baker RJ, Kramer S (1992) Characterizing changes in auditory filter bandwidth as a function of level. In Y Cazals, K Horner, L Demany (eds) Auditory Physiology and Perception. Oxford: Pergamon Press.

Rosen S, Fourcin A (1986) Frequency selectivity and the perception of speech. In BCJ Moore (ed.) Frequency Selectivity in Hearing. London: Academic Press.

Rosen S, Howell P (1991) Signals and Systems for Speech and Hearing. London: Academic Press.

Rosen SM, Fourcin AJ, Moore BCJ (1981) Voice pitch as an aid to lipreading. Nature 291: 150–2.

Ruggero MA (1992) Responses to sound of the basilar membrane of the mammalian cochlea. Curr Opin Neurobiol 2: 449–56.

Ruggero MA (1994) Cochlear delays and traveling waves: Comments on 'Experimental look at cochlear mechanics'. Audiology 33: 131–42.

Ruggero MA, Rich NC (1987) Timing of spike initiation in cochlear afferents: dependence on site of innervation. J Neurophysiol 58: 379–403.

Ruggero MA, Rich NC (1991) Furosemide alters organ of Corti mechanics: evidence for feedback of outer hair cells upon the basilar membrane. J Neurosci 11: 1057–67.

Ruggero MA, Rich NC, Recio A (1993) Alteration of basilar membrane response to sound by acoustic overstimulation. In H Duifhuis, JW Horst, P van Dijk, SM van Netten (eds) Biophysics of Hair Cell Sensory Systems. Singapore: World Scientific.

Ruggero MA, Rich NC, Recio A, Narayan SS, Robles L (1997) Basilar-membrane responses to tones at the base of the chinchilla cochlea. J Acoust Soc Am 101: 2151–63.

Ruggero MA, Rich NC, Robles L, Recio A (1996) The effects of acoustic trauma, other cochlea injury and death on basilar membrane responses to sound. In A Axelsson, H Borchgrevink, RP Hamernik, PA Hellstrom, D Henderson, RJ Salvi (eds) Scientific Basis of Noise-Induced Hearing Loss. Stockholm: Thieme.

Ruggero MA, Robles L, Rich NC (1992) Two-tone suppression in the basilar membrane of the cochlea: mechanical basis of auditory-nerve rate suppression. J

Neurophysiol 68: 1087–99.

Ryan A, Dallos P (1975) Absence of cochlear outer hair cells: effect on behavioral auditory threshold. Nature 253: 44–6.

Ryan AF, Dallos P (1984) Physiology of the cochlea. In JL Northern (ed.) Hearing Disorders. Boston: Little, Brown.

Sachs MB, Abbas PJ (1974) Rate versus level functions for auditory-nerve fibers in cats: Tone-burst stimuli. J Acoust Soc Am 56: 1835–47.

Sachs MB, Kiang NYS (1968) Two-tone inhibition in auditory nerve fibers. J Acoust Soc Am 43: 1120–8.

Salvi RJ, Arehole S (1985) Gap detection in chinchillas with temporary high-frequency hearing loss. J Acoust Soc Am 77: 1173–7.

Scharf B (1970) Critical bands. In JV Tobias (ed.) Foundations of Modern Auditory Theory. New York: Academic Press.

Scharf B (1978) Loudness. In EC Carterette, MP Friedman (eds) Handbook of Perception. Volume IV. Hearing. New York: Academic Press.

Scharf B, Hellman RP (1966) Model of loudness summation applied to impaired ears. J Acoust Soc Am 40: 71–8.

Schoeny Z, Carhart R (1971) Effects of unilateral Ménière's disease on masking level differences. J Acoust Soc Am 50: 1143–50.

Schouten JF (1940) The residue and the mechanism of hearing. Proc Kon Ned. Akad Wetenschap 43: 991–9.

Schouten JF (1970) The residue revisited. In R Plomp, GF Smoorenburg (eds) Frequency Analysis and Periodicity Detection in Hearing. Leiden, The Netherlands: Sijthoff.

Schroder AC, Viemeister NF, Nelson DA (1994). Intensity discrimination in normal-hearing and hearing-impaired listeners. J Acoust Soc Am 96: 2683–93.

Schroeter J, Poesselt C (1986) The use of acoustical test fixtures for the measurement of hearing protector attenuation, Part II. Modeling the external ear, simulating bone conduction and comparing test fixture and real-ear data. J Acoust Soc Am 80: 505–27.

Schwander TJ, Levitt H (1987) Effect of two-microphone noise reduction on speech recognition by normal-hearing listeners. J Rehab Res Devel 24: 87–92.

Seewald RC (1992) The desired sensation level method for fitting children: Version 3.0. The Hearing Journal 45: 36–41.

Sek A, Moore BCJ (1995) Frequency discrimination as a function of frequency, measured in several ways. J Acoust Soc Am 97: 2479–86.

Sellick PM, Patuzzi R, Johnstone BM (1982) Measurement of basilar membrane motion in the guinea pig using the Mössbauer technique. J Acoust Soc Am 72: 131–41.

Shackleton TM, Carlyon RP (1994) The role of resolved and unresolved harmonics in pitch perception and frequency modulation discrimination. J Acoust Soc Am 95: 3529–40.

Shailer MJ, Moore BCJ (1983) Gap detection as a function of frequency, bandwidth and level. J Acoust Soc Am 74: 467–73.

Shailer MJ, Moore BCJ (1985) Detection of temporal gaps in band-limited noise: effects of variations in bandwidth and signal-to-masker ratio. J Acoust Soc Am 77: 635–9.

Shailer MJ, Moore BCJ (1987) Gap detection and the auditory filter: Phase effects using sinusoidal stimuli. J Acoust Soc Am 81: 1110–17.

Shailer MJ, Moore BCJ, Glasberg BR, Watson N, Harris S (1990) Auditory filter shapes at 8 and 10 kHz. J Acoust Soc Am 88: 141–8.

Shamma SA (1985) Speech processing in the auditory system. II: Lateral inhibition and the central processing of speech evoked activity in the auditory nerve. J Acoust Soc Am 78: 1622–32.

Shannon RV (1976) Two-tone unmasking and suppression in a forward masking situation. J Acoust Soc Am 59: 1460–70.

Shaw EAG (1974) Transformation of sound pressure level from the free field to the eardrum in the horizontal plane. J Acoust Soc Am 56: 1848–61.

Shaw WA, Newman EB, Hirsh IJ (1947) The difference between monaural and binaural thresholds. J Exp Psychol 37: 229–42.

Sher AE, Owens E (1974) Consonant confusions associated with hearing loss above 2000 Hz. J Speech Hear Res 17: 669–81.

Siebert WM (1970) Frequency discrimination in the auditory system: place or periodicity mechanisms. Proc IEEE 58: 723–30.

Simon HJ, Yund EW (1993) Frequency discrimination in listeners with sensorineural hearing loss. Ear Hear 14: 190–9.

Skinner MW, Fourakis MS, Holden TA, Holden LK, Demorest ME (1996) Identification of speech by cochlear implant recipients with the multipeak (MPEAK) and spectral peak (SPEAK) speech coding strategies. I. Vowels. Ear Hear 17: 182–97.

Skinner MW, Miller JD (1983) Amplification bandwidth and intelligibility of speech in quiet and noise for listeners with sensorineural hearing loss. Audiology 22: 253–79.

Slepecky N, Hamernik R, Henderson D, Coling D (1982) Correlation of audiometric data with changes in cochlear hair cell stereocilia resulting from impulse noise trauma. Acta Otolaryngol 93: 329–40.

Small AM (1959) Pure-tone masking. J Acoust Soc Am 31: 1619–25.

Smoorenburg GF (1972a) Audibility region of combination tones. J Acoust Soc Am 52: 603–14.

Smoorenburg GF (1972b) Combination tones and their origin. J Acoust Soc Am 52: 615–32.

Smoorenburg GF (1992) Speech reception in quiet and in noisy conditions by individuals with noise-induced hearing loss in relation to their tone audiogram. J Acoust Soc Am 91: 421–37.

Smoski WJ, Trahiotis C (1986) Discrimination of interaural temporal disparities by normal-hearing listeners and listeners with high-frequency sensorineural hearing loss. J Acoust Soc Am 79: 1541–7.

Snell KB, Ison JR, Frisina DR (1994) The effects of signal frequency and absolute bandwidth on gap detection in noise. J Acoust Soc Am 96: 1458–64.

Soede W, Berkhout AJ, Bilsen FA (1993) Development of a directional hearing instrument based on array technology. J Acoust Soc Am 94: 785–98.

Soede W, Bilsen FA, Berkhout AJ (1993) Assessment of a directional microphone array for hearing-impaired listeners. J Acoust Soc Am 94: 799–808.

Sommers MS, Humes LE (1993) Auditory filter shapes in normal-hearing, noise-masked normal and elderly listeners. J Acoust Soc Am 93: 2903–14.

Spiegel MF (1981) Thresholds for tones in maskers of various bandwidths and for signals of various bandwidths as a function of signal frequency. J Acoust Soc Am 69: 791–5.

Spoendlin H (1970) Structural basis of peripheral frequency analysis. In R Plomp, G F Smoorenburg (eds) Frequency Analysis and Periodicity Detection in Hearing. Leiden: Sijthoff.

Srulovicz P, Goldstein. JL (1983) A central spectrum model: a synthesis of auditory-nerve timing and place cues in monaural communication of frequency spectrum. J Acoust Soc Am 73: 1266–76.

Staffel JG, Hall JW, Grose JH, Pillsbury HC (1990) N_0S_0 and N_0S_π detection as a function of masker bandwidth in normal-hearing and cochlear-impaired listeners. J Acoust Soc Am 87: 1720–7.

Steeneken HJM, Houtgast T (1980) A physical method for measuring speech-transmission quality. J Acoust Soc Am 69: 318–26.

Steinberg JC, Gardner MB (1937) The dependency of hearing impairment on sound intensity. J Acoust Soc Am 9: 11–23.

Stelmachowicz PG, Jesteadt W, Gorga MP, Mott J (1985) Speech perception ability and psychophysical tuning curves in hearing-impaired listeners. J Acoust Soc Am 77: 621–7.

Stelmachowicz PG, Lewis DE, Larson LL, Jesteadt W (1987) Growth of masking as a measure of response growth in hearing-impaired listeners. J Acoust Soc Am 81: 1881–7.

Stern RM, Trahiotis C (1995) Models of binaural interaction. In BCJ Moore (ed.) Hearing. New York: Academic Press.

Stevens SS (1935) The relation of pitch to intensity. J Acoust Soc Am 6: 150–4.

Stevens SS (1957) On the psychophysical law. Psych Rev 64: 153–81.

Stevens SS, Newman EB (1936) The localization of actual sources of sound. Am J Psychol, 48: 297–306.

Stone MA, Glasberg BR, Moore BCJ (1992) Simplified measurement of impaired auditory filter shapes using the notched-noise method. Brit J Audiol 26: 329–34.

Stone MA, Moore BCJ, Wojtczak M, Gudgin E (1997) Effects of fast-acting high-frequency compression on the intelligibility of speech in steady and fluctuating background sounds. Brit J Audiol 31: 257–73.

Summers IR (1991) Electronically simulated hearing loss and the perception of degraded speech. In DL Wise (ed.) Bioinstrumentation and Biosensors. New York: Marcel Dekker.

Summers IR, Al-Dabbagh AD (1982) Simulated loss of frequency selectivity and its effects on speech perception. Acoust Lett 5: 129–32.

Ter Keurs M, Festen JM, Plomp R (1992) Effect of spectral envelope smearing on speech reception. I. J Acoust Soc Am 91: 2872–80.

Ter Keurs M, Festen JM, Plomp R (1993) Effect of spectral envelope smearing on speech reception. II. J Acoust Soc Am 93: 1547–52.

Terhardt E (1974a) Pitch of pure tones: its relation to intensity. In E Zwicker, E Terhardt (eds) Facts and Models in Hearing. Berlin: Springer.

Terhardt E (1974b) Pitch, consonance and harmony. J Acoust Soc Am 55: 1061–9.

Thibodeau LM, Van Tasell DJ (1987) Tone detection and synthetic speech discrimination in band-reject noise by hearing-impaired listeners. J Acoust Soc Am 82: 864–73.

Thornton AR, Abbas PJ (1980) Low-frequency hearing loss: Perception of filtered speech, psychophysical tuning curves, and masking. J Acoust Soc Am 67: 638–43.

Tobias JV, Zerlin S (1959) Lateralization threshold as a function of stimulus duration. J Acoust Soc Am 31: 1591–4.

Turner CW, Burns EM, Nelson DA (1983) Pure tone pitch perception and low-frequency hearing loss. J Acoust Soc Am 73: 966–75.

Turner CW, Fabry DA, Barrett S, Horwitz A R (1992) Detection and recognition of stop consonants by normal-hearing and hearing-impaired listeners. J Speech Hear Res 35: 942–9.

Turner CW, Henn CC (1989) The relation between vowel recognition and measures of frequency resolution. J Speech Hear Res 32: 49–58.

Turner CW, Robb MP (1987) Audibility and recognition of stop consonants in normal and hearing-impaired subjects. J Acoust Soc Am 81: 1566–73.

Turner CW, Zwislocki JJ, Filion PR (1989) Intensity discrimination determined with two paradigms in normal and hearing-impaired subjects. J Acoust Soc Am 86: 109–15.

Tyler RS (1986) Frequency resolution in hearing-impaired listeners. In BCJ Moore (ed.) Frequency Selectivity in Hearing. London: Academic Press.

Tyler RS (1993) Cochlear Implants: Audiological Foundations. San Diego: Singular.

Tyler RS, Hall JW, Glasberg BR, Moore BCJ, Patterson RD (1984) Auditory filter asymmetry in the hearing impaired. J Acoust Soc Am 76: 1363–8.

Tyler RS, Lindblom B (1982) Preliminary study of simultaneous-masking and pulsation-threshold patterns of vowels. J Acoust Soc Am 71: 220–24.

Tyler RS, Summerfield AQ, Wood EJ, Fernandes MA (1982) Psychoacoustic and phonetic temporal processing in normal and hearing-impaired listeners. J Acoust Soc Am 72: 740–52.

Tyler RS, Wood EJ, Fernandes MA (1982) Frequency resolution and hearing loss. Brit J Audiol 16: 45–63.

Tyler RS, Wood EJ, Fernandes MA (1983) Frequency resolution and discrimination of constant and dynamic tones in normal and hearing-impaired listeners. J Acoust Soc Am 74: 1190–9.

Van Buuren RA, Festen J, Houtgast T (1996) Peaks in the frequency response of hearing aids: evaluation of the effects on speech intelligibility and sound quality. J Speech Hear Res 39: 239–50.

Van Buuren RA, Festen JM, Plomp R (1995) Evaluation of a wide range of amplitude-frequency responses for the hearing impaired. J Speech Hear Res 38: 211–21.

Van Dijkhuizen JN, Festen JM, Plomp R (1991) The effect of frequency-selective attenuation on the speech-reception threshold of sentences in conditions of low-frequency noise. J Acoust Soc Am 90: 885–94.

Van Rooij JCGM, Plomp R (1990) Auditive and cognitive factors in speech perception by elderly listeners. II: Multivariate analyses. J Acoust Soc Am 88: 2611–24.

Van Tasell DJ, Crain TR (1992) Noise reduction hearing aids: release from masking and release from distortion. Ear Hear 13: 114–21.

Van Tasell DJ, Fabry DA, Thibodeau LM (1987) Vowel identification and vowel masking patterns of hearing-impaired subjects. J Acoust Soc Am 81: 1586–97.

Verschuure J, Dreschler WA (1996) Dynamic compression in hearing aids. In B Kollmeier (ed.) Psychoacoustics, Speech and Hearing Aids. Singapore: World Scientific.

Verschuure J, Van Meeteren AA (1975) The effect of intensity on pitch. Acustica 32: 33–44.

Viemeister NF (1972). Intensity discrimination of pulsed sinusoids: The effects of filtered noise. J Acoust Soc Am 51: 1265–9.

Viemeister NF (1979) Temporal modulation transfer functions based on modulation thresholds. J Acoust Soc Am 66: 1364–80.

Viemeister NF, Wakefield GH (1991) Temporal integration and multiple looks. J Acoust Soc Am 90: 858–65.

Villchur E (1973) Signal processing to improve speech intelligibility in perceptive deafness. J Acoust Soc Am 53: 1646–57.

Villchur E (1974) Simulation of the effect of recruitment on loudness relationships in speech. J Acoust Soc Am 56: 1601–11.

Villchur E (1977) Electronic models to simulate the effect of sensory distortions on speech perception by the deaf. J Acoust Soc Am 62: 665–74.

Von Békésy G (1960) Experiments in Hearing. New York: McGraw-Hill.

Wakefield GH, Nelson DA (1985) Extension of a temporal model of frequency discrimination: Intensity effects in normal and hearing-impaired listeners. J Acoust Soc Am 77: 613–19.

Walden BE, Schwartz DM, Montgomery AA, Prosek RA (1981) A comparison of the effects of hearing impairment and acoustic filtering on consonant recognition. J Speech Hear Res 24: 32–43.

Wallach H (1940) The role of head movements and vestibular and visual cues in sound localization. J Exp Psychol 27: 339–68.

Ward WD (1954) Subjective musical pitch. J Acoust Soc Am 26: 369–80.

Weber DL (1983) Do off-frequency simultaneous maskers suppress the signal? J Acoust Soc Am 73: 887–93.

Webster JC, Schubert ED (1954) Pitch shifts accompanying certain auditory threshold shifts. J Acoust Soc Am 26: 754–60.

Wegel RL, Lane CE (1924) The auditory masking of one sound by another and its probable relation to the dynamics of the inner ear. Phys Rev 23: 266–85.

Weiss M (1987) Use of an adaptive noise canceller as an input preprocessor for a hearing aid. J Rehab Res Devel 24: 93–102.

Wier CC, Jesteadt W, Green DM (1977) Frequency discrimination as a function of frequency and sensation level. J Acoust Soc Am 61: 178–84.

Wightman FL, Kistler DJ (1989) Headphone simulation of free field listening. I: stimulus synthesis. J Acoust Soc Am 85: 858–67.

Wightman FL, McGee T, Kramer M (1977) Factors influencing frequency selectivity in normal and hearing-impaired listeners. In EF Evans, JP Wilson (eds) Psychophysics and Physiology of Hearing. London: Academic Press.

Wilson BS, Finley CC, Lawson DT, Wolford RD, Eddington DK, Rabinowitz WM (1991) Better speech recognition with cochlear implants. Nature 352: 236–8.

Wilson RH, Carhart R (1971) Forward and backward masking: interactions and additivity. J Acoust Soc Am 49: 1254–63.

Wittkop T, Hohmann V, Kollmeier B (1996) Noise reduction strategies in digital binaural hearing aids. In B Kollmeier (ed.) Psychoacoustics, Speech and Hearing Aids. Singapore: World Scientific.

Woolf NK, Ryan AF, Bone RC (1981) Neural phase-locking properties in the absence of outer hair cells. Hear Res 4: 335–46.

Yates GK (1990) Basilar membrane non-linearity and its influence on auditory nerve rate-intensity functions. Hear Res 50: 145–62.

Yates GK (1995) Cochlear structure and function. In BCJ Moore (ed.) Hearing. San Diego: Academic Press.

Yost WA (1974) Discrimination of interaural phase differences. J Acoust Soc Am 55: 1299–303.

Yost WA, Dye R (1988) Discrimination of interaural differences of level as a function of frequency. J Acoust Soc Am 83: 1846–51.

Yost WA, Wightman FL, Green DM (1971) Lateralization of filtered clicks. J Acoust Soc Am 50: 1526–31.

Yund EW, Buckles KM (1995a) Enhanced speech perception at low signal-to-noise ratios with multichannel compression hearing aids. J Acoust Soc Am 97: 1224–40.

Yund EW, Buckles KM (1995b) Multichannel compression hearing aids: Effect of number of channels on speech discrimination in noise. J Acoust Soc Am 97: 1206–23.

Zeng FG, Turner CW (1991) Binaural loudness matches in unilaterally impaired listeners. Q J Exp Psychol 43A: 565–83.

Zurek P M (1981) Spontaneous narrowband acoustic signals emitted by human ears. J Acoust Soc Am 69: 514–23.

Zurek PM, Delhorne LA (1987) Consonant reception in noise by listeners with mild and moderate sensorineural hearing impairment. J Acoust Soc Am 82: 1548–59.

Zurek PM, Formby C (1981) Frequency-discrimination ability of hearing-impaired listeners. J Speech Hear Res 24: 108–12.

Zwicker E (1958) Über pschologische und methodische Grundlagen der Lautheit. Acustica 8: 237–58.

Zwicker E (1961) Subdivision of the audible frequency range into critical bands (Frequenzgruppen). J Acoust Soc Am 33: 248.

Zwicker E (1970) Masking and psychological excitation as consequences of the ear's frequency analysis. In R Plomp, GF Smoorenburg (eds) Frequency Analysis and Periodicity Detection in Hearing. Leiden: Sijthoff.

Zwicker E, Fastl H (1990) Psychoacoustics – Facts and Models. Berlin: Springer-Verlag.

Zwicker E, Flottorp G, Stevens SS (1957) Critical bandwidth in loudness summation. J Acoust Soc Am 29: 548–57.

Zwicker E, Scharf B (1965) A model of loudness summation. Psychol Rev 72: 3–26.

Zwicker E, Schorn K (1978) Psychoacoustical tuning curves in audiology. Audiology 17: 120–40.

Zwicker E (1980) A device for measuring the temporal resolution of the ear. Audiol Acoust 19: 94–108.

Zwislocki J (1953) Acoustic attenuation between the ears. J Acoust Soc Am 25: 752–9.

Zwislocki JJ (1960) Theory of temporal auditory summation. J Acoust Soc Am 32: 1046–60.

Zwislocki JJ (1969) Temporal summation of loudness: An analysis. J Acoust Soc Am 46: 431–41.

Zwislocki JJ, Jordan HN (1986) On the relations of intensity jnds to loudness and neural noise. J Acoust Soc Am 79: 772–80.

Glossary

This glossary defines most of the technical terms that appear in the text. Sometimes the definitions are specific to the context of the book and do not apply to everyday usage of the terms. The glossary also defines some terms not used in the text, but which may be found in the literature on hearing. Terms in italic within definitions are themselves entries in the glossary.

Absolute threshold The minimum detectable level of a sound in the absence of any other external sounds. The manner of presentation of the sound and the method of determining detectability must be specified.

Acoustic reflex A contraction of muscles in the middle ear which reduces the transmission of sound through the middle ear, mainly at frequencies below 1000 Hz.

Active mechanism A mechanism within the cochlea that amplifies the response of the *basilar membrane* to weak sounds, enhances the sharpness of tuning, and introduces *non-linearity*. It depends on the function of the *Outer hairs cells,* and is easily damaged.

AGC see *Automatic gain control.*

Amplitude The instantaneous amplitude of an oscillating quantity (e.g. sound pressure or voltage) is its value at any instant, whereas the peak amplitude is the maximum value that the quantity attains. Sometimes the word peak is omitted when the meaning is clear from the context.

Amplitude modulation (AM) The process whereby the amplitude of a carrier is made to change as a function of time.

Apex The inner tip of the spiral-shaped cochlea; the opposite end from the *base.*

Articulation Index (AI) A measure of the proportion of the speech spectrum that is audible for a given listening situation and a given listener. Each spectral region is given a weighting according to its contribution to intelligibility. The AI varies between 0 and 1.

Attack time The time taken for the output of an *automatic gain control* circuit to get within 2 dB of its steady value when the input level is abruptly increased (usually by 25 dB).

Audiogram A graph showing the *absolute threshold* for *pure tones* as a function of frequency. It is usually plotted as hearing loss (deviation from the average threshold for young normally hearing people) in decibels as a function of frequency, with increasing loss plotted in the downward direction.

Auditory filter One of an array of bandpass filters that are assumed to exist in the peripheral auditory system. The characteristics of the filters are often estimated in masking experiments.

Aural harmonic A frequency *component* generated by *non-linearity* in the auditory system in response to a sinusoidal input. Its frequency is an integer multiple of the frequency of the input.

Automatic gain control (AGC) system An electronic circuit whose gain changes over time so as to reduce the range of levels at the output relative to the range at the input; the gain decreases as the input level increases.

Automatic volume control (AVC) system A form of *automatic gain control* in which the *gain* changes slowly with time. The effect can be similar to adjusting a volume control by hand.

AVC See *Automatic volume control.*

Azimuth The angle of a sound relative to the centre of a listener's head, projected on to the *horizontal plane*. It is represented by θ in Figure 7.1.

Bandwidth A term used to refer to a range of frequencies. The bandwidth of a bandpass filter is often defined as the difference between the two frequencies at which the response of the filter has fallen by 3 dB (i.e. to half power). It can also be defined in terms of the *equivalent rectangular bandwidth (ERB)*.

Base The end of the cochlea closest to the oval window and stapes.

Basilar membrane A membrane inside the cochlea that vibrates in response to sound and whose vibrations lead to activity in the auditory pathways (see Chapter 1).

Beamformer A system in which the outputs of two or more microphones are processed and combined to give a specific directional characteristic.

Beats Periodic fluctuations in peak amplitude which occur when two sinusoids with slightly different frequencies are superimposed.

Bel A unit for expressing the ratio of two powers. The number of bels is the logarithm to the base 10 of the power ratio.

Best frequency See *Characteristic frequency*.

BF See *Characteristic frequency*.

BILD See *Binaural intelligibility level difference*.

Binaural A situation involving listening with two ears.

Binaural intelligibility level difference (BILD) The decrease of the *speech reception threshold* (SRT) in noise when the speech is spatially separated from the noise, relative to the SRT when both speech and noise come from the same position in space.

Binaural masking level difference (BMLD or MLD) This is a measure of the improvement in detectability of a signal which can occur under binaural listening conditions. It is the difference in threshold of the signal (in decibels) for the case where the signal and masker have the same phase and level relationships at the two ears and the case where the interaural phase and/or level relationships of the signal and masker are different.

CB See *Critical bandwidth*.

Characteristic frequency (CF), Best frequency (BF) The frequency at which the threshold of a given single neurone is lowest, i.e. the frequency at which it is most sensitive. Characteristic frequency is also used to describe the frequency to which a given place on the *basilar membrane* is most sensitive.

Cochlear echoes See *evoked oto-acoustic emissions*.

Cochlear hearing loss A hearing loss produced by damage to the structures inside the cochlea.

Combination tone A *tone* perceived as a component of a complex stimulus which is not present in the sensations produced by the constituent components of the complex when they are presented alone. Also used to describe a physical frequency component present in the output of a nonlinear system, but absent from the input, when the input consists of two or more sinusoids.

Complex tone A *tone* composed of a number of sinusoids of different frequencies.

Component One of the sinusoids composing a complex sound. Also called a *frequency component*.

Compound action potential (CAP) A gross measure of the response of the auditory nerve to clicks or short tone bursts.

Compression limiter A type of *automatic gain control* circuit with a high *compression threshold* and short *attack* and *recovery times*. It is used to prevent over-amplification of intense sounds.

Compression ratio A property of an *automatic gain control* circuit. It is the change in input level (in decibels) required to achieve a 1 dB change in output level (once the *compression threshold* is exceeded).

Compression threshold The input level at which the gain of an *automatic gain control* circuit is reduced by 2 dB, relative to the gain applied in the region of linear amplification.

Compressive non-linearity A *non-linearity* in which the output grows by a smaller factor than the input when the input is increased. For example, if the input is doubled, the output increases by less than a factor of two.

Compressor A type of *automatic gain control* circuit in which the gain changes fairly rapidly when the input level changes. The gain decreases as the input level increases, so the range of levels at the input is compressed to a smaller range at the output.

Conductive hearing loss A hearing loss produced by reduced transmission of sound through the outer and/or middle ear.

Cone of confusion A surface defining all points in space that lead to a given interaural time difference or a given interaural intensity difference.

Constant velocity tuning curve See *Tuning curve.*

Critical bandwidth A measure of the 'effective bandwidth' of the auditory filter. It is often defined empirically by measuring some aspect of perception as a function of the bandwidth of the stimuli, and trying to determine a 'breakpoint' in the results. However, such breakpoints are rarely clear. In this book the term *ERB* is used in preference to critical bandwidth.

Cycle That portion of a periodic function that occurs in one *period*.

Decibel One-tenth of a bel, abbreviated dB. The number of dB is equal to ten times the logarithm (base 10) of the ratio of two intensities, or 20 times the logarithm of the ratio of two amplitudes or pressures.

Dichotic A situation in which the sounds reaching the two ears are not the same.

Difference limen(DL) Also called the just-noticeable difference (JND) or the differential threshold. The smallest detectable change in a stimulus. The method of determining detectability must be specified.

Diotic A situation in which the sounds reaching the two ears are the same.

Diplacusis Binaural diplacusis describes the case when a tone of fixed frequency evokes different pitches in the left and right ear.

Directional microphone A microphone whose sensitivity to sounds varies with the direction of the sounds.

Directivity A measure of the sensitivity of a microphone to sounds coming from the direction giving maximum response, relative to the sensitivity to sounds from other directions.

Distortion-product otoacoustic emissions One or more frequency components emitted from the ear in response to two or more primary tones. The distortion products are not present as frequency components in the input signal.

DLC (difference limen of a complex) The smallest detectable difference in repetition rate between two successive complex tones.

DLF (difference limen for frequency) The smallest detectable difference in frequency between two successive pure tones.

Dynamic range The range of sound levels over which a system operates in a specified way. For example, for a single neurone in the auditory nerve it is the range of sound levels between the threshold and the level at which *saturation* occurs. In the case of auditory perception at a given frequency, it refers to the range of sound levels between the threshold for detection and the level at which the sound becomes uncomfortably loud.

Duplex theory A theory proposed by Lord Rayleigh which assumes that sound localisation depends on the use of interaural time differences at low frequencies and interaural intensity differences at high frequencies.

Elevation The angle of a sound relative to the centre of a listener's head, projected on to the *median plane*. It is represented by δ in Figure 7.1.

Envelope The envelope of any function is the smooth curve passing through the peaks of the function.

Equal-loudness contours Curves plotted as a function of frequency showing the sound pressure level required to produce a given *loudness level*.

Equivalent rectangular bandwidth (ERB) The ERB of a filter is the bandwidth of a rectangular filter that has the same peak transmission as that filter and that passes the same total power for a *white noise* input. The ERB of the *auditory filter* is often used as a measure of the *critical bandwidth*.

ERB See *Equivalent rectangular bandwidth*.

ERB scale A scale in which the frequency axis has been converted into units based on the ERB of the auditory filter. Each ERB corresponds to a distance of about 0.89 mm on the basilar membrane.

Evoked oto-acoustic emissions Sounds emitted from the ear in response to sounds applied to the ear. The emissions are thought to be generated by the *active mechanism* in the cochlea.

Excitation pattern A term used to describe the distribution of activity produced by a given sound at different places (corresponding to different *characteristic frequencies*) in the auditory system. Sometimes the term is used to describe the effective level of excitation (in decibels) at each CF. Psychoacoustically, the excitation pattern of a sound can be defined as the output of the auditory filters as a function of centre frequency.

Expansive non-linearity A *non-linearity* in which the output grows by a greater factor than the input when the input is increased. For example, if the input is doubled, the output increases by more than a factor of two.

F0 See *Fundamental frequency.*

Fast Fourier Transform (FFT) A mathematical technique for calculating the amplitudes and phases of the frequency components in a sample of a sound of finite duration.

FFT See *Fast Fourier Transform.*

Filter A device with an input and an output whose response varies with frequency. For example, a bandpass filter shows a relatively large response to sinusoids whose frequencies fall within its *passband,* and shows a smaller response to frequencies outside the passband.

FMDL (frequency modulation detection limen) The smallest amount of *frequency modulation* needed to distinguish a frequency-modulated tone from a steady tone.

Formant A *resonance* in the vocal tract which is usually manifested as a peak in the spectral envelope of a speech sound.

Fourier analysis A mathematical technique for determining the *amplitudes* and *phases* of the sinusoidal frequency components in a complex sound.

Free field A field or system of waves free from the effects of boundaries.

Frequency For a sine wave the frequency is the number of *periods* occurring in one second. The unit is cycles per second, or hertz (Hz). For a complex periodic sound the term 'repetition rate' is used to describe the number of periods per second (p.p.s.).

Frequency component See *Component.*

Frequency modulation (FM) The process whereby the frequency of a carrier is made to change as a function of time.

Frequency-threshold curve See *Tuning curve.*

Frontal plane The plane lying at right angles to the horizontal plane and intersecting the upper margins of the entrances to the ear canals. See Figure 7.1.

Fundamental frequency The fundamental frequency of a periodic sound is the frequency of that sinusoidal component of the sound that has the same *period* as the periodic sound.

Gain The gain of a system (for example, a filter or an amplifier) is the magnitude of the output divided by the magnitude of the input. For example, if the output is ten times the input, the gain is said to be 10. The gain is often expressed in decibels.

Harmonic A harmonic is a component of a complex tone whose frequency is an integer multiple of the *fundamental frequency* of the complex.

Harmonic distortion Sinusoidal components present at the output of a nonlinear system when a single sinusoid is present at the input. The components have frequencies that are integer multiples of the frequency of the input.

Homogeneity A property of a linear system whereby if the input magnitude is changed by a certain factor, then the output magnitude changes by that same factor.

Horizontal plane The plane passing through the upper margins of the entrances to the ear canals and the lower margins of the eye sockets. See Figure 7.1.

Hz See *Frequency.*

IFFT See *Inverse Fast Fourier Transform.*

Inner-hair cells (IHCs) Specialised cells lying between the *basilar membrane* and the *tectorial membrane.* They are transducers that convert mechanical vibration into electrical neural responses (action potentials or spikes) in the auditory nerve.

Input-output function A plot of the magnitude of the output of a system as a function of the magnitude of the input.

Intensity This is the sound power transmitted through a given area in a sound field. Units such as watts per square metre are used. The term is also used as a generic name for any quantity relating to amount of sound, such as power or energy, although this is not technically correct.

Inter-modulation distortion When the input to a system consists of two sinusoids and the output contains frequency components other than the two sinusoids, the extra components are said to result from inter-modulation distortion. This only happens in a non-linear system.

Inter-spike interval histogram A histogram of the time intervals between successive nerve spikes. The peaks in the histogram indicate the time intervals that occur most often.

Inverse Fast Fourier Transform (IFFT) A mathematical technique for calculating the waveform of a sound from the amplitudes and phases of its frequency components.

Kemp echoes See *Evoked oto-acoustic emissions.*

Level The level of a sound is specified in decibels in relation to some reference level. See *Sensation level* and *Sound pressure level.*

Limiter See *Compression limiter.*

Linear A linear system is a system which satisfies the conditions of *super-position* and *homogeneity* (see Chapter 1).

Loudness The subjective impression of the magnitude of a sound. It is defined as the attribute of an auditory sensation in terms of which sounds may be ordered on a scale extending from quiet to loud.

Loudness level The loudness level of a sound, in phons, is the sound pressure level in decibels of a sinusoid of frequency 1 kHz which is judged by the listener to be equivalent in loudness.

Loudness recruitment See *Recruitment.*

Loudness summation An expression reflecting the idea that the loudness of sounds depends on summing the *specific loudness* occurring in different critical bandwidths or *ERBs*. It is sometimes used to describe the observation that, for a fixed overall intensity, a sound appears louder when its spectrum covers a wide frequency range than when its spectrum covers a narrow frequency range.

MAA See *Minimum audible angle.*

Magnitude estimation A method used to investigate the relationship between the physical magnitude of a stimulus (e.g. the intensity of a sound) and its subjective magnitude (e.g. its loudness). A series of stimuli with differing magnitudes is presented, and the subject is asked to assign a number to each stimulus, reflecting its subjective magnitude.

Magnitude production A method used to investigate the relationship between the physical magnitude of a stimulus (e.g. the intensity of a sound) and its subjective magnitude (e.g. its loudness). The subject is asked to adjust the magnitude of a stimulus so that the subjective impression of its magnitude corresponds to a number given by the experimenter. This is repeated for a series of numbers.

Masked audiogram See *Masking pattern.*

Masking Masking is the amount (or the process) by which the threshold of audibility for one sound is raised by the presence of another (masking) sound.

Masking level difference (MLD) See *Binaural masking level difference.*

Masking pattern, masked audiogram A graph of the detection threshold of a sinusoidal signal, plotted as a function of the signal frequency, determined in the presence of a fixed masking sound. Sometimes, the thresholds are expressed as amount of masking (in decibels).

Mean-square value A quantity related to the *power* of a signal. It is obtained by squaring the instantaneous value of the signal (for example, deviation of sound pressure from the mean atmospheric pressure) and taking the average of the squared values over time.

Median plane The plane containing all points that are equally distant from the two ears. See Figure 7.1.

Middle-ear reflex A contraction of muscles in the middle ear which reduces the transmission of sound through the middle ear, mainly at frequencies below 1000 Hz.

Minimum audible angle (MAA) The smallest detectable change in angular position of a sound source, relative to the subject's head.

Modulation Modulation refers to a change in a particular dimension of a stimulus. For example, a sinusoid may be modulated in frequency or in amplitude.

Monaural A situation in which sounds are presented to one ear only.

Noise Noise in general refers to any unwanted sound. *White noise* is a sound whose power per unit bandwidth is constant, on average, over the range of audible frequencies. See also, *pink noise*.

Non-linearity A property of a system that is not *linear,* i.e. does not obey the conditions of *superposition* and *homogeneity*.

Occlusion effect An effect occurring when the ear canal is blocked. The person's own voice sounds unnaturally loud and boomy.

Octave An octave is the interval between two tones when their frequencies are in the ratio 2:1.

Omni-directional microphone A microphone equally sensitive to sounds from all directions.

Organ of Corti A complex structure lying between the *basilar membrane* and the *tectorial membrane*. It contains the inner and outer hair cells.

Outer hair cells (OHCs) Specialised cells lying between the *basilar membrane* and the *tectorial membrane*. They play an important role in the *active mechanism* of the cochlea.

Partial A partial is any sinusoidal frequency component in a complex tone. It may or may not be a *harmonic*.

Passband The range of frequencies passed by a bandpass filter. Usually, it is specified as the range over which the response of the filter falls within certain limits.

Passive mechanism The mechanism that gives rise to tuning on the *basilar membrane* in the absence of the *active mechanism*. It is revealed when the active mechanism ceases to function, for example, after death. The passive mechanism depends on the basic mechanical properties of the basilar membrane and surrounding structures.

Period The period of a periodic waveform is the smallest time interval over which the waveform repeats itself. For a sinusoid, it corresponds to the reciprocal of the *frequency*.

Periodic waveform A waveform that repeats itself regularly as a function of time.

Phase The phase of a periodic waveform is the fractional part of a period through which the waveform has advanced, measured from some arbitrary point in time. It may be expressed in degrees or radians; $180°$ $= \pi$ radians.

Phase locking The tendency for nerve firings (spikes) to occur at a particular phase of the stimulating waveform on the basilar membrane.

Phon The unit of *loudness level*.

Pink noise This is a noise whose *spectrum level* decreases by 3 dB for each doubling of frequency.

Pitch The attribute of auditory sensation in terms of which sounds may be ordered on a musical scale.

Power A measure of energy per unit time. It is difficult to measure the total power generated by a sound source, and it is more common to specify the magnitudes of sounds in terms of their intensity, which is the sound power transmitted through a unit area in a sound field.

Power function A mathematical expression in which the magnitude of a quantity y is proportional to the magnitude of a quantity x raised to a power α: $y = C \times x^{\alpha}$, where C is a constant. The loudness of a sinusoid in *sones* is often assumed to be a power function of intensity, with $\alpha = 0.3$.

Presbyacusis (also called presbycusis) The hearing loss that is associated with ageing.

Psychometric function A plot of performance (e.g. percentage correct) in a detection or discrimination task as a function of the size of the stimulus to be detected or discriminated.

Psychophysical tuning curve (PTC) A curve showing the level of a narrowband masker needed to mask a fixed sinusoidal signal, plotted as a function of masker frequency.

Pure tone A sound wave whose instantaneous pressure variation as a function of time is a sinusoidal function. Also called a 'simple tone'.

Rate-versus-level function A plot of the firing rate of a single neurone as a function of the sound level applied to the ear.

Recovery time The time taken for the output of an *automatic gain control* circuit to get within 2 dB of its steady value when the input level is abruptly decreased (usually by 25 dB).

Recruitment This refers to a more rapid than usual growth of loudness with increase in stimulus level, which occurs in people with cochlear hearing loss.

Release time See *Recovery time.*

Residue pitch Also known as virtual pitch, low pitch and periodicity pitch. The low pitch heard when a group of *partials* is perceived as a coherent whole. For a harmonic complex tone, the residue pitch is usually close to the pitch of the *fundamental* component, but that component does not have to be present for a residue pitch to be heard.

Resonance An enhancement of the intensity of a sound that occurs when its frequency equals or is close to the natural frequency of vibration of an acoustic system or air-filled cavity. The word is also used to describe the process by which the enhancement occurs.

Retrocochlear hearing loss A hearing loss caused by damage to the auditory nerve and/or higher levels of the auditory pathway.

rms See *Root-mean-square.*

Root-mean-square (rms) value A quantity obtained by squaring the instantaneous value of a waveform (for example, deviation of sound pressure from the mean atmospheric pressure), taking the average of the squared values over time, and then taking the square root of the average.

Saturation The phenomenon whereby at medium to high sound levels a neurone no longer changes its rate of firing in response to increases in sound level.

Scala tympani One of the two outer chambers of the cochlea. It lies on the opposite side of the basilar membrane from the *organ of Corti.*

Scala vestibuli One of the two outer chambers of the cochlea. It lies on the same side of the basilar membrane as the *organ of Corti.*

Sensation level (SL) The level of a sound in decibels relative to the threshold level for that sound for the individual listener.

Sensorineural hearing loss A general term used to describe hearing loss caused by damage to the cochlea and/or the auditory nerve and higher levels of the auditory pathway.

Simple tone See *Pure tone.*

Sine wave, Sinusoidal vibration, Sinusoid A waveform whose variation as a function of time is a sine function. This is the function relating the sine of an angle to the size of the angle.

Sone A unit of subjective loudness. A 1 kHz sinusoid presented binaurally in *free field* from a frontal direction is defined as having a loudness of one sone when its level is 40 dB SPL. The loudness in sones roughly doubles for each 10-dB increase in sound level above 40 dB SPL.

Sound pressure level (SPL) This is the level of a sound in decibels relative to an internationally defined reference level. The latter corresponds to an intensity of 10^{-12} W/m^2, which is equivalent to a sound pressure of 20 μPa.

Spatial filter See *beamformer.*

Specific loudness A term used in loudness models to denote the loudness evoked by a sound in each *critical bandwidth* or each *ERB.*

Specific loudness pattern A plot of *specific loudness* as a function of frequency, usually with frequency expressed on a critical-bandwidth scale or *ERB scale.*

Spectrogram A display showing how the short-term *spectrum* of a sound changes over time. The abscissa is time, the ordinate is frequency and the amount of energy is indicated by the lightness or darkness of shading. Spectrograms are often used in the analysis of speech sounds.

Spectrum The spectrum of a sound wave is the distribution in frequency of the magnitudes (and sometimes the phases) of the components of the wave. It can be represented by plotting *power, intensity, amplitude,* or *level* as a function of frequency.

Spectrum level This is the level of a sound in decibels measured in a 1-Hz wide band. It is often used to characterise sounds with continuous spectra such as noises. A *white noise* has a long-term average spectrum level that is independent of frequency. A *pink noise* has a spectrum level that decreases by 3 dB for each doubling of frequency.

Speech intelligibility index (SII) See *Articulation index.*

Speech reception threshold (SRT) A measure of the level of speech required to achieve a given degree of intelligibility (for example 50%

correct). When measured in the presence of background noise, the SRT is often expressed as the speech-to-background ratio, in decibels.

Speech-shaped noise Noise whose spectrum matches the long-term average spectrum of speech.

Spike A single nerve impulse or action potential.

SPL See *Sound pressure level.*

Spontaneous otoacoustic emissions Sounds emitted from the ear in the absence of any external sound source. They are thought to be generated by the *active mechanism* in the cochlea.

SRT See *Speech reception threshold.*

Stereocilia Small hair-like structures that project from the tops of the *inner* and *outer hair cells.*

Superposition A property of a linear system whereby the response to two or more inputs presented simultaneously (e.g. two sinusoids with different frequencies) is the sum of the responses to the inputs presented individually.

Suppression The process whereby excitation or neural activity at one characteristic frequency is reduced by the presence of excitation or neural activity at adjacent characteristic frequencies.

Tectorial membrane A gelatinous structure lying above the *stereocilia* of the *inner* and *outer hair cells.*

Temporal integration The phenomenon whereby performance on a specific task improves as the duration of the stimulus is increased. It is often used to describe the fact that the intensity of a sound at the absolute threshold for detection decreases with increasing duration.

Temporal modulation transfer function (TMTF) The modulation depth required for detection of sinusoidal *amplitude modulation* of a carrier, plotted as a function of modulation frequency.

Timbre That attribute of auditory sensation in terms of which a listener can judge that two sounds similarly presented and having the same loudness and pitch are dissimilar. Put more simply, it relates to the quality of a sound.

Time invariant Description of a system or mechanism whose properties do not vary over time.

Tinnitus The perception of a sound in the absence of any external sound applied to the ear.

TMTF See *Temporal modulation transfer function.*

Tone A sound wave capable of evoking an auditory sensation having *pitch.*

Tonotopic organisation A property of the auditory system that *characteristic frequency* (CF) is represented in an orderly spatial arrangement. For example, the CF of the *basilar membrane* varies monotonically with position along the membrane. In the auditory nerve, CF varies smoothly with the position of neurones within the nerve.

Tuning The property of a system that it responds best to a limited range of sinusoidal frequencies.

Tuning curve For the *basilar membrane,* this is a graph of the sound level required to produce a fixed response at a specific point (constant velocity or constant amplitude), plotted as a function of frequency. For a single nerve fibre it is a graph of the lowest sound level at which the fibre will respond, plotted as a function of frequency. This is also called a *frequency-threshold curve* (FTC). See also *Psychophysical tuning curve.*

Two-tone suppression A phenomenon observed on the *basilar membrane* and in single neurones of the auditory nerve whereby the response to a tone close to the *characteristic frequency* is reduced by a second tone at a higher or lower frequency.

Virtual pitch See *Residue pitch.*

Waveform A term used to describe the form or shape of a wave. It may be represented graphically by plotting instantaneous amplitude or pressure as a function of time.

Weber fraction The smallest detectable change in a stimulus, ΔS, divided by the magnitude of that stimulus, S.

Weber's law A 'law' stating that the smallest detectable change in a stimulus, ΔS, is proportional to the magnitude of that stimulus, S. In other words, $\Delta S/S$ = constant. The law holds reasonably accurately for the intensity discrimination of white noise. For sinusoids, $\Delta S/S$

decreases somewhat with increasing sound level, which is called the 'near miss' to Weber's law.

White noise A noise with a *spectrum level* that does not vary as a function of frequency.

Index